Clinical Neuropsychology of Attention

Clinical Neuropsychology of Attention

Adriaan H. van Zomeren
Wiebo H. Brouwer

NEW YORK   OXFORD
OXFORD UNIVERSITY PRESS
1994

Oxford University Press

Oxford   New York   Toronto
Delhi   Bombay   Calcutta   Madras   Karachi
Kuala Lumpur   Singapore   Hong Kong   Tokyo
Nairobi   Dar es Salaam   Cape Town
Melbourne   Auckland   Madrid

and associated companies in
Berlin   Ibadan

Library of Congress Cataloging-in-Publication Data
Zomeren, A. H. van (Adriaan H.), 1940–
Clinical neuropsychology of attention / Adriaan H. van Zomeren, Wiebo H. Brouwer.
p.   cm.   Includes bibliographical references and index.
ISBN 0-19-506373-2
1. Clinical neuropsychology.   2. Attention.   3. Neuropsychological tests.   4. Brain damage—Diagnosis.
I. Brouwer, Wiebo H.   II. Title.
[DNLM: 1. Attention—physiology.   2. Neuropsychology.
BF 321 Z86c 1994]
RC386.6.N48Z65   1994   616.8—dc20
DNLM/DLC   for Library of Congress   93-17824

9 8 7 6 5 4 3 2 1

Printed in the United States of America
on acid-free paper

Preface

This book is an attempt at integration. We have been working for many years in the field of attentional impairments after head injury. During this period we began to realize that an overview of theories of attention and pathological phenomena in neurological patients might be useful to our clinical colleagues. In particular, it became clear that the terminology in the area of attention is confusing, as all investigators have their favorite terms, depending largely on their backgrounds (neurology, cognitive psychology, psychophysiology, etc.). Hence this book is an attempt to present a conceptual scheme to help understand the evidence obtained in many different areas of clinical research on attention. We have tried to link areas that were traditionally separated and to analyze the relationships between concepts from various theoretical backgrounds. It is for the readers of this monograph to judge whether our attempt at integration has been successful.

The scope of the book is broad: the topics range from event-related potentials to driving automobiles, and from head injury to dementia. Thus we were confronted with the dilemma of depth versus breadth. On the one hand, experts may find that "their" topics have been covered incompletely or superficially, but on the other hand, clinicians and researchers from widely different settings may find something of interest. Faced with this dilemma, we always tried to decide what to include by using clinical relevance as a criterion. The book is first of all meant to be used by colleagues in clinical neuropsychological and rehabilitation settings.

Despite our wish to keep the scope as wide as possible, we were forced to skip one important sector: child neuropsychology. It seemed beyond our abilities to cover the subject of attentional impairments in children, especially attention deficit disorder with hyperactivity. As a whole library could be filled with books on this topic, and as neither author has experience in this field, it seemed wise to accept this limitation.

We would like to thank one man in particular. This is Arthur Benton, who at the New Orleans conference of the International Neuropsychological Society in 1988 introduced us to the publisher, with the suggestion that we should write a book like this. In fact, the initial informal agreement was made over a plate of crayfish from the Cajun kitchen. Although integrating our experiences and ideas in one volume had been in the back of our minds for some time, this encouraging move by one of the "fathers" of neuropsychology was exactly the little push we needed to begin writing.

Next, we thank the various colleagues who commented on earlier drafts of several chapters: Rob Haaxma (Chapter 3), Rudolf Ponds (Chapter 5), Willem Alpherts and Seth Boonstra (Chapter 7), Marie Vanier (Chapter 8), and Paul Eling (references). Chapter 10, on cognitive rehabilitation, is an extension of a text that the first author wrote in cooperation with Luciano Fasotti. We are particularly grateful to Jordan Grafman and Dorothy Gronwall for reviewing the entire manuscript. Rolf Saan and Marthe Koning-Haanstra should also be thanked for taking on the lion's share of the clinical work in the Neuropsychology Unit, allowing the first author to concentrate on writing.

We express our appreciation to the people who gave us secretarial help: Tineke Bijzitter, Eveline Eimers and Harriet Roffel; or technical assistance: Coen Dobma, Bernie Duym, and Lukas Dijck. We are very grateful to Leacy O'Hanlon who removed numerous "quirky turns of phrase" from the Dutch-flavored English of our first draft. Finally, Jeffrey W. House was a stimulating publisher, whose critical remarks were most helpful in the preparation of the final manuscript.

We are pleased to present this monograph as a product of the State University of Groningen, and in particular, of the department of Neurology in the University Hospital and the Department of Psychology.

Groningen   Ed van Zomeren
July 1993   Wiebo Brouwer

Contents

Clinical Neuropsychology of Attention

1

Introduction

What is attention? This basic question cannot yet be answered at this point in our discussion. Attention cannot be reduced to a single definition, nor can it be linked to a single anatomical structure or assessed with a single test. Moreover, it is increasingly clear that cognitive rehabilitation of attentional impairments must rely on a combination of approaches.

The phenomenology of attention is broad. The word is used in a variety of ways, some colloquial, others limited to scientific investigation. In daily language, attention is primarily used to denote directed and selective perception, as when referring to someone "paying attention" to a particular source of stimulation. This use of the word suggests a quantitative as well as a selective aspect of attention, as if a given situation requires a certain amount of attention to be paid. Colloquial use of the word attention may also suggest effort, for example, when it is said that a person is concentrating hard on a task. Finally, attention as used by laymen may also contain a time element, often with a negative connotation: attention falters, that is, an individual will stop attending if the source of stimulation becomes boring to him.

While these aspects of direction, selectivity, quantity, effort, and time are reflected in the terminology of academic psychology and neurophysiology, investigators from these disciplines have often shown a tendency to stick to narrow definitions, excluding any aspects of attention not relevant to their own studies. This has had an unfortunate but predictable outcome; Moray (1969) noted that the terminology in the field of attention was at best confusing and at worst a mess. Fifteen years later Donchin (1984) again warned his colleagues of the vagueness of the general term "attention," and of the risks involved in uncritical use of it. He stressed that it was only a metaphor, "a term that has really not been defined sufficiently, but that is used to label a very complex set of processes." With these warnings in mind, the theoretical foundation and the philosophical background of attentional concepts will be discussed at length in the next chapter.

As stated in the preface, this book will attempt to present a useful overview to clinical neuropsychologists, and in particular, to describe impairments of attention on the *behavioral level*, or more precisely at the task level, and their consequences for everyday activities. For that reason, psychophysiology and electrophysiology will play modest roles in this book. More emphasis will be placed on focused attention, divided attention, and sustained attention as they can be operationalized in tasks. Flexibility will also be discussed, and while this may be seen as a higher-order aspect of attention—a control mechanism—it can be described or defined in terms of task performance. Important theoretical issues in the book are strategies of attention, and supervisory attentional control. These concepts are relatively new and have not yet formed the basis for much neuropsychological research. Still, their theoretical importance is such that they are discussed in all chapters.

The relationship between cognitive psychology and clinical neuropsychology as they bear on attention is explored. Until now some distance has existed between these two disciplines. Fortunately, the gap has begun to close, as cognitive psychologists have developed an interest in pathological phenomena. Even before this, however, clinical psychologists had begun to realize that the generation of so-called "organic tests" meant to differentiate between psychiatric and brain-damaged patients did not produce good results. Consequently, investigators from the two fields began to work in closer harmony, often in pairs, developing tests that were more specific and better founded theoretically. Splendid examples of this approach are Gronwall and Sampson (1974) and Wilson and Baddeley (Wilson et al., 1985). We hope that our work and writings, including the present volume, will fit into this historical development.

The combining of cognitive psychology and neuropsychology leads to the question of the clinical usefulness of theoretical models. The next chapter reviews many models in the boxes-and-arrows tradition, a tradition that has been regarded by some as reductionistic, sterile, and academic. We want to stress that in our view the ultimate test of a model should be its usefulness in applied psychology—in this case, clinical work. For the clinician they are expedients that should enhance the quality of clinical work, be it assessment, cognitive rehabilitation, or advising patients in practical matters such as the resumption of work and driving. Many psychologists working in a clinical setting must have concluded that theoretical models are of little help in the face of practical problems. Still, a clinical neuropsychology without theoretical foundations is inconceivable, and there seems to be no better alternative than to continue using the available models in the hope that repeated confrontations with clinical phenomena will eventually improve them.

The coming and going of models in cognitive psychology is another problem. Developments have been rapid, particularly under the influence of the information-processing approach; as soon as clinical neuropsychologists have become familiar with one model, a newer one is reported at conferences of cognitive psychologists. Again, there seems to be no choice for neuropsychology but to follow these developments critically and to judge the clinical merits of each new theory. This has more or less been the attitude of the present authors. So, if somewhere in this book we express our hopes about the possible contribution of connectionism to neuropsychology, we should not be viewed as "dedicated followers of fashion" (Davies et al., 1966). Hope is not synonymous with uncritical belief, and as long as we are working with real patients we will not be seduced by the charms of boxes, arrows, and networks—unless they can help us in the assessments of deficits and the making of practical decisions concerning our patients.

STRUCTURE OF THE BOOK

The structure of this book is determined largely by neurologic nosology. A series of discussions of clinical categories, ranging from head injury to epilepsy, follows two theoretical chapters. We have assumed that readers will be interested mainly in attentional deficits in certain patient groups, rather than one particular impairment as it is seen in various patient groups. Still, the structure of the chapters is such that specific sections, for example, "Focused Attention," can be easily located in various chapters without consulting the index.

When reviewing the literature on attentional impairments in neurologic patient groups, we discovered that research interests vary greatly for these groups. For example, stroke patients have mainly been studied with regard to the phenomenon of hemi-inattention, while research on epileptic patients has emphasized so-called lapses of attention. As a result, there is considerable variation between chapters in the number of pages allocated to each area of research, although we have tried to apply systematically the theoretical framework described in Chapter 2.

Chapter 2 serves as the theoretical foundation for the rest of the book. It gives a conceptual overview, providing readers with the theoretical framework required for the more clinical chapters. A definition of attention, to the extent that we have dared to make one, can be found in this chapter.

Chapter 3 explores the relationships between aspects of attention and cerebral anatomy and physiology.

Chapters 4 to 7 describe impairments of attention in four basic neurologic conditions that affect the majority of patients seen by neuropsychologists: head injury, Alzheimer's disease, Parkinson's disease and epilepsy. For practical reasons the topics of cerebrovascular accident (CVA) and neoplasm are not covered in separate chapters as the effects of these kinds of lesions vary widely according to their size and site. Moreover, studies of attentional deficits in these patients have been scarce, and the patients have been combined in groups referred to as "brain-damaged," particularly in the literature before 1970. Research interest in patients with CVA has been focused mainly on hemi-inattention and extinction. These topics are discussed in Chapters 3 and 8.

Of all the chapters, *Chapter 8* is the most practically oriented. Here we give an overview of available assessment techniques, ranging from simple observation to more sophisticated techniques with a clear theoretical background. We argue that the final choice of methods and tests should be determined by one's clinical setting, that is, the specific questions that must be answered regarding a particular patient. Although a few general guidelines can be proposed, the complexity of the subject "attention" is such that any final test battery should be tailored to each specific clinical population and its specific problems.

Chapter 9 addresses the behavioral and social consequences of attentional impairments. It gives a brief description of the effects of deficits in attention on daily life. In the course of preparing this chapter, we were confronted with the fact that performance on attention tests has too infrequently been related to real-life situations. As a result of this scarcity of empirical data, the chapter is to some extent contemplative in nature and partly based on our own clinical experiences. Also discussed in this chapter is the problem of delimiting "attention" where it borders on intelligence and social skills, especially social perception.

Finally, *Chapter 10* deals with the efficacy of "attention training" techniques that have emerged from the cognitive rehabilitation boom. The book closes with a glossary of essential definitions and concepts.

2

Theories and Concepts of Attention

Attention may be said to be qualified by selection and quantified by intensity. Theories of attention differ in their emphasis on selection and intensity, but in most recent theories selection is more prominent. In global terms (Kahneman, 1973), selection occurs either on the basis of enduring dispositions, as when attention is automatically drawn to a cry, or on the basis of momentary intentions, as when concentrating on details of a construction. Because what is selected has a greater likelihood of further cognitive processing, thus affecting behavior, attention holds an important position.

A common metaphor for attention is the spotlight system found in theaters. A spotlight is selective (beamwidth) and has intensity. What is outside the spotlight is hardly noticed. We will use this metaphor frequently to illustrate the differences between theoretical approaches. While it may seem more appropriate for visually applied attention than for attention to auditory messages or memory representations, we will use it in a general sense, in which the spotlight is a metaphor for selection enhancement possible at different levels of perceptual, cognitive, and motor representation. Theories of attention specify how the movement and intensity of the spotlight are regulated and sustained.

EARLY HISTORY OF ATTENTION

The concept of attention is much older than academic psychology. As early as 400 B.C. Greek orators sought to improve their skills by applying memory rules, such as: "This is the first thing: if you pay attention, the judgment will better perceive the things going through it" (Yates, 1966). This quotation suggests a view of attention as a consciously controlled process enhancing perception and involving certain costs (*paying* attention).

Still, the following centuries produced little in the way of a better understanding of attention. Philosophers and physicians such as Augustine (354–430) and Avicenna (Abu Ali al-Husain ibn-Sina, 980–1037) tried to analyze the relationship between the senses and the soul, but they never considered the states and processes that influence and direct the work of these senses. Leibniz (1646–1716), the German mathematician, logician, and philosopher, was the first to describe explicitly some phenomena that can truly be called "attentional."

He pointed out that not every perception results in awareness. On the contrary, the bulk of our perceptions do not seem to enter consciousness. Leibniz argued that a process called "apperception" must be added to perception to produce conscious awareness. In his essays Leibniz (1765) sought to analyze attentional phenomena he observed in daily life. For example, he pointed out that perception of stimuli can be active, that is, our attention is voluntarily focused on a certain stimulus, "an act of will"; or it can be passive, that is, a stimulus captures our attention automatically, although we are absorbed in some unrelated activity. Elements of this are seen in the distinction between selection on the basis of enduring dispositions or momentary intentions made earlier.

Leibniz also described a phenomenon illustrating the close connection between memory and attention: when someone speaks to us at a moment when we are attending to something else, we may ask "What?" and then answer the question before it has been repeated. Leibniz suggested that this phenomenon indicates that the seemingly unattended question was nevertheless stored in memory and could be attended to subsequently (Leahey, 1980).

In the meantime, the Scientific Revolution had changed the world. Kepler, Galileo, and Newton conceived of the world as a great machine understandable by simple mechanical-mathematical laws. As Leahey (1980) put it: "In the nineteenth century the mechanical analogy overthrows the angelic view of human reason and mechanizes psychology." Psychology was officially born in the nineteenth century, a child of philosophy and physiology. Philosophers had hitherto considered consciousness a feature that distinguished humans from all other animals. By the mid-nineteenth century, however, the philosophy of consciousness had become rather static, while the science of physiology was booming. Von Helmholtz was measuring nerve conduction velocity in frogs and humans with remarkable success. It was at this time that Wilhelm Maximilian Wundt began his study of medicine and became an experimental physiologist. He received an assistantship from Von Helmholtz and in 1862 gave his first course, "Psychology as a Natural Science." In 1875 he received a chair in philosophy at Leipzig where he opened his Psychological Institute—and the first two years of its existence, he paid for it out of his own pocket.

Wundt saw psychology as the study of consciousness. His belief that introspection and experiment were the means for acquiring knowledge in the field reflects the academic background of his era. *Reaction time* (RT) played an important role in his experiments, but he was inevitably confronted with the problem of attention. It became clear that RT was not only determined by sensory modality, stimulus intensity, and mode of responding, but also by internal factors in the subject. It seems that Wundt's interest in this internal, or personal, factor was partly inspired by a practical problem at the Greenwich Observatory, reported in 1794, called the "personal equation." Astronomers had noted that there were relatively large individual differences in the accuracy of recording transit times of stars, that is, the exact moment when a star passed the cross hairs in the field of a telescope. The discrepancy between the head astronomer's measurement and that of one of his assistants even resulted in the latter's dismissal. If this story of Wundt's inspiration is true, it is the first example of a practical problem inspiring experimental psychological research.

Wundt himself did not use the word attention in this context. Rather, he explained the influence of the internal factor in terms of Leibniz's *apperception*. Apperception is a process resulting in a clear perception of a mental content. Through apperception, perceptions and mental data (e.g., memories, fantasies, or symbolic transformations) are drawn into clear introspective consciousness. Wundt defined attention as the feeling that accompanies the act of apperception. In Wundt's views, both apperception and attention referred more to the intensity aspect of attention than to selection. This emphasis on intensity was also prominent in the thinking of Titchener, a British student of Wundt who later emigrated to the United States (Cornell University). For him, attention not only determined the contents of consciousness, but also influenced the quality of conscious experience. In the heyday of introspective psychology, academic psychologists agreed on the importance of this elusive internal factor. "The doctrine of attention is the nerve of the whole psychological system, and that as men judge it, so shall they be judged before the general tribunal of psychology" (Titchener, 1908). Nevertheless, definitions of attention given in the second half of the nineteenth century showed considerable variation: it was defined as a mental state, as an accommodation of consciousness, a force starting within the Ego, an inhibitory power, a consciousness passing from passivity to activity, and an act of will (Leahey, 1980; see also Pillsbury, 1908; and Geissler, 1909). More

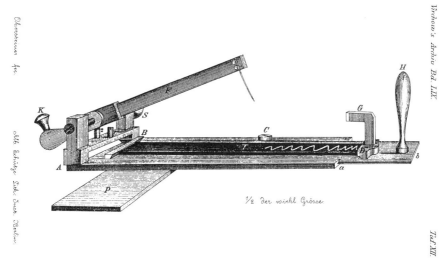

Figure 2-1 One of the many ingenious devices invented in the second half of the nineteenth century by investigators of psychological phenomena. This apparatus for recording reaction times was developed by Obersteiner (1874) in cooperation with his friend Exner, who introduced the term "reaction time." By means of a handle (*H*) a sooted glass strip was slowly pulled out of the apparatus, until the catch (*G*) released the steel spring (*F*), this giving out a loud tone. Due to the vibration of the spring, a steel pin attached to it was writing sinuses on the sooted strip, providing a time base. The subject was instructed to push the button (*K*) as quickly as possible when hearing the tone, lifting the pin from the glass strip and ending the recording. Obersteiner reported that many of his patients were frightened by the device.

specific ideas also existed about the mechanism of attention. According to Obersteiner (1879), attention was an "inhibitory power." He proposed that "in perception, thinking, and action the same inhibitory faculty is in action." His metaphor for attention was a kind of inverse spotlight (p. 453): When an artist wishes to call special attention to some object in his picture, he does so by means of color, illumination, and so on. But there are limits imposed by his materials. To achieve his aim, he places the surroundings or other objects more or less in shadow, and the principal object to which he wishes to attract the eye stands out in a corresponding manner. A similar result is effected in a mental picture by the power of attention (see Figure 2-1).

The variety of definitions of attention sheds a somewhat ironic light on the extensively quoted remark of William James: "Everyone knows what attention is," which preceded his definition of attention (James, 1890, p. 416):

> It is the taking possession by the mind, in clear and vivid form, of one out of what seems several simultaneously possible objects or trains of thought. Focalization, concentration, of consciousness are of its essence. It implies withdrawal from some things in order to deal better with others.

While recognizing the importance of attention, psychology in the early twentieth century found it hard to develop the concept further. Titchener remarked that the discovery of attention was something like the discovery of a hornet's nest: the first touch brought out a whole swarm of insistent problems. The literature of the time illustrates that the introspectionist struggle with these problems was in vain and led to a continuous shrinkage of the concept such that only a sterile entity remained, quite remote from James' rich definition, which involved selectivity, intensity, perception, and cognition.

In retrospect, the most insistent problems appeared to be twofold (Sanders, 1963). Emphasis was given to the intensity aspect of attention without explaining how intensity serves selectivity of thinking and behavior. So attention was reduced to the level of a mere attribute of a sensation or thought, a clearness of its consciousness experience. The second problem had to do with the distinction between attention on the one hand, and perception and cognition on the other. Of course, this is a real problem if one looks critically at definitions of attention such as those offered by Obersteiner and James. As late as 1969, Moray (p. 2) stated that James' writing on attention "compares rather poorly . . . with the experimental precision of Titchener." But when Titchener's students attempted to isolate all perceptual and cognitive processes, what remained tended to be sterile and devoid of function, certainly in the context of the dynamically and behaviorally oriented views inherent in the radically new approaches to psychology emerging at that time.

Psychoanalysis preferred to explain behavior in terms of energy, unconscious conflicts, and defense mechanisms. *Gestalt psychology* and *Behaviorism* shared the conviction that the operations that relate output to input conform to a simple and straightforward set of rules. One of the leading Gestalt psychologists, E. Rubin (1921), published a paper entitled "The nonexistence of attention." He argued that selectivity and direction of attention are purely the result of the structural organization of the perceived field, and that the laws governing attention are thus in fact nothing more than the structural laws of visual perception. So, not surprisingly, these schools discarded the concept of attention.

It is remarkable that attention survived in more practically oriented fields. In neurology, especially in the study of higher cerebral functions often called *behavioral neurology*, attention was connected with the phenomena of epilepsy, confusional states, and hemi-inattention (e.g., Poppelreuter, 1917). Occasionally, psychologists working in clinical neurological settings studied aspects of attention in patients who had sustained closed head injuries (Conkey, 1938; Ruesch, 1944b). Here, as well as in other areas of *applied psychology*, attention was treated as an individual ability, the ability to concentrate, which a person could possess to a greater or lesser extent. In industrial and educational psychology in particular, tasks were used that were considered "attention tests." Most of these were visual search tasks in which subjects had to search in a rapid and accurate manner for certain letters, digits, or figures, such as the Bourdon Dot Cancellation Task (Bourdon, 1895) and the French *Test de Deux Barrages*. The term attention was also used for the common factor in a variety of tests requiring unfamiliar mental manipulations of symbolic stimuli (Woodrow, 1939; Wittenborn, 1943), tests, which, according to modern terminology, would require working memory and supervisory attentional control (see below). The common factor in both types of tasks appears to be that both would require concentration and mental effort, approximating the definitions of attention given by James.

ATTENTION AFTER WORLD WAR II

A Unitary Mechanism?

Aandacht, the Dutch word for attention, means, etymologically, what one thinks of. This literal meaning is included in the definition of attention given by William James and cited above as the resulting "clear and vivid" perceptions and thoughts. But by using the phrase "taking possession by the mind," James added to this the suggestion of a selective endogenous mechanism facilitating the processing of part of the available information at the cost of the remainder. As we related, Titchener's school of psychology, the last bastion of attention in early twentieth century academic psychology, took the selective element out of attention. However, after World War II, when attention returned to academic psychology, *selectivity* became its most important element.

After psychology had gone through the wringers of behaviorism and gestalt psychology, all references to consciousness were initially avoided and emphasis was given to selection on the basis of enduring dispositions. Attention was ascribed a "tuner" function for perception, but what did the tuning was not specified. Only with the rise of cognitive psychology and its use of the computer metaphor, did selection on the basis of momentary intentions—the other side of our global dichotomy—become an object of study.

The study of selection based on enduring dispositions has moved from global neurophysiological theories (applicable to many species and modalities) about the orienting reflex (see Chapter 3) to highly specific theories about the physical characteristics governing the salience of visual features. Some of these developments will be described below in the section on visual selective attention. The dominant theories in this area are early selection theories, wherein selection of stimuli for attention is based on preattentive and preconscious mechanisms and is specific to a modality. Interestingly, because of this emphasis on early selection, such theories are not about attention, at least not in the terms of William James, but rather about preattentive selective processes. Stimuli selected by these processes are subsequently given attention. The early selection theories leave the process of attention itself unexplained.

In retrospect, one might say that the use of the word "attention" for selection based on momentary intentions as well as enduring dispositions has been the cause of much confusion. This confusion is aggravated, since attention also has the connotation of a central process associated with individual ability. The use of one term may suggest that the same attentional ability selects information and sustains its processing in many different situations and modalities. The expectation that persons with signs of impaired attention in one mental task will also have difficulties in another if both require selecting or sustaining "one out of several simultaneously possible objects or trains of thought," is based on this notion. Until now there has been far too little systematic research in the area of individual differences; according to Davies and colleagues (1984) the evidence is not encouraging from the "unitarian" point of view. They conclude their chapter on individual differences by stating that "the most successful theoretical accounts of individual and group differences are likely to be nonunitary in nature and to incorporate features from all types of theories" (p. 434). The types of theories they refer to are discussed below, with the exception of those at the neurophysiological level, which are described in Chapter 3. We will return to the issue of individual differences later in this chapter.

The Information Processing Approach

The investigator's basic means for acquiring data in the "information processing approach" is mental chronometry. The influence of variations in task demands on reaction time provides material used to validate theories of information processing. A related method is the presentation of stimuli during a fixed short period to study accuracy. With these methods there is a strong tendency to use discrete stimuli and responses; clearly defined stimuli are presented in an on-and-off fashion requiring a simple, timed motor or perceptual response. Such chronometric methodology revealed that in processing symbolic stimuli a slow serial stage of processing for a certain class of cognitive operations ("limited capacity" processing) often follows an earlier stage of parallel information processing ("unlimited capacity" processing). The process of selecting from simultaneous sources of information, by enhancing the processing of material from some sources and/or by suppressing information from others, is referred to as selective attention. Selective attention may operate at two points in time: *before* the limited capacity processing occurs, protecting this system against overload, or *during* limited capacity processing.

In some theories, the primary locus of selection is perceptual, that is, preceding the recognition of objects and meanings. This is called *early selection*. Investigators studying visual (spatial) selective attention tend to prefer early selection theories, while many general theories of attention and information processing where response choice and cognitive decisions are made on the basis of recognized objects and meanings favor late selection. Attention in the second meaning, during limited capacity processing, is closer to James' definition of attention as an endogenous activity of the mind. Early selection theories are thus more concerned with pre-attentional processes that lead to the selection of some stimuli for attention. We will first describe general theories of attention before proceeding to the more specific theories of visual selective attention.

General Theories

After World War II, experimental psychology was strongly influenced by communication theory. Psychologists began to view the mind as an information processing system, and included concepts such as channel capacity and bits of information in their theories. This telecommunication metaphor inspired a whole generation of structural models in which a chain of events occurred between the

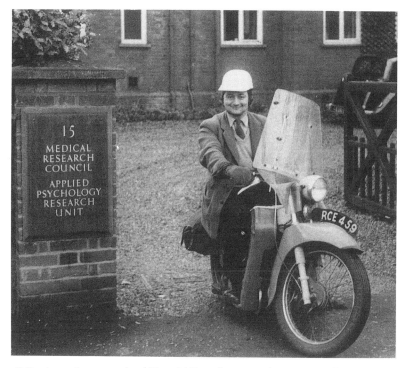

Figure 2-2 An action portrait of Donald Broadbent, made in 1958 when he was still an untenured staff member of the Applied Psychology Unit at the University of Cambridge. He later became director of the same institute but continued riding his motorcycle. His book *Perception and Communication*, published in 1958, played a major role in the information-processing approach in psychology. By courtesy of Dr. Broadbent.

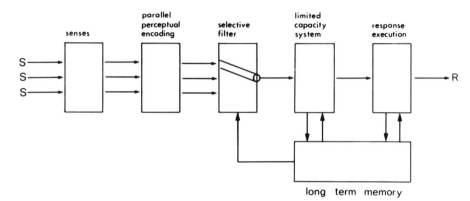

Figure 2-3 Broadbent's filter model in a slightly modified version. Processing of information occurs in parallel up to the filter, and is serial afterward. Both the limited capacity system and the response execution system are interacting with long-term memory. *S*, stimulus; *R*, response.

familiar *S* (stimulus) and *R* (response) signs that had been left as a heritage of behaviorism. The models invariably depicted a stream of information going from left to right, *S* marking the input side and *R* marking the output side. The best-known of these was the filter model devised by Broadbent (1958) (see Figures 2-2 and 2-3). These models postulated an early stage in which stimulus attributes such as loudness, color, intensity, and even symmetry in patterns were automatically processed in parallel. It was assumed that these attributes were coded in parallel by means of inborn or wired-in characteristics of the central nervous system. Stimulus identification and response selection took place in subsequent stages. Operations were assumed to occur in a serial and stepwise manner beyond the selective filter.

Attention is incorporated in these models in two ways, via the concepts of selectivity and capacity. All investigators assumed that, after the initial parallel stage, the system gave priority to a minor part of the information coming in, more or less ignoring the rest. Broadbent postulated a filter that excluded irrelevant information on the basis of crude physical features like color, localization, or pitch, enabling the system to deal efficiently with task-relevant signals. In terms of the spotlight metaphor, one could say that the information passing through the filter came into the spotlight of attention, the spotlight being the limited capacity channel. The filter was assumed to be located behind the first parallel stage of stimulus encoding. Later investigators demonstrated experimentally that a filter with an absolute blocking of irrelevant information could not explain how subjects were distracted from a task by seemingly irrelevant stimuli such as the faint sound of an ambulance siren outside. For that reason, later theorists (Deutsch and Deutsch, 1963; Treisman, 1964) contended that "ignored" information was merely attenuated, but still processed by the system in a crude or superficial way. This appears to be a biologically sensible mechanism as it enables animals and humans to react to signals heralding danger even when they are fully concentrated on a task. Broadbent (1971) himself adapted his original model by introducing an attenuation filter, and by assuming the existence of a second mechanism called "pigeonholing," which referred to relative thresholds of responses on the output side of the system. The attenuation filter could be seen as a kind of inverse spotlight in the sense of Obersteiner's metaphor of attention as inhibition. Still, the development of these serial models of information processing had reached a deadlock. Norman (1969) stated his criticism of a two-stage theory of selective attention as follows:

> The problem with this is simply that it is difficult to see how Treisman can both have a saving in the number of signals that must be analyzed (an attenuated signal, after all, acts like it is hardly there at all) and an analysis of all signals when it is convenient (the attenuated signal is still there, after all).

The problem was partly solved by Shiffrin and Schneider (1977) who presented a *two-process model* of information processing. Their model must be viewed against the background of a change in metaphor. The older, structural models were inspired by rigid hardware systems in telecommunication, but in the meantime the computer metaphor had become more popular. A computer acts as a flexible system, which includes a pragmatic selective mechanism on the basis of its software. Shiffrin and Schneider incorporated this concept of flexible selectivity into their model while retaining the possibility of hard-wired selection on the basis of enduring dispositions.

These authors extended a distinction that had been made before between *automatic* and *conscious* processing of information. Some tasks, particularly when they are overlearned or well-trained, seem to be executed completely automatically—implying that the execution of such a task is not dependent on a conscious choice, and not impaired by the concurrent execution of another task. In contrast, new or unfamiliar tasks require "our full attention" and a conscious effort. Their execution is strongly impaired when they must be combined with other activities. Automaticity may be inborn for the processing of basic perceptual features of stimuli, but is based on learning for the remainder. Shiffrin and Schneider convincingly demonstrated how visual search and memory comparison can become automatic by learning in a situation with consistent and predictable *S-R* relationships. In such a situation conscious or controlled processing develops into automatic processing as a result of practice on the task.

Automatic processing occurs in parallel, and therefore the capacity of this mode of processing is almost unlimited. On the other hand, controlled processing is thought to proceed in a serial manner because of its strong interference with and from other tasks, and because its efficiency is strongly dependent on time-pressure. Generally speaking, the duration of controlled processes is a linear function of the number of hypothetical cognitive steps to be taken in a task. The area of controlled processing more or less overlaps with "conscious" decision-making and with nonroutine decision processes in "working memory" (WM). This was a computer-inspired concept (Baddeley and Hitch, 1974; Baddeley, 1986) to which we return later in this chapter. Shiffrin and Schneider emphasized the paramount role of automatic information processing, while at the same time demonstrating that a hypothetical attention director can select information from any source in any stage between *S* and *R* in order to process this material consciously in further stages (see Figure 2-3).

These same authors described two kinds of attentional problems: focused attention deficits (FADs) and divided attention deficits (DADs) (see Figure 2-4).

A *focused attention deficit* occurs when a response produced by automatic processing interferes with a response produced by controlled processing. For example, when driving a new car where the positions of windshield wiper and turn indicator controls are located opposite to their positions in the previous vehicle, the windshield wipers will often be turned on accidentally. It does not always come to the actual turning on of the wipers, but the tendency is experienced and may only be overcome by more controlled processing. In terms of our earlier distinction, FADs could be described as attention controlled by enduring dispositions, but in this case the enduring dispositions have been acquired through previous experience, and because of that they may vary greatly between individuals.

Sometimes the response drawn by an automatic process is "stop, look, and listen." One might call this an automatic attention response, as when someone calls your name. Using the spotlight metaphor, the spotlight is suddenly given a jerk in an unexpected direction because of an automatic attention response. Essentially, a FAD is a disruption of ongoing controlled processing by automatic processing. For example, when driving it is generally wise to look ahead, but when someone addresses the driver he may almost automatically turn his head to the speaker. This is why city buses have signs for passengers stating, "Please don't talk to driver while bus is in motion."

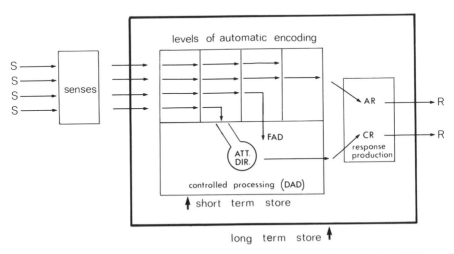

Figure 2-4 The two-process model of information processing as described by Shiffrin and Schneider. *ATT. DIR.*, attention director; *AR*, automatic response, in this case compatible with *CR*, controlled response; *FAD*, focused attention deficit, a result of automatic processing intruding in the domain of controlled processing; *DAD*, divided attention deficit, when rate of controlled processing is too low. Note that *short-term store* is an activated part of *long-term store*. (Adapted from Shiffrin and Schneider, 1977, with permission.)

A *divided attention deficit* (DAD) results from the limited capacity of the system for controlled processing. This is clearly a case of attention by momentary intentions. If too much task-relevant information is presented too quickly, the system can no longer cope. Hence, relevant signals will be missed, or the required series of responses cannot be carried out. DAD is also a familiar problem in daily life, for example, when trying to understand a complex argument or in the early stages of learning a new skill. The system's limitations become apparent in particular when it tries to carry out two tasks or two elements of an unfamiliar skill simultaneously, dividing the capacity for controlled processing between two sources of information and two kinds of responses. In the spotlight metaphor, controlled processing may be conceptualized as the sequential movement of a spotlight over a series of subproblems, moving from stimulus to response, while each subproblem, as in a filming process, requires the application of light for a considerable duration.

Summary. In modern general theories of attention the need for selective attention is explained by the limited capacity of central stages of information processing. In structural theories, selection works as a process of attenuation of part of the input on the basis of physical features and, at the output side of the system, as a process of selectively modulating thresholds for responding. In Shiffrin and Schneider's two-process theory, attention is not located at a fixed stage in the *S-R* chain and no separate selective mechanisms are postulated. At any level of processing, early or late, when a representation is given controlled processing, it is attended. When it is not given controlled processing it is not attended. Because controlled processing is a slow and capacity-limited process, limitations of attention occur when a task requires many controlled operations per unit time. Attention through controlled processing can best be understood in terms of a software analogy. The cognitive actions required for this selectivity are regulated through the currently active control-program in working memory and can only be interrupted by the outcome of automatic processes which proceed independent of working memory.

The strength of this approach lies in the precise quantitative predictability of performance of relatively simple cognitive tasks with an element of time pressure, the intuitively appealing explanation of deficits of focused and divided attention in such tasks and the well defined relationship between selective and intensive aspects of attention (see the section on resource theories). A relative weakness of the approach is that it does not take into account the large differences that appear to exist between modalities. In the auditory system, for example, there is little possibility for peripheral filtering of information, except by putting a finger into one ear—as we do when making a phone call in a noisy room. In the visual and tactual systems, such filtering is quite easily achieved by directing the orientation of the eyes or fingers. Spatial aspects of selective attention are underrepresented in general theories. These central issues are addressed in the literature on visual selective attention, discussed in the next section.

Another weakness of the information processing approach is that higher order aspects of attention, such as the planning and regulation of goal-directed activity, are not taken into account. The cognitive schema theory, described later, does a better and more realistic job of this, but it is too imprecise for quantitative predictions of performance.

Theories of Visual Selective Attention

There are a number of spatial constraints in visual selective attention. One important spatial constraint is that the eyes can only see in one direction so that all information from behind is missed. More seriously, however, the retinal area most sensitive for identifying detail is limited to a small area around the fovea, or to only a few degrees of visual angle (LaBerge and Brown, 1989). The major part of the brain's capacity to process visual information is used for information from this small area. Besides this highly sensitive foveal area, there is a much larger peripheral area (both eyes together extend 180–200 degrees in the horizontal direction and about 130 degrees in the vertical direction). Visual function of the peripheral area is enough for global orientation in space, but details can only be examined after the head and/or eyes align the foveal area with the projected object. So, a very reasonable assumption is that head and eye movements are the instrumental elements of the mechanism for allocating the brain's visual information processing capacity to a visual stimulus. In our spotlight metaphor, head and eyes direct the orientation of the spotlight.

According to Theeuwis (1992; also Engel, 1977) this global way of selecting and analyzing certain parts of the visual environment by head and/or eye movement is strongly controlled by top-down strategies, as in deciding to look first to the left and then to the right before crossing a street. This could be described as selection on the basis of momentary intentions, a different strategy when wanting to turn left than when wanting to turn right. But the cognitive schema specifying this strategy may have been formed during extensive prior experience with the activity and therefore it has elements of an enduring disposition as well. Being continental Europeans, we experience this dualistic character when visiting the United Kingdom where traffic drives on the left side of the road. When crossing as pedestrians, we consciously know we have to look right first but our enduring disposition to look left first is quite hard to inhibit. Common to both conflicting tendencies is that they are top-down selective strategies.

When a highly salient object is encountered, even outside the range specified by the top-down strategy, this object may capture control and elicit an eye movement toward it. This can certainly be described as selection on the basis of enduring dispositions and, in addition, it is also a bottom-up process (in contrast to the just described top-down processes). Salience is determined by factors like temporal onset, proximity to the fovea and size, whereas fine structure is unimportant (Boff et al., 1986).

Van der Heiden (1991), questioned the necessity for the limited capacity assumption with regard to central visual perception, citing neurophysiological evidence (Barlow, 1985) with regard to the number of retinal ganglion cells (approximately 2,000,000) and the number of cortical cells involved in visual information processing (a factor 100 more). In his view the limited capacity factor in the system are the eyes. Remarkably though, theories of visual selective attention are not about the regulation of head and eye movement. Instead they are about the selection process occurring within a single fixation of the eyes. The reasoning behind this is that eye movements should not be considered the selection process itself, but merely a consequence of the attentional selection processes preceding actual eye-shifts. According to Posner and Cohen (1984), when a saccade is made toward a particular location, attention moves to that location *before* its onset. Attention is thought to have two functions here, namely, specifying the beamwidth of the area, for example, only the small central part, or a wider area, and the precuing of a small area within that area for extraefficient processing. This restriction to information processing within a fixation eliminates a lot of (unknown) individual and situational differences in scanning strategies. This is considered necessary to be able to obtain accurate estimations of beamwidth and intensity. On the negative side, this experimental restriction leads to the use of very artificial situations, which may strongly limit the generalization of results to everyday activities. For example, the strategic control of head and eye movements in the light of task requirements is an important aspect in traffic. Also, in clinical neuropsychology, the importance of eye movements as an indicator of failing search strategies was recognized by Luria (1973). It is hoped that in the near future more attention will be given to the study of eye movements and their top-down attentional control. The theoretical approach that may be most relevant here is the cognitive schema theory described later.

Selective Attention Within a Fixation

In daily life, a shift in attention is usually followed by an overt movement of the eyes. It has been repeatedly demonstrated in experimental situations that a shift in attention can occur without eye movement. The spotlight metaphor implies that directing attention in visual space is necessary before selective response to a visual target is possible. This is particularly so in searching for targets which can be distinguished from their surroundings only on the basis of a conjunction of separable features, as, for example, a green T in a field of blue T's and green X's (Treisman and Gelade, 1980). The *feature integration theory* (FIT) of attention suggests that attention must be directed serially to each stimulus in a display, in this case by a sequential spatial scan, comparable to controlled processing. This is based on the linear relation (some 10 to 30 ms per item, depending on experimental details) between the reaction time and the number of stimuli in a visual display. "Thus focal attention provides the "glue" that integrates the initially separable features into unitary objects (Treisman and Gelade, 1980, p. 98)."

Prior to the slow serial feature integration process, the visual scene has been coded in parallel along a number of separable dimensions, such as color, orientation, spatial frequency, brightness, and direction of movement. This conclusion is based on the finding that reaction time is not influenced by the number of elements in a display when targets are distinguished from distractors on the basis of a separable feature only, for example, color. Such stimuli are said to "pop out." In general, experimental evidence has been quite supportive of the FIT, but there are some exceptions to the claim that the search for conjunction targets is performed serially. According to Theeuwis (1992, p. 30): "Under certain circumstances, e.g., large display sizes or when searching for conjunctions involves a special type of feature, e.g., movement and depth, search functions become relatively flat."

FIT is primarily concerned with attention on the basis of momentary intentions in the case of relatively unfamiliar objects and does not imply that all conjunctions of features require attention. Theeuwis (1992, p. 98) claims that

> attention is necessary for the *correct* perception of conjunctions, although unattended features are also conjoined prior to conscious perception. The top-down processing of unattended features is capable of utilizing past experience and contextual information. Even when attention is directed elsewhere, we are unlikely to see a blue sun in a yellow sky.

Further, Theeuwis (1992, p. 30) notes that "The alternative theories for the FIT all incorporate some top-down mechanism on the parallel preattentive stage so that targets which are very dissimilar to the target do not have the same probability of entering the attentive stage, as do nontargets which are more similar to the target." This dissimilarity may be in the physical sense but possibly also in the semantic sense as is suggested by the results of Shiffrin and Schneider (1977) on automatic processing described earlier.

Neuropsychological evidence also supports the possibility of deep semantic processing of stimuli without prior localization and attention. McGlinchey-Berroth and colleagues (1992) demonstrated that patients with unilateral (left-sided) neglect could profit from picture primes in the (neglected) left visual field, which facilitated RT in a subsequent lexical decision task. However, these patients were unable to perceive similar left-sided stimuli in a discrimination task. The interpretation of the linear increase of RT with display size could be in terms of the time needed to move (the spotlight of) attention from one position to the next but also in terms of the time necessary to engage attention on a stimulus and check the conjunction. Several studies have been aimed at the question of how fast attention moves. The original claim that "the spotlight of attention" moves with constant velocity through visual space (e.g., Posner, 1980) is not supported by recent studies (Kwak et al., 1991; Shyi and Chen, 1992). The latter authors conclude "that shifting the focus of attention in the visual space should best be characterized as discrete movement that is time-invariant with respect to the travel distance." Moreover, they found evidence that a larger attentional focus may move faster in visual space than a small one.

More detailed study of the "movement" of attention, in particular the processes of engaging and disengaging attention to and from a stimulus has been carried out in the so-called covert orienting paradigm (Posner, 1980). In covert orienting experiments, a cue specifying the most probable location of the subsequent target significantly influences detection of and reaction time to that target. The positive effect of covert orienting is shown as decreased reaction time to targets presented at the cued location, and its negative effect is shown as increased reaction time to targets at an uncued location. Also, events occurring at the cued location "give rise to enhanced electrocortical activity . . . and can be reported at a lower threshold . . . . This covert shift of attention appears to function as a way of guiding the eyes to the appropriate area of visual field" (Posner, 1989, p. 5).

Two different methods are used for producing a covert shift of attention. Either a peripheral cue is given at the location where the subsequent relevant event will probably occur, or a central cue is given which symbolizes or points to the relevant location. The first method could be taken as an example of attention drawn by enduring dispositions, a form of automatic orienting of attention, and the second as attention drawn by momentary intentions, a voluntary (controlled) form of attention. There is neuropsychological evidence that suggests the brain mechanisms involved in these two forms of covert orienting are different, as patients with so-called unilateral neglect (see Chapter 3) are particularly impaired in the automatic orienting of attention and less so in the voluntary form (Ladavas, 1992). This suggests that the primary problem these patients have is not with attention as such (in the "William James connotation" of an active mental process, in this case the voluntary form of covert orienting), but rather with preattentive processes selecting salient stimuli for attention. This becomes a major problem when a cue is presented ipsilateral to the side of the lesion just prior to presentation of a relevant stimulus in the visual field, contralateral to the lesion. In this case, the right parietal patients tested by Posner and coworkers (1982) often did not react at all to relevant stimuli in the left visual field. This is an example of the clinical phenomenon of extinction where a stimulus in the not neglected area is said to draw attention like a "magnet." According to Posner (1989), the most important problem patients with unilateral neglect (following right parietal lesions) have, is in disengaging attention from stimuli in the not-neglected area of the visual field.

Most theories of visual selective attention assume that location plays a unique role in the selection of information for further processing. Posner's account of covert orienting suggests that a spatial cue facilitates processing, since all attentional resources are concentrated on a relatively small portion of the visual field, and increases the processing speed of objects appearing at that location. Even more striking, in Treisman and Gelade's FIT, locating a target on the basis of a conjunction of features is a prerequisite for its identification. Theories of general attention, on the other hand, of which Shiffrin and Schneider's (1977) is the most important, hold that location is just one selection dimension, albeit a very effective one. Visual selection can be guided by any type of cue as long as it provides discriminative power to separate targets from nontargets.

A strong clinical argument for a special role of spatial cues in the selection of information for further processing is provided by the existence of the *neglect* syndromes. In its pure form, a patient with visual-spatial neglect fails to report, respond, or orient to novel or meaningful stimuli presented to the side opposite a brain lesion (Heilman et al., 1985). However, evidence from electrophysiological studies and priming studies (McGlinchey-Berroth et al., 1992) demonstrates that neglected stimuli are clearly represented in the patient's brain, even at a rather high level of abstraction, but that these representations appear to be inaccessible.

It is possible that this inaccessibility is related to the fact that spatial cues act as an index required for assessing the activated memory representation. Van der Heiden's (1991) recent theory of postcategorical filtering appears to fit this notion. In spite of being a neuropsychological theory based on recent physiological insights about a separation of processing channels in the brain for identity and position, it emerged from the field of normal experimental psychology and has not yet been applied to clinical neuropsychology.

Van der Heiden's theory does not easily fit into the early or late selection dichotomy, which we found convenient for classifying theories of attention. In line with late selection theories, it suggests that visual information is automatically registered and processed in parallel up to the level of identification before selection takes place. In line with early selection theories, it suggests that attention operates via spatial locations: retrieval of the identity code can only occur by the means of positioning the object. The essentials of the theory are schematically represented in Figure 2-5.

Van der Heiden gives a neurophysiological underpinning to his theory by referring to a fundamental distinction within the "new" visual system involving the geniculate nuclei. The "old" system involved the superior colliculi as described in Chapter 3. Two subsystems may be distinguished from the retinal level up to the visual association cortex: the *parvo* system (small cells) and *magno* system (large cells) (Livingstone and Hubel, 1988). From the primary and sec-

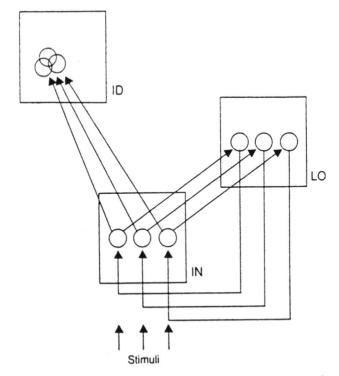

Figure 2-5 Van der Heiden's model of postcategorical filtering. Sensory information enters the input module (*IN*). Identity (*ID*) and location (*LO*) are processed in separate modules, with massive feedback from the location module to the input module. (From Van der Heiden, 1991, with permission.)

ondary visual cortices, the magno system projects onto the parieto-occipital cortex and the parvo system onto the temporo-occipital cortex. Visual information is initially organized in an "input module" (the striate cortex) in the form of a "primary sketch," uninterpreted features not yet localized in space. The information is transmitted through an identity channel (parvo) and a location channel leading to the parieto-occipital cortex (magno). Thus visual selective attention works by way of feedback between the input model and the parieto-occipital location module and the input module.

The postulated existence of the location module within the parieto-occipital cortex is compatible with data showing that lesions in this area are most often associated with the neglect syndrome (Heilman et al., 1985). Still, the issue is open to question. A weak point in the theory as it now stands is that it does not account for the differential contributions of left and right hemispheres to spatial attention. The neglect syndrome is much more general and profound with right rather than left hemisphere lesions (see Heilman et al., 1985 for a review). Otherwise, the theory offers a satisfactory explanation for neglect phenomena. It is a retrieval theory (information is available but not accessible), making it understandable how quite elaborate representations of stimuli could exist without drawing attention to define its meaning (e.g., the results of the semantic priming study described above).

Bisiach and Luzatti's observation (1978) regarding neglect of left-sided details may also be interpreted in terms of a retrieval problem (Baddeley and Lieberman, 1980). When two patients with neglect of the left were asked to imagine that they stood on a well-known plaza in Milan viewing the cathedral and describe what they would see, they failed to describe buildings to their left. Subsequently they were asked to imagine that they stood on the same plaza with their back to the cathedral. Now they described the initially omitted buildings but failed to describe buildings on the other side of the square.

The Cognitive Schema Theory

The emphasis on the role of automatic information processing and automatic responding inevitably raises the question of control over automatisms. This

Figure 2-6 Schema-driven information processing as conceived by Shallice. Arrows represent activating input, except for contention scheduling; these inputs are primarily mutually inhibitory. The term *effector system* refers to specific purpose processing units, involved in schema operation for both action and thought schemas. (Adapted from Shallice, 1982, with permission.)

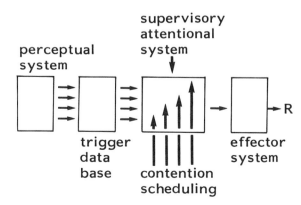

question was addressed by Shallice (1982), who presented a theoretical model of human behavior in which all activity, mental and overt, is viewed as the unfolding of mental schemas. These schemas specify the interpretation of external input and subsequent action. Specific trigger conditions in the external input are required for a schema to become active and subsequently determine behavior. Often, however, many triggers will be present at the same time, and hence many schemas could be activated simultaneously, resulting in disrupted or chaotic behavior. Shallice postulated two adaptive mechanisms to regulate the mutual power relationships between schemas: contention scheduling and supervisory attentional control (see Figure 2-6).

Contention scheduling is an automatic conflict resolution process that selects one of the conflicting schemas according to priorities and environmental cues and gives it precedence at any given moment. When a schema is active it is assumed to bias the elicitability of other schemas by lateral inhibition of incompatible schemas and lateral facilitation of compatible ones. This process makes it less probable that incompatible schemas leading to chaotic behaviors will be selected. At the same time, subsequent triggers may be anticipated, at least if they fit compatible schemas.

In contention scheduling, schema selection is solely regulated by external triggers and the lateral biasing of elicitability. The latter aspect is based on dependencies between the schemas. These have been developed through experience and are represented by associative connections between their representations in long-term memory. A compatible schema is one, experienced previously, which has led to successful performance in a similar context. Thus, contention scheduling is optimally suited for routine behavior in well-known circumstances. The other adaptive mechanism, *supervisory attentional control*, is called upon in nonroutine situations. In contrast to contentional scheduling schemas are not biased on the basis of associative relationships represented in long-term memory but instead on the basis of a strategy active in working memory. Supervisory attentional control may be viewed as a voluntary top-down modulation of the excitability of schemas (most likely by inhibition). It is thought that the supervisory attentional control cannot select schemas in a direct manner but must proceed by influencing the excitability of schemas. Because of this, it is possible for unwanted schemas to become active in spite of the supervisory attentional control, as seen in the classical Stroop test.

According to De Jong (1991), we have only vague notions about the manner in which schema selection by the supervisory attentional control might occur. Most authors do agree that this selection occurs on the basis of activity in working memory. This also provides the link that allows experimental psychologists to control subjects' behavior by verbal instruction when they are performing unfamiliar mental tasks. Applying the supervisory attentional control concept to the spotlight metaphor requires some imagination. One could imagine a largely automatic spotlight system that is triggered by some automatic movement detection device to follow the most salient visible object on a stage. The same spotlight is necessary, however, for lighting an area on the stage where there is currently little action, but where a very important action is likely to develop within a short time. The reaction of the spotlight to the currently most active person on the stage may be prevented by temporarily inhibiting the current supply of the movement-following system. But this inhibition must be immediately lifted when the scene of the action has shifted. Using this metaphor, anticipation, inhibition, and flexibility are important elements of supervisory attentional control. The anticipatory character is primarily provided by the plan behind the cognitive strategy. Inhibition and flexibility are characteristic of the regulation of this strategy in accordance with the dynamics of the task requirements.

Both the cognitive schema theory and the information processing approach have confronted investigators with close connections between attention and memory (Baddeley, 1993). The role of previous experiences and associations in long-term memory has already been mentioned repeatedly. Both the Shiffrin and Schneider model and the Shallice model contain features that are related to the concept of working memory as postulated by Baddeley and Hitch (1974). This concept refers to the functional analysis of temporary storage and manipulation during information processing, incorporating a central executive for complex decision and control processes, and a number of subsidiary slave systems thought to be involved in specific processing (Baddeley, 1986). In his chapter on the central executive element of working memory, which he more or less models according to the supervisory attentional control concept, Baddeley gives a description of the situations wherein this element is strongly put to the test (Baddeley, 1986, p. 228):

> including: (a) tasks that involve planning or decision making, (b) situations in which the automatic processes appear to be running into difficulties and some form of troubleshooting is necessary, (c) where novel or poorly learned sequences of acts are involved, (d) where the situation is judged to be dangerous or technically difficult, and (e) where some strong habitual response or temptation is involved.

The central executive in this description is comparable to the concept of "supervisory attentional control" and plays a similar role in the theoretical explanation of attention. One might express the close connection between short-term memory and attentive behavior by stating that we are, in fact, attending with our working memory (Baddeley, 1993). The Shallice model clearly has some features in common with the Shiffrin and Schneider model. The latter emphasized that all information processing begins with automatic processing and proceeds by using existing associative connections in long-term memory. Likewise, Shallice points out that routine schemas are activated in any mental activity. Even in a new task there will always be familiar components in either the input or the motor output, or both. Further, the Attention Director in the Shiffrin and Schneider model is able to read out information from any stage in automatic processing, just as supervisory attentional control is able to suppress routine programs anywhere between stimulus and response. There is a difference of emphasis, however. The Shallice model is basically concerned with the selection of and switching between schemas, while the Shiffrin and Schneider model is concerned with the execution of activities specified by these schemas.

Capacity and Processing Resources

Capacity theories of attention originated with the observation of interference between tasks that are executed simultaneously. In such theories it is assumed that psychological processes require processing structures, as well as the commitment of a certain amount of processing resources. It is further assumed that these resources are limited. Different psychological processes can vary in the amount (and type) of resources they require, as may be revealed by the pattern of interference seen in a particular combination of tasks (Wickens, 1984, p. 63):

> The concept of processing resources is proposed as a hypothetical intervening variable to account for variations in the efficiency with which time-sharing can be carried out; that is the degree to which two tasks can be performed concurrently as well as each can be performed in isolation.

According to capacity theories, the selectivity of attention is a result of the limited availability of a processing resource. The latter may be viewed as an intensity aspect of attention. If more resources become available, attention may be applied more intensely or, alternatively, with the same intensity over a wider range.

Salthouse (1988, p. 258) observed that "the bulk of references to the concept of processing resources could be encompassed within three categories organized around the *metaphors of time, energy and space.*" These categories will be elaborated below. In Shiffrin and Schneider's theory, the available processing *time* is an important factor limiting performance in a divided attention task requiring controlled processing, a slow serial activity. Therefore, one might say that the resource which limits divided attention here is the amount of available time for processing. Taking this reasoning one step further, the time required for a controlled process, as estimated with mental chronometric methods, gives a direct estimation of attentional capacity.

Obersteiner (1879) suggested using the duration of reaction time (RT) as a measure of attention in the very first issue of the journal *Brain*. Related ideas can be found in the works of Wells and colleagues (1921) and McComas (1922). However, as RT will be determined in part by the perceptual and motor characteristics of the person reacting, it is difficult to separate these peripheral elements from attention. Modern psychology has developed methods for eliminating this confounding by using, for example, Sternberg's paradigm of speeded memory scanning (Sternberg, 1975) and Shiffrin and Schneider's (1977) visual search tasks. In this paradigm, the slope of the linear function relating RT to memory set size identifies a purely central RT component indicating the rate of information processing.

One problem emerging when the rate of processing is taken as a measure of attention is its dependency on the nature of the symbolic stimulus material presented which might involve visual search, mental arithmetic, mental rotation, sentence comprehension or any other cognitive activity. Is the task at hand a test of attention, or a test of perception, intelligence, semantic memory, or what? This view also implies that attention is not a unitary concept, as noted above, but something which has to be assessed separately for different cognitive areas. This implication will be discussed below in more detail.

Assuming that a subject is doing the best he can, the individual rate of processing in a certain task could be considered a measure for the individual's maximum capacity of attention in that area. Shiffrin and Schneider (1977) have shown that this measure can also explain performance and deficits in divided attention, as long as no real time-sharing is possible between the two tasks involved. However, possibilities for parallel processing increase when the two tasks are from entirely different areas. Of course prior experience with the tasks also plays a role, particularly if this has led to automatization. Automatic processing is parallel processing, almost by definition.

The electrical power supply of a spotlight system is an example of the way in which resources could be imagined as *energy*. The number of spotlights that can be used simultaneously is not only limited by the number of separate lights (and hands moving them), but also by the power supply providing the energy. In this metaphor, the maximum capacity of the power supply stands for the processing resources. Kahneman (1973) proposed a psychological theory based on the energy metaphor in which all non-structural interference between tasks was explained by a central energy "mental effort" limitation. In his view, mental effort, a scarce commodity, must be allocated by the processing system to a variety of tasks or subtasks. The availability of mental effort is not a fixed property in an individual but may vary somewhat with his/her arousal level (see Chapter 3).

Resources in competition for *space* are difficult to visualize using the spotlight metaphor. One might think of two different theaters in which separate plays are being performed having to share the same set of spotlights. In principle, the activities in the two theaters are independent, but if one play requires all the spotlights, the play in the other theater has to stop. A more naturalistic metaphor would be to view the surface of the stage as the resource; if it is smaller, fewer separate spots of lights can be projected without interference. Kinsbourne and Hicks (1978) presented a similar concept in which resources are thought to reflect competition for a "functional cerebral space."

When the resource theories were applied for predicting interference between various types of cognitive tasks, it appeared that explanations in terms of only one resource, be it time, energy or space, failed. For example, it can be shown that there is strong interference between the simultaneous demands of a visual motor tracking task and a mental rotation task. This can also be demonstrated for verbal learning tasks and mental computation. Taken separately, these results agree with a single resource theory. The difficulty for such a theory arises when tracking tasks are combined with verbal learning tasks. It then appears that both tasks can be time-shared perfectly. The possibilities for time-sharing vary between situations and individuals. Individuals often appear able to time-share very easily between two or more tasks, as when driving while thinking and singing.

Wickens (1984) produced a multiple-resource model by combining various types of tasks and studying interference (Figure 2-7). Interpreting this model in terms of the spatial metaphor, the coarse outlines of a "brain model" with

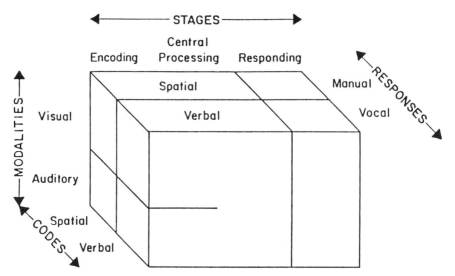

Figure 2-7   The dimensional structure of human processing resources proposed by Wickens. The absence of a complete separation of auditory and visual resources through the perceptual-central processing stages indicates uncertainty as to whether the benefit of cross-modality presentation is preserved in central processing. (From Wickens, 1984, with permission.)

separate loci for spatial and verbal processing and for different modalities may be observed in the figure. In this respect, Wickens (1984, p. 90) states:

> Two tasks with demands in close proximity within this functional space share re-sources—neural processing mechanisms—and will interfere with each's perfor-mance. Where this space contains discontinuities (as between cerebral hemispheres or processing modalities), adoption of a multiple-resources conception becomes quite plausible.

A general criticism of capacity models is that they may be based on circular reasoning. Identification of resources and their limited availability is mainly derived from the patterns of interference between various tasks and interference is explained by the limited availability of resources. Basically, this criticism can only be overcome by measuring the commitment of processing resources inde-pendently of task performance. These measures will presumably be of a phys-iological or anatomical nature. The circularity criticism applies particularly to the space and energy metaphors. In the time metaphor, independent assessment of processing resources may be obtained in some elementary tasks by using mental chronometric methods. The conceptualization of processing resources in terms of time is usually more difficult, however, as differences in performance attributable to attentional, perceptual and cognitive processes are difficult to distinguish.

Notwithstanding these criticisms, the multiple-resource models are a useful heuristic for parsimoniously describing a large body of evidence on interference effects in dual tasks. A second appeal of capacity models of attention, particularly the energy versions, is that they have a certain face-validity with regard to subjectively felt functional limitations of attention which tend to change from situation to situation and which are only partially under voluntary control (mental effort). "Lulled into a pleasant state of drowsiness by his teacher's voice, the schoolboy does not merely fail to pay attention to what the teacher says; he has less attention to pay (Kahneman, 1973, p. 3).

ATTENTION AS AN INDIVIDUAL TRAIT

In our discussion of the question of attention as a unitary mechanism, we referred to Davies and colleagues' (1984) chapter on individual and group differences in healthy populations. These authors stated that there is a paucity of basic data on attention concerning the range of individual variation in performance, the reliability of performance in any task, and the extent to which performance scores in different tasks intercorrelate. The limited number of studies they could find nevertheless allowed them to conclude:

> With respect to individual differences, there is little or no support for a general time-sharing ability or for a general vigilance ability; and the existence of a general selective-attention ability seems unlikely.

Stankov (1983, 1988) and De Jong (1991) discussed the factor-analytic evidence for separate factors of focused or divided attention and came to similar conclusions. If scores on tests of attention intercorrelated highly, it was often on the basis of task similarities not related to the variation of the requirement to focus, divide, or sustain attention, such as stimulus or response modality or area of skill or knowledge. If factor structure reflects the structure of abilities, then it appears that individual attentional abilities can not be easily categorized in terms of focused, divided, and sustained attention.

In a sense this conclusion is not surprising, as there are large differences between tasks within these broad classes, in terms of stimulus and response modalities and in terms of the required mental operations. If someone easily gets drowsy when understimulated and only becomes very alert under high task pressure, it is quite likely that this discrepancy will also show up in his performance scores on two sustained attention tasks that differ widely with respect to the rate of information presentation. Yet, both types of tasks are common in sustained attention research (Parasuraman and Davies, 1977).

The number of studies designed to measure individual differences and correlations between various attentional test scores is very limited. It is not at all clear at this moment how many distinct focused, divided, and sustained attention abilities exist. The paradigms of visual selective attention described above provide a number of potentially interesting possibilities for investigating individual differences in the area of focused attention. Neuropsychological research with patient groups suggests that separate abilities might exist for voluntary (endogenous) and reflexive (exogenous) covert orienting (Ladavas, 1992). It would be interesting to see if this dissociation also occurs in normals. One might conjecture that the endogenous type loads higher than the exogenous type on a visual analysis factor as measured from performance on tests like the Embedded Figures Test.

Turning to *divided attention*, our research in healthy adults illustrates dissociations between performance in task blocks with high and low attentional requirements, suggesting genuine attentional abilities and considerable individual variation with respect to each one. We conducted a number of divided attention studies in which two continuous visual motor tasks were performed separately and in combination (Ponds et al., 1988; Brouwer et al., 1989, 1990, 1991). The difficulty of each of the tasks to be combined in the divided attention condition was individually determined on the basis of single-task performance. The correlation between divided attention costs (performance loss relative to single task) and single-task performance appeared to be negligible in healthy adults, while both could be assessed with reasonable reliability. We also demonstrated that the divided attention cost scores provide information not available in the single-task scores: specific negative effects of normal aging could be shown on the former but not the latter. These results point to a specific ability with regard to integrating visual-motor skills rather than to a general time-sharing ability and therefore agree with the conclusions drawn by Davies and colleagues (1984).

A comparable dissociation was observed in the area of *sustained attention* when a monotonous low event rate auditory vigilance task was administered to a normal control group (Van Zomeren et al., 1984; Brouwer, 1985). Each subject was tested twice on separate occasions three months apart. Substantial performance decrement in the later part of the vigilance task only occurred in subjects who became drowsy as defined by independent, on-line EEG analysis. The average detection performance of subjects who were going to be drowsy and those who were not, was approximately the same in the early part of the vigilance task. Therefore, information indicating individual differences in the ability to sustain attention was available from the subjects' performance in the later but not the earlier part of the task. Although the study had other aims the task it employed probably revealed reliable individual differences in ability to sustain attention in monotonous, low event rate situations; three of the four subjects who showed much drowsiness on the first test occasion, did so again three months later.

By and large, the existing evidence concerning individual differences in attention might better fit a "vertical mental faculty" framework (Fodor, 1983) than the horizontal framework suggested by the clustering in terms of focused, divided, and sustained attention. The vertical mental faculty framework, also described as modularity, assumes that the mind consists of a number of independent cognitive systems or modules, each relating to a specific mental area, as, for example, verbal and visuospatial information processing. The term vertical implies that each system may encompass subordinate perceptual, cognitive, motivational, and mnestic processes within that area. Modules are assumed to be structurally and functionally independent of each other, as indicated, for example, by either selective destruction or sparing of one cognitive function relative to others as a result of brain dysfunction. [A spectacular demonstration of sparing occurs in so-called "idiots savants" (see Gardner, 1983)]. By implication, selective processes are part of one module and will be largely independent of similar processes in other modules. Hence as many varieties of attention can exist as there are modules. In terms of our metaphor, the quality of the spotlight systems would be independent in the many different theaters in which mental acts are performed. Modality specific theories of attention and multiple resource theories (Wickens et al., 1981; Wickens, 1984), which imply separate attentional capacities for different task categories (e.g., verbal vs spatial tasks), fit reasonably well into this type of thinking.

Fortunately, this is not the whole story. A further, interesting role for attention, but now in a general sense, emerges when a problem cannot be solved within a vertical faculty or when two separate vertical faculties working in parallel lead to conflicting responses. Fodor (1983) saw the role of attention as a horizontal cognitive faculty that comes into play when vertical faculties fail and an alternative information processing route has to be found. Attention cannot penetrate into the processes within a vertical faculty but it can assess their products and translate these into a code serving as an input for a processor in a different module. There is considerable evidence to support supervisory attentional control from the cognitive schema theory as a good candidate for this general faculty or ability.

De Jong (1991) discussed all the older factor analytic studies in the area of attention and partly reanalyzed their data. An important early study was published by Wittenborn (1943). According to him, a test of attention should correlate as little as possible with factors identified previously and should not require intellectual skills and experience. Performance should be determined primarily by "a continuous sustained application of mental effort" (p. 20). Starting with these guidelines, he constructed six tests that appear to require sustained mental flexibility. In each test a number of letters or digits were presented vocally, which had to be verified within a short time limit. For instance, in "Triplet Numbers," three digits were presented, one after the other and the task was to write a plus sign when the first digit was the largest and the second one the smallest, but also when the three digits were in ascending order. No response was required in all other cases. In a study involving 175 army recruits, the scores on these 6 tests and 12 more from Thurstone's battery for primary mental abilities, were factor-analyzed, and it appeared that the tests constructed for assessing attention indeed loaded on a separate factor.

De Jong (1991) argued that Wittenborn's attention tests put a strong load on *working memory* and *mental flexibility* and might be described as tests primarily of the central executive aspect of working memory (supervisory attentional control). He further noted that scores from cancellation tasks which are often used for assessing attention in a clinical setting, do not load on Wittenborn's attention factor, but on a separate factor labeled *perceptual speed*. De Jong further observed that subsequent factor-analytic studies of attention or related concepts appeared to confirm the distinction between perceptual speed and the working memory aspect of supervisory attentional control. So, the distinction between attention as speed of information processing and as supervisory attentional control appears to be relevant as far as individual differences in a healthy population are concerned. The qualification has to be made, however, that speed of information processing must be specified according to the area in which it occurs (e.g., visual or verbal). Supervisory attentional control would probably also vary according to area (Shallice, 1988).

The many different connotations of attention, to both laymen and psychologists (Parasuraman and Davies, 1984), the low correlation between performance on different attention tasks, and the "boundary disputes" with perception, problem solving and memory, all demonstrate that *attention certainly cannot be viewed as a single individual trait*. It is meaningless to say that a person's attention is poor, without further elaboration, and without mentioning the test on which that judgment is based. Relevant general aspects appear to be supervisory attentional control and speed of processing, but these are still very broad categories. More specific attentional abilities have not yet been well investigated. This is an important task for the future. In this endeavor, theories of attention and sound psychometric practice are of equal importance.

We stress this latter point because experimental psychology, and particularly information processing psychology, tends to show a lack of interest in the basic psychometric issues of validity and reliability. It is often implicitly assumed that the elementary processes investigated by means of mental chronometry are so universal that they will appear in a variety of tasks, including classic psychological tests and everyday tasks, and as such they are treated as a kind of "natural" abilities. To quote Robert Sternberg (1985), who is quite favorably disposed to the information processing approach: "It is not immediately obvious that performance in real-world settings can be reduced to task performance on very simple tasks" (p. 19).

A colorful illustration of the relevance of this (under)statement may be observed in the investigation of fitness to drive in patients suspected of suffering from Alzheimer's disease. More than once, we have seen such patients leave our laboratory and perform complicated driving maneuvers impeccably when merging with the traffic on the busy road outside the building, despite the fact that just before they had scored far below the normal range on almost every test of information processing and attention administered to them, tests that had been selected because they supposedly tap basic processes intrinsic to the task of driving. Of course, this does not prove that Alzheimer patients are fit drivers, but it is a warning against overly simplistic extrapolation of psychological test scores to everyday practice.

ATTENTION AS A DYNAMIC COGNITIVE STATE

An alternative to viewing attention as an individual trait is to view it as the dynamic cognitive state preceding and promoting selective behavior in a specific situation or task. This dynamic state could be conceived as a distribution of activation value over schemas and actions. The quality of attention is then judged by the "fine tuning" of the generated behavior to the task requirements. If attention is not viewed as a controlling variable but as a controlled variable, theories of attention would have to explain the characteristics and dynamics of this state under the influence of task variables, organismic variables, and environmental stressors.

Given the concept of attention as a controlled variable, the meaning of what constitutes an impairment of attention also changes. Impaired attention implies that a person's cognitive state does not meet the requirements of the environment. But this can only be said for situations in which the activation value of that representation of the stimuli which should be selected is not strong enough. The limiting factors could be investigated for any type of situation. These could vary greatly, for example, from partial deafness to low intelligence. Correlations in performance scores in two situations would be expected only where they have common limiting factors, as when both require fast mental rotation, for instance. The multitude of explanations and patterns of impairment are not a problem for this concept of attention, as the findings do not affect the validity of the concept. Attention in these terms means nothing more nor less than the cognitive state, a pattern of distribution of activation over schemas and elements preceding selective behavior.

Does this "definition" of attention mean that all cognitive psychology is psychology of attention? The answer to this depends on how far one stretches the meaning of the term "cognitive state." We can only suggest that cognitive psychology is considered psychology of attention for those research areas that are traditionally described as attention. This usually involves tasks in which the selectivity and intensity requirements of the cognitive state (the required state) can be specified and determined by the task goals, and in which the actual state, or the deviations from the required state, can be derived in a straightforward way from performance. For example, the areas of intelligence and creativity would not fall under the psychology of attention, as these abilities are supposed to deal with new situations for which no prescribed cognitive state exists. Also, in these cases the sources of information over which intensity is distributed might tend to be internal, and therefore difficult to derive from performance in any straightforward manner.

ATTENTION, BRAIN, AND COGNITION

We will be cautious in relating attention to brain mechanisms, primarily because the level of description in our discourse is psychological. The exception to this is Chapter 3, where discussions at the anatomical and physiological level may be found.

As mentioned earlier, the information processing metaphor has been dominant in cognitive psychology since about 1950. In this view the human brain is regarded as an adaptive, general-purpose, symbol-manipulating system (Newell and Simon, 1972; Michon et al., 1976; Lachman et al., 1979). Following from this is the idea that one-to-one relationships between structural characteristics of the brain and behavior are not to be expected. Nursing such expectations would be comparable to hoping to understand the input/output characteristics of an operational digital computer system from its hardware components only, forgetting that there is a program level in between. In this framework, psychology is the study of mind, that is, defining the structure of the "program" that transforms basic symbolic representations from sensory systems to central and motor representations and how these transformations develop in an adaptive manner. With regard to the latter, particular emphasis is placed on the recursive property of the system: its ability to change its own program. Such change is based on evaluations of the effects of the pattern of active representations in the previous program state, as delivered by the sensory systems. In other words, the system is able to learn from its "experience." The homunculus character of the metaphor is precluded in this manner. Ultimately the whole program of the system is written by the environment, that is, by the "survival of successful mental states" and, in the very long run, by the survival of successful species.

Superficially, this approach does not leave much room for *neuro*psychology as there is no theoretical sense in relating brain to behavior. Neuropsychology would be just a field of applied psychology, a field in which the structure of the mind and the learning abilities of various neurologic patient groups are described without any obvious implications for the understanding of brain processes. Similarly, the information processing metaphor has little relevance of psychophysiology, just as local heat emission from the circuits of a digital computer system says very little about the nature of the processing going on.

Such a view does not deny the practical importance of neuropsychology i.e., for establishing disability and in providing guidelines to rehabilitation workers. It is on these merits that tests of attention in clinical neuropsychology should be primarily judged. Nevertheless, neuropsychologists believe that there is more between the ears than information. Luckily for our professional identity, sound arguments can be raised to defend the position that there is a special and important theoretical contribution to psychology from neuropsychology. That regular and repeatable relationships have been found between performance on cognitive tasks and neurologic patient characteristics cannot be denied. Numerous examples can be found in any handbook of clinical neuropsychology. Shallice (1988) formulates the value of neuropsychology for the understanding of normal function as follows:

> Given the task of the organisation of the cognitive system, the first attraction of neuropsychological evidence is that the effects that occur can be both large and counterintuitive. . . . One appears to be receiving a privileged view into the structure of the information-processing system. . . . As neurological disease affects every part of the brain—if with different incidence rates—the disorders that have been described will probably encompass damage to nearly all the cognitive mechanisms. "Inverting" the set of disorders that exist might enable us to map the subcomponents of mind.

This type of argument is usually made by citing very specific impairments, but it can also be made with regard to very general ones like slow information processing. A recent example in which evidence from neuropsychology may be used to validate psychological notions concerns *connectionism* (Schneider, 1987; Smolensky, 1988). In connectionism, psychological processes are described in terms of parallel interaction of many nodes in a network. Knowledge is not represented or localized in any specific part of a network but at a number of

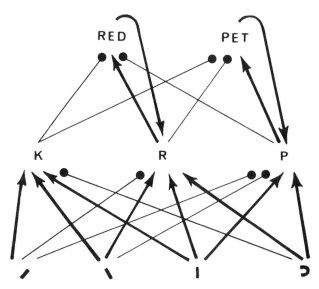

Figure 2-8   A network for the recognition of words, described by Atkinson and associates. The bottom level contains features: ascending diagonal, descending diagonal, vertical line, and right-facing curve. The middle level contains letters. Connections with arrowheads are excitatory: if the feature is activated, activation spreads to the letter. Connections with a solid circle at the end are inhibitory: when a feature is connected to a letter by an inhibitory connection, activating the feature decreases activation of the letter. On the top level words can be activated or inhibited by connections from the middle level. However, top-down activation is postulated here, symbolized by recurring arrows. Top-down activation explains why letters are more easily recognized in a logical context: for example, a letter is easier to perceive when presented as part of a word than when presented alone. (From Atkinson et al., 1990, with permission.)

nodes and in the pattern and complexity of their interconnections. Consequently, loss of any specific node or connection does not make a specific piece of knowledge disappear, but it might make the knowledge contained within the entire network slightly more difficult to access. In the case of well-learned knowledge assumed to be redundantly represented, this could show up as a longer recognition latency, and in the case of weakly represented knowledge as a temporal retrieval deficit. This concept fits rather well with the behavioral efficiency loss characterized as "graceful degradation" that is seen in certain cases of brain damage and in aging (Brouwer, 1985; Salthouse, 1988). In this important respect, performance data from neurologic patients are more compatible with the results from simulations involving parallel distributed networks than those involving computational models. See Figure 2-8.

Moreover, network models can deal better with the capacity problem in terms of a space metaphor. The space available in the network, or in the damaged structures of the brain, dictates the limitations of information processing, even assuming that psychological processes largely proceed in parallel throughout the network. Another attractive feature of these models is their self-organizing character: sensory input may change the patterns of connections and the results.

This characteristic implies that the network can learn from its experiences. As mentioned above, the homunculus in the central executive of the computer-inspired models no longer plays a role in the network models. At present this is a theoretical advantage rather than a practical one since existing network models are better suited to explaining performance in simple tasks like the recognition of words or pictures (e.g., McClelland and Rumelhart, 1985) than in the complex cognitive tasks that gave rise to the concept of supervisory attentional control. It was this concept in particular that engendered the criticism of homunculism.

Ultimately, a theory of brain and behavior relationships should make it possible to understand how given structural limitations of the brain limit the efficiency of information processing in such a way that a specific behavioral symptom arises. A description of the performance of patients suffering from well-defined deficits in well-designed cognitive tasks is required for testing such a theory. "Well-designed" in this case refers to experimental and psychometric criteria.

TYPES OF ATTENTION TASKS

A review of impairments of attention associated with the most important adult neurological disorders is presented in Chapters 4 through 7. The available evidence from clinical research will be categorized on the basis of task characteristics: focused attention, divided attention, and sustained attention. In view of our previous arguments, we will be particularly concerned with explanations of limitations of attention in these tasks in terms of supervisory attentional control and speed of information processing. We will also look for the possibility of modality- and/or area-specific limitations of attention. This requires us to give a broad account of the available evidence for each type of neurologic disorder. First, attention tasks in general and then the three different classes of tasks distinguished above will be defined in an atheoretical manner. These definitions will be broad and a large variety of tasks will be discussed both within and between neurologic groups. The precise choice of tasks within each class and the interpretation of performance scores has depended heavily on the theoretical or practical questions the investigators had in mind.

The key features of attention are *selectivity* and *intensity*. An attention task is one in which the difficulty of the selection requirements, or the intensity of the mental activity required, is systematically varied. It is assumed that the magnitude of the effect such variations have on performance tells something about a person's limitations of attention. It follows from this that a task with a constant selection or intensity requirement, when used alone, cannot be considered an attention task. This will be demonstrated with a test that is widely used in clinical neuropsychology, the Continuous Performance Test (CPT) (Rosvold et al., 1956).

Letters of the alphabet are visually presented in the CPT for a few hundred milliseconds at a regular rate of about one per second. The subject is instructed to respond only to a given critical stimulus, that is, in one version to the letter

X and in an other version to the letter X only if it follows the letter A. The duration of the task can be from 5 to 15 minutes. According to our description of an attention task, the short version of the CPT, with response to all X's, is not a test of attention. An attentive person could be inaccurate and slow (and variable in speed) on this task because of either sensory or motor impairments, or even illiteracy. The task only becomes an attention test when the effect of increased selection or concentration is assessed by comparing performance in the easy and difficult versions, or by comparing performance during the first 5 minutes with that in the 10th to 15th minute. Scores indicating an impairment of attention should always be based on the difference between performance in the situation requiring the greatest attention and that requiring the least. This boils down to the statement that a test of attention must consist of at least two conditions or subtests.

Selectivity requirements in an attention task may be varied in many different ways, as may intensity requirements. However, the tasks that have been previously used may be sorted into a small number of main types which largely correspond to the areas of research we have distinguished. The selectivity aspect has been approached with tasks that can be broadly classified as involving either *focused attention* or *divided attention*. "The former require attention focused on one source or kind of information to the exclusion of others, for example, one of several competing sensory inputs or information channels or one of several stimulus dimensions or attributes. The latter require attention to be divided or shared between two or more sources or kinds of information, or two or more mental operations" (Davies et al., 1984). It should be clear that the subject is still highly selective in both categories; while he is attending to the task at hand, most of the stimulation his sensory receptors receive goes unnoticed. A difference between the two categories is that in focused attention tasks there are usually irrelevant stimuli ("distractors"). These extra stimuli must be ignored. By contrast, all stimuli are relevant in divided attention tasks, but they may come from different sources and require different responses.

Sustained attention tasks "require attention to be directed to one or more sources of information over long and generally unbroken periods of time for the purpose of detecting and responding to small changes in the information being presented" (Davies et al., 1984). In such tasks, the loss of performance over time and the variability of performance are supposed to indicate the loss or instability of concentration, the intensity aspect of attention. Studies of sustained attention may concern three different aspects: time-on-task effects, intraindividual variability, and lapses of attention. *Time-on-task effects* result in performance decrements over time, which distinguish them from practice effects that produce changes in the opposite direction. The first classical studies in this field were directly inspired by wartime surveillance problems (Mackworth, 1950). It had been noted that military personnel showed a troublesome decrease of vigilance in monotonous watchkeeping situations such as radar or sonar monitoring within 20 minutes after starting a shift. *Intraindividual variability* refers to the fluctuations in an individual's efficiency that generally occur during any continuous task. For example, reaction time varies somewhat from trial to trial.

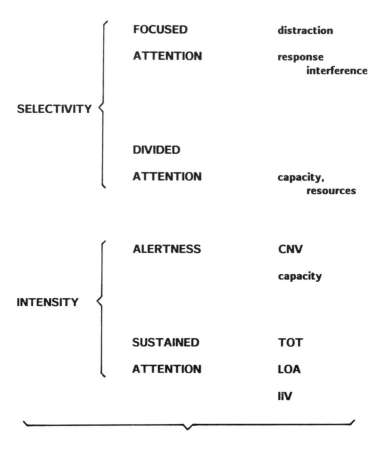

Figure 2-9   A schedule of the theoretical framework for this book. *Supervisory Attentional Control* can modulate both the selectivity and the intensity dimension. In the right-hand column secondary concepts are listed. Capacity features at the levels of both *Divided Attention* and *Alertness*, as capacity probably varies with level of alertness. *CNV*, contingent negative variation; *TOT*, time on task; *LOA*, lapses of attention; *IIV*, intraindividual variability.

A special kind of variability is indicated by the term *lapses of attention*. These are sudden dips in level of performance lasting a few seconds at the most.

Figure 2-9 presents the theoretical framework for this book. We do not regard the schema as carved in stone, however. For one thing, the concepts listed are not completely independent of each other and may show some overlap. However, in our experience the framework has a certain usefulness and may help in getting an overview of this complicated area of cognitive psychology.

3

Anatomy and Physiology of Attention

"Attention" refers to a collection of states, processes, and abilities. It is impossible to relate all of its various aspects to separate cerebral structures. Furthermore, a working definition of attention in the fields of neurophysiology and neuroanatomy depends on the specificity of the questions posed. Several definitions of attention were given in Chapter 2. Some fail to specify the processes involved, while others are quite specific. Broadly speaking, a distinction can be made between definitions based on a capacity concept and those based on a mechanistic concept. According to the *capacity concept*, task performance depends on the commitment of just one or a few diffuse attentional resources. As a working definition, this concept relates to the effects of general brain damage rather than specific lesions. The emphasis is primarily on "mass effects" occurring in large areas of the brain (e.g., left versus right hemisphere and posterior versus anterior). More specific localization would be superfluous. The connecting "theory" relating psychology and anatomy might be a variation of a neural network theory (less brain → fewer neurons → diminished resources). The only specific lesions of interest are those affecting systems that modulate the spread of activation in the associative network, for example, the classical ascending reticular activating system (see below).

From a *mechanistic* viewpoint the opposite is seen in focused visual attention. The concept of covert orienting is very specific with regard to process: a focus of attention is attached to, disconnected from or moved to a specific location. This very specific process might depend on a very specific piece of "cerebral hardware," so it makes sense to study the brain in detail. In this case, the theory relating psychology with anatomy would be mechanistic, a one-to-one mapping of a psychological mechanism on anatomy.

Interestingly, both approaches use the same type of behavioral assessment methodology—reaction time (RT) tasks. This can be seen in the case of mental slowness. Given the proper stimuli and instructions, almost any neuropsychological impairment can be expressed in a RT task as slow information processing. Data on the existence and severity of the impairment are related to the design of the task. Where attention is conceived of as a resource emanating from the volume of a neural network (a spatial metaphor), there is greater interest in the general slowness associated with certain diffuse brain disorders and indicated by meta-analysis of RT data. On the other hand, in the study of specific attentional mechanisms, it is necessary to know precisely which task variable makes the patient with a circumscribed lesion extremely slow. The problem is that most neuropsychologists would like to use the latter approach, but their patients' brains are not very cooperative. The effects of many types of brain damage are quite diffuse. Even when lesions are well-defined, they seldom conform to "mental faculties." It is very difficult to specify exactly which "real" elementary psychological processes can be mapped to brain mechanisms or locations (see Chapter 2). Hence it is seldom possible to relate a particular RT score to a specific brain injury or dysfunction. The exception seems to be when the effect is very task-specific, the lesion or dysfunction is clearly localized and well-documented, and the effect clearly exceeds the normal variation.

Still, both approaches have merit. Neuroanatomy and neurophysiology may contribute to an understanding of how the brain sometimes functions as a system with diffuse relationships between structure and function, fitting the capacity concept, and conversely of how a small, strategically placed lesion may have specific but far-ranging effects, fitting the mechanistic concept. Most modern literature on the relationships between neuroanatomy, neurophysiology, and neuropsychology focuses on specific effects, as does this chapter for the most part.

By 1800 the view had taken hold that mental activity is mediated by the cerebral cortex, a belief that was reinforced by Broca's and Wernike's discovery of cortical areas essential for language. This emphasis on the cortex led to neglect of the role of subcortical structures, which were seen as subordinates of the cortex, responsible for a few vital but humble tasks like the execution of automatic movements or the regulation of respiration. This view of the brain was essentially hierarchical and implied a rigid top-down control in which lower structures depended on the activity of higher ones. After 1950 this hierarchical concept was challenged by studies revealing the essential role of brainstem structures in mental activity (Moruzzi and Magoun, 1949). It became clear that one of the lower parts of the brain was, in fact, modulating the state of activation of the cortex. In later years, a striking interdependence of higher and lower structures was documented which made the hierarchical view of the brain untenable. As Hebb (1958) stated, without the support of the lower structures, cortical processes cease, as far as behavior is concerned. Luria (1973) described mental processes in terms of a vertical organization of functional systems. In this view, higher brain structures have a modulating influence on lower ones, but are themselves dependent on the activities of the lower structures. Despite the understanding that the brain is an integrated system, it is useful to highlight the cerebral structures that are essential for attentional mechanisms one by one, starting at a low level, the mesencephalon or midbrain.

MESENCEPHALON

Our brains consist of 1100 to 1400 g of excitable tissue that is actively reaching out for stimulation and that enables us to interact with our environment (Droogleever-Fortuyn, 1979). However, the thresholds for reacting to environmental stimulation vary strongly with the background state of wakefulness, from stage IV sleep to hyperalertness. The scale between these two extremes is called the level of alertness, which may be defined as a generalized state of receptivity to stimulation and preparedness to respond (Posner, 1975; Posner and Rafal, 1987). [Alertness defined in this way refers to the normal states of consciousness, occurring in healthy subjects. Abnormal states of consciousness, like coma of varying depth, could be considered as very low levels of alertness, but it should be noted that there is a very important qualitative difference between coma and sleep: a sleeper can be awakened to normal consciousness almost instantaneously, but a comatose patient cannot be awakened.]

Changes in alertness are even observable in lower animals like fishes and birds. This indicates that it does not take much brain to attend, or more accurately, that these phenomena must have their neuroanatomical substrate in the phylogenetically oldest parts of the human brain. Research in the last half-century has indeed demonstrated that a system for the regulation of alertness exists in the core brain of all vertebrate species. In the mesencephalic brainstem there is a column of medially placed cells with structural and functional characteristics that clearly distinguish it from its anatomical environment. First, this column has a netlike appearance under the microscope, showing an intricate latticework of nerve cells called the *reticular formation*. This formation does not consist of isolated neurons with long axons, but of nerve cells connected to each other by short processes. Excitation spreads over the net of this neural structure gradually, changing its level of activity little by little (Luria, 1973).

Macroscopically, the reticular formation (RF) is inconspicuous; in fact, it is that part of the mesencephalic brainstem that remains when all ascending and descending tracts and specific nuclei have been defined. Still, these few grams of tissue are the cornerstone of a subcortical system that is responsible for the maintenance of alertness (Moruzzi and Magoun, 1949; Jasper, 1954; Nauta, 1964). The RF exerts an excitatory influence on the whole brain by means of a nonspecific projection system, the ascending reticular activating system (ARAS). This system consists of the RF plus nonspecific afferents that arise from it, ascend through the intralaminar nuclei of the thalamus, and then fan out to various parts of the brain, particularly the cortex. The ARAS plays a decisive role in activating the cortex and regulating the state of its activity. The importance of the system was stressed by Luria (1973), who described it as the first functional unit of the brain, responsible for regulating tone, waking, and mental states. See Figure 3-1.

The activity of the RF itself is mainly determined by sensory input. As the main afferent paths ascend through the brainstem and approach the thalamus, branches turn away from the mainstream and enter the RF. In accordance with the special histological character of the formation, the effect of this sensory stimulation is not specific, but results in a pooling of excitatory effects. The ARAS then transmits this excitation through its diffuse projection system to the cortex. This implies that any sensory stimulation will affect the cortex in two ways: as a specific input, relayed through thalamic nuclei, and as a contribution in the nonspecific activating system.

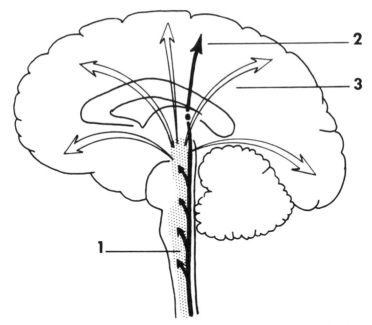

Figure 3-1 The ascending reticular activating system (ARAS). *1*, reticular formation; *2*, specific projection via thalamus; *3*, diffuse projecting system.

The fact that excitation is pooled in the RF might lead to the inference that the level of alertness is determined by a simple energetic model: the more input, the higher the level of activation in the brain. This view is definitely wrong, for a tired person can fall asleep in a noisy and brightly illuminated room. Moreover, a sudden reduction of sensory stimulation will not result in decreased alertness. On the contrary, a paradoxical effect occurs. If someone is working in his study and the air-conditioning suddenly stops humming, he will look up from his task and show an orienting reaction with a puzzled expression. Likewise, the sudden disappearance of a light in the peripheral visual field will catch our attention rather than lower our level of alertness. These phenomena indicate that although alertness is certainly maintained by stimulation from the outside world, additional factors may cause changes in alertness.

It is almost impossible to indicate the upper and lower ends of the RF. In fact, the netlike tissue can still be traced in the medulla oblongata and the spinal cord. In an upward direction, the RF enters the thalamus and fills the spaces between specific thalamic nuclei. In addition, an important branch turns away to enter the hypothalamus, thus providing a link between alertness and viscero-autonomic phenomena (Pribram and McGuinness, 1975). Still, a useful distinction can be made between the upper and lower ARAS at the level of the mesencephalon. This distinction is related to a distinction at the behavioral level between tonic and phasic changes in alertness. Sharpless and Jaspers (1956) demonstrated that tonic changes are mediated by the lower ARAS. The drowsiness provoked by low-event-rate task situations, for example, is explained in terms of decreased collateral sensory input in the lower half of the reticular formation. On the other hand, phasic changes in alertness are mediated by the upper ARAS or the nonspecific thalamic projection system. In other words, even in the functioning of the brainstem, the vertical organization manifests itself with the upper part effecting short-term changes and the lower part effecting long-term changes in alertness.

AROUSAL OR THE ORIENTING REACTION

An elementary attentional mechanism is the sudden increase in alertness known as *arousal*. This phasic change has various names, depending on the discipline. Electrophysiologists usually call it activation, while biologists and psychologists often refer to it as the *orienting reaction* or arousal reaction. Arousal is a very complex phenomenon, described by Luria and Homskaya (1970) as a complex functional system including a series of somatic, sensory, vegetative, EEG, and other components. At the behavioral level the orienting reaction is marked by a sensory preparation for the perceptual analysis of stimuli; animals will prick up their ears and turn their heads toward the source of stimulation. Luria (1973) views this pattern of changes as a mobilization of the organism to meet possible surprises. Arousal can be considered as a multicomponent reflex, as it proceeds without a conscious decision to attend.

While having a certain autonomy, all components of the orienting reaction obey common laws: they appear upon presentation of stimuli that are new or have a specific signal value; they have a nonspecific character and do not depend on the modality of the stimulus, and they disappear in proportion to repetition. According to Pribram and McGuinness (1975), arousal is controlled by *two reciprocal systems* that converge on the *amygdala*. This almond-shaped nucleus in the pole of the temporal lobe is part of the limbic system, and might thus supply the emotional tone of arousal. Both systems originate in the frontal cortex, converge on the amygdala, and finally influence hypothalamic structures related to arousal. The first of these systems has its cortical component in the dorsolateral frontal cortex, and has a facilitating effect on arousal. The second system originates in the orbitofrontal cortex and represents an extensive inhibitory pathway. This reciprocal innervation allows a sensitive modulation of the arousal mechanism. The frontoamygdala influence may be conceived of as a finely tuned determinant, controlling visceroautonomic arousal initiated by the hypothalamic mechanism during orienting.

Pribram and McGuinness' arousal model includes another subcortical element. In their view, the *hippocampus* plays an important role in the arousal or orienting reaction. The hippocampus, a long structure in the medial part of the temporal lobe, has an inhibitory influence on the reticular formation. The hippocampus is essential for storage of information, and therefore it has a key role in distinguishing between "old" and "new" stimuli. It is assumed that the function of the hippocampus is to compare and match an incoming pattern of stimuli with an internal model. If stimulus and model match, the hippocampus continues to inhibit the RF. But if a mismatch occurs, the stimulus is considered "novel" and the hippocampus releases the RF, resulting in arousal.

The orienting response must be divided into two phenomena: a general arousal effect (phasic alertness) and a selective orienting of attention to the source of information (Posner and Rafal, 1987). This *selective orienting* is of special importance to vision, where it has a subcortical circuit of its own. At the back of the mesencephalic brainstem, just before the cerebellum, there are two small knobs known as the superior colliculi. This part of the midbrain tectum has served throughout most of vertebrate evolution as the primary visual center of the brain. Like the reticular formation, it is a phylogenetically very old structure. It receives direct input from the optic tract. At the level of the thalamus this tract splits, sending its main branch to the lateral geniculate body, a thalamic nucleus projecting on the area striata of the visual cortex. However, a separate branch enters the superior colliculus, which itself projects on the neocortex. The fibers from the colliculus do not end in the visual cortex itself, but in a nearby cortical region. Thus, the visual system apparently has two channels ascending to the cerebral cortex (Livingstone and Hubel, 1988), an old and a young one, phylogenetically speaking. It is believed that the old channel is involved in the visual component of the orienting reaction, particularly in spatial orienting. In a way, this is a primitive but efficient system, enabling rapid orienting to "something" happening in our field of vision. The system implies "panoramic vision" (Denny-Brown and Fischer, 1976) in which events are noted, even in the periphery of the visual field. This results in head and eye movements, and finally in foveal fixation, the aligning of the fovea with the source of stimulation. Only then do the occipital lobes of the geniculostriate system take over to discriminate and identify the target (Posner and Rafal, 1987). The presence of this double visual system dictates a sequence in the perception of sudden visual events: first locate, then see.

HABITUATION

A repeated sensory event tends to lose its capacity to produce arousal rapidly. The result is known as *habituation*, or negative adaptation (Hebb, 1958). This is another basic biological effect and it is fundamental for an efficient interaction with our environment. If no habituation occurred, any source of stimulation would keep alerting us, making goal-directed behavior impossible. In addition, we would be unable to sleep, even in a situation with a very low stimulation level. But there is one absolute requirement for habituation to occur: the repeated stimulus must have no signal value or emotional connotation. For example, we do not habituate to a constant pain. Another example would be the sound of a leaking tap keeping us awake at night; even though this stimulation is perfectly regular and constant, we do not habituate to it if we experience the sound as irritating—leaving us no other choice than getting up and turning off the tap more firmly.

One of the characteristics of habituation due to repetition of a stimulus is the progressive restriction of cerebral sites involved in the orienting reaction. Paradoxically, this restriction involves primarily the sites where arousal neurons are located, and does not encompass either sensory pathways or the primary sensory projection systems, where responses continue to be recorded in the habituated organism (Pribram and McGuinness, 1975). Stated otherwise, in habituation the diffuse effect of a stimulus on the brain disappears gradually, while the specific projection remains. Proof of this effect is also found in evoked potentials in sleeping subjects: even if sounds do not awake them, potentials evoked by these sounds can be recorded from their cortex. For an awake subject this implies that he still hears stimuli that he is no longer listening to. This is a very important characteristic, enabling an organism to monitor its environment without paying conscious attention to it. It explains why the sudden disappearance of a monotonous stimulation can alert us and cause an orienting reaction. Truly complete habituation would render an organism unable to note such a sudden disappearance: someone who is reading in his study would not discover that the clock has stopped ticking, or the air-conditioning stopped humming. This preattentive or automatic monitoring of stimulation, even if we are habituated to it, also enables us to detect subtle changes in it. For example, the car driver on the highway is not listening to the constant sound of his cars' engine, but he will be alarmed when this sound gets a disquieting extra component.

It is conceivable that habituation may vary in its differentiation, in accordance with the distinction between upper and lower ARAS. Haider (1964) contends that the lower portions of the ARAS are capable of habituation for a given sense modality but not for highly differentiated qualities of stimulation.

BASAL GANGLIA AND LIMBIC SYSTEM

The basal ganglia are a collection of subcortical gray nuclei surrounding the thalamus. The largest of these is the *caudate nucleus*, a long-tailed structure of which the anterior portion (the head of the nucleus) is situated against the forehorn of the lateral ventricle. When it extends posteriorly, it becomes very slender, forming a tail that passes along the thalamus and then curves down into the medial part of the temporal lobe. Here it ends in the *amygdala*, which is considered by some investigators as being itself one of the basal ganglia. Two other nuclei, the *putamen* and the *globus pallidus*, lie close to each other between the thalamus and the insula. They are separated from the thalamus by an important bundle of white fibers, the internal capsule that contains sensory and motor tracts ascending to and descending from the cortex. See Figure 3-2.

Until recently, the basal ganglia were seen as a subcortical part of the motor system. This view is concisely phrased by Marsden (1982): the basal ganglia are responsible for the automatic execution of learned motor plans. Luria (1973) states that the kinetic organization of movements depends on the combined activity of the basal ganglia and the premotor area. Lesions in the subcortical nuclei or in the premotor cortex therefore result in kinetic apraxia, a disorganization of the smooth, consecutive transition of single movements.

Since 1970, however, evidence has accumulated that this view is too limited; the basal ganglia not only have a motor function, but also contribute to selectivity in perceiving and responding. Luria (1973) cited the hippocampus and the caudate nucleus as "essential structures for the elimination of responses to irrelevant

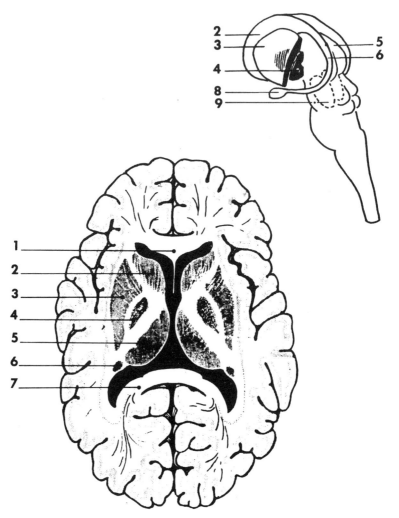

Figure 3-2 The basal ganglia, shown in a horizontal plane and in a three-dimensional view from the left. *1*, genu of corpus callosum; *2*, head of caudate nucleus; *3*, putamen; *4*, globus pallidus; *5*, thalamus; *6*, tail of caudate nucleus; *7*, splenium of corpus callosum; *8*, amygdala; *9*, substantia nigra.

stimuli, enabling an organism to behave in a strictly selective manner. A lesion of these structures is a source of the breakdown of selectivity of behavior, which is in fact more a disturbance of selective attention than a defect of memory." Teuber (1976) also reported that disorders of the basal ganglia produced more than purely motor difficulties, that is, characteristic perceptual and cognitive deficits. Denny-Brown and Yanagisawa (1976), like Luria, ascribed a role to the basal ganglia in selective responding. In their view, the basal ganglia have all aspects of a "clearinghouse" that accumulates samples of ongoing cortical activity and, on a competitive basis, can facilitate any one and suppress others. This view is based on research with experimental lesions in animals. Damasio and colleagues (1980) presented clinical evidence for the same interpretation, pointing out that lesions in the basal ganglia may cause unilateral neglect, or hemi-inattention in humans (see Chapter 6). They concluded that the basal ganglia, in combination with frontal and parietal cortical areas, comprise a system subserving attention.

Mainly on the basis of experiments in primates, Alexander and colleagues (1986) postulated that the basal ganglia have a level of organization and functional specificity paralleling that of the cerebral cortex itself. In their view, it is obvious that the basal ganglia should no longer be seen as "centers" or structures having a role independent of the cortex and thalamus, with which they have intimate and well-organized afferent and efferent connections. Alexander and colleagues viewed the basal ganglia as having components in five separate circuits: motor, oculomotor, dorsolateral prefrontal, lateral orbitofrontal, and anterior cingulate. Each of these five basal ganglia-thalamocortical circuits appears to receive input from several separate but functionally related cortical areas, traverse specific portions of the basal ganglia and thalamus, and then project back upon the same cortical areas providing input to the circuit, thus forming partially closed loops. Although Alexander and colleagues described these circuits in great anatomical and physiological detail, they were cautious about the functions of the circuits in the human brain: "The precise role of the basal ganglia in disturbances of higher functions in humans is still controversial because of the often associated neuropathological changes occurring in other structures." The oculomotor circuit is involved in the distribution of visual spatial attention, while the lateral orbitofrontal circuit might be involved in switches in behavioral set (Fuster, 1980).

On the basis of their connections with other brain structures, the basal ganglia can be divided into an afferent group and an efferent group. The caudate nucleus and the putamen, called together the striatum, must be seen as the afferent or receptive part (Carpenter, 1976). The striatum receives excitatory input from the intralaminar thalamic nuclei, and in Hassler's view (1978) this part of the basal ganglia is integrated in the nonspecific thalamocortical pathway. Hence the caudate nucleus and the putamen are functionally related to the RF. Hassler believes that they have a gating function for sensory information that is relayed by the thalamus to the cortex, and therefore play a major role in selective attending. Electrical stimulation of the putamen in cats results in enhanced alertness, emotional reaction, and intentional action to one outer event, and at the same time causes all other environmental stimuli and simultaneously intentional actions to fade and dim. In other words, this stimulation produces selective attending.

In describing the activity of ARAS, a distinction can be drawn between specific and nonspecific projection of sensory stimulation to the cortex. Interestingly, it has now become clear that the afferent part of the basal ganglia is integrated in the nonspecific projection. According to Hassler, under normal conscious conditions each cortical region receives two sets of impulses during perception. One set comes through the thalamocortical projection of the different sensory pathways, the other from the nonspecific loop through the basal ganglia. These latter impulses might determine the degree of awareness. Only if both sets of impulses arrive at a distinct cortical region do the neuronal processes fulfill the preconditions for a conscious perception. The case of habituation illustrates the importance of the double set of impulses: while a repeated stimulus continues to evoke activity in the specific projecting system, activity in the nonspecific system gradually disappears and the subject is no longer aware of the repeated stimulus.

Even if one accepts a gating function for the basal ganglia, however, the question remains how these subcortical nuclei can discriminate between relevant and irrelevant stimulation. Inevitably, some cortical influence must be assumed. While the intralaminar thalamic nuclei have an excitatory effect on the striatum, the frontal cortex has important inhibitory connections with the basal ganglia. It is conceivable, therefore, that the selection of sensory stimulation is realized by an integrated frontostriatal system (Luria, 1973). The model of basal ganglia function as proposed by Alexander and colleagues (1986), with its five basal ganglia-thalamocortical circuits, specifies the frontal cortical areas integrated in closed loops that enable intensive interactions between cortex and basal ganglia.

The globus pallidus seems to be the *efferent* part of the basal ganglia. Many investigators consider the substantia nigra, a pigmented nucleus in the mesencephalic brain stem, as another basal ganglion (DeLong, 1974; Côté and Crutcher, 1985). Globus pallidus and substantia nigra are the major outflow nuclei of the basal ganglia, having excitatory effects via the ventral thalamus on the premotor areas anterior to the primary motor cortex.

Finally, an important aspect in the organization of the basal ganglia is the relation between the afferent and the efferent part. In Hassler's view, the afferent part is essential for selective attending to sensory stimulation, while the globus pallidus is essential for a motor orientation to stimulation coming from outside the present focus of attention. It seems that the putamen, as part of the afferent system, can suppress the activity of the pallidum by inhibitory projections (Hassler, 1978). As briefly mentioned above, this has been demonstrated with electrical stimulation of the various nuclei in cats, but also during stereotaxic operations in humans. Electrical stimulation, 15–50 Hz, of the putamen in cats immediately arrests the animals' ongoing activity. Their eyes open and pupils dilate which are well-known signals of arousal and part of the orienting reaction.

THE CEREBRAL CORTEX

There are three roles for the neocortex in attention:

1. The cerebral cortex itself serves as a source of input for the brainstem RF as a regulator of level of activation.
2. The cortex is the final analyzer of signals that are or are not attended to.
3. The cortex supplies a representation of the outside world for localizing novel stimuli that provoke arousal.

The role of the cortex as *activator* is largely dependent on a number of connections forming the descending reticular activating system. In many respects this descending system is the mirror image of the ARAS. Luria (1973) points out, that the descending fibers have a well-differentiated cortical organization. Whereas the most specific bundles of these fibers, raising or lowering the tone of the sensory or motor systems, arise from the primary projection zones of the cortex, the more general activating influences on RF arise primarily from the frontal regions. Its descending fibers run from the orbital and medial frontal cortex to nuclei of the thalamus and the brainstem. These form a system that permits the higher levels of the cortex, that participate directly in the formation of intentions and plans, to recruit the lower systems and modulate their work making the most complex forms of conscious activity possible. According to Luria's theory, the principal function of these brain zones is not communication with the outside world, but regulation of the general state and control over inclinations and emotions. Mesulam (1985) likewise stresses that the frontal lobes may be particularly important in the regulation of, what he calls, the overall attentional tone.

The importance of the activating role of the cerebral cortex is clearly illustrated by the fact that it can induce a high level of activation, even in situations with a very low level of sensory stimulation, like a dark and silent bedroom. A person may stay wide awake despite a lack of sensory input, simply with activation of cortical origin. To put it more plainly, thoughts can keep us awake, and in fact often do. The high frequency of insomnia in the healthy population illustrates how anxious thoughts about tomorrow, or feelings of guilt about the past, may stimulate the brainstem RF via the nonspecific descending activating system.

The cerebral cortex also functions as an *analyzer*, or better, a collection of analyzers of sensory input. As pointed out before, on a very basic level the cortex is monitoring continuous stimulation, even when a subject is habituated to it and no longer attending to it consciously. This monitoring can therefore be characterized as preattentive. A subtle but sudden change will be noted, and even the sudden disappearance of a monotonous stimulation will cause an orienting reaction. Of course, both events can be considered as cases of novelty, or mismatch between stimulation and internal template. Obviously, the cortical analysis of mismatch triggers hippocampal activity releasing the reticular formation (Pribram and McGuinness, 1975). It is plausible that the neocortex containing the projection areas of the three main senses (vision, hearing, and the sensory function) plays a dominant role in the continuous analysis of sensory stimulation. In other words, the whole cortex behind the central fissure, indicated by Luria as the brain unit for receiving, analyzing, and storing of information, enables the monitoring of the environment in order to detect change and novelty.

The process of preattentive monitoring has been studied in some detail with electrophysiological methods, particularly in the auditory domain. Näätänen (1988) described a component in the auditory event-related potential called *mismatch negativity* (MMN) (Figure 3-3). When a subject is presented with a monotonous series of clicks, and when his attention has been attracted elsewhere by instruction, a subtle change in the clicks will nevertheless result in an orienting reaction. Electrophysiologically, this reaction is preceded by MMN some 200 ms after presentation of the deviant stimulus. The striking thing is that physical stimulus features are apparently fully processed, irrespective of the direction of

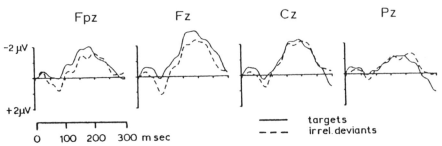

Figure 3-3 Mismatch negativity (*MMN*). Difference waves for 4 electrode positions, obtained when the ERP evoked by frequently occurring tones was subtracted from the ERP to infrequently occurring deviant tones. The dotted lines are based on the situation when *no* attention had to be given to the tones, and the solid lines on the condition in which the deviant tones had to be counted silently. The MMN is similar in both conditions, indicating that it is independent from attention. Note that MMN is visible quite early, that is, within 100 ms after stimulus onset. (Adapted from Näätänen, 1988, with permission from the author and Elsevier Science Publishers, Amsterdam.)

attention. Stated otherwise, MMN is independent from attention. Näätänen stresses that all auditory stimuli receive a rapid and complete processing of their physical features, a processing that is truly automatic. It is assumed that the neuronal traces involved in MMN production form the neurophysiological basis for the short-duration sensory memory called the preattentive store, or the echoic memory in audition (Neisser, 1967). This storage mechanism may be located in the auditory cortex. By magnetoencephalographic recordings it has been possible to localize the MMN generator, or at least a significant part of it, in the primary auditory cortex. The storage mechanism must contain a memory trace that represents the standard stimulus very accurately, since even slightly deviant stimuli elicit an MMN. It appears that the local MMN generator is an attention-switch mechanism for responding to physical stimulus change. Its output represents a "call" from the preattentive mechanism to focus attention.

Finally, the neocortex serves as a *localizer* of stimuli that evoke an orienting reaction. Although the monitoring function of the cortex guarantees attention to change and novelty, the organism can only react adequately to stimuli once they are localized in space. The parietal association cortex is an important area in this context, providing an internal representation of the body with respect to the outside world (both auditorily and visually) (Mesulam, 1985). Of course, the parietal cortex does not perform localization independent of other cerebral areas. As noted above, also the phylogenetically older visual system, involving the superior colliculi is involved in directing attention and the eyes to the source of stimulation (Buchtel).

INTEGRATED THEORIES

Understanding of the brain as a highly integrated system has promoted the view that attention is subserved by combinations of cerebral structures. In behavioral neurology such combinations are frequently described as "networks." This implies, unfortunately, that neurology and psychology are using the word network in different ways. In the psychological models of connectionists (Schneider, 1987), networks are made up of a multitude of equivalent neuronlike elements. These models were inspired by neuroscience, but their resemblance with brain function is to be found on the level of cells or layers of cells. In contrast, behavioral neurology favors networks that are made up of a few macroscopic structures. Although confusing, the use of the word network by behavioral neurologists to describe brain mechanisms of attention has the advantage that it stresses the concerted and integrated action of different structures. We will describe three integrated theories featuring such networks that have been proposed in the past decade (Mesulam, 1981; Stuss and Benson, 1986; Posner and Petersen, 1990). Presenting these integrated theories here will compensate for our foregoing discussion of the anatomical structures involved in attention as if they were functionally distinct entities.

The Frontal-Diencephalic-Brainstem System (Stuss and Benson)

Stuss and Benson (1984, 1986) outlined a comprehensive network that appears to account for a variety of attention disorders encountered in clinical work, particularly in acute conditions. The system is tripartite; it comprises the ARAS in the brainstem, the diffuse thalamic projection system and the frontal-thalamic gating system.

In this model, the ARAS provides tonic levels of alertness. The diffuse thalamic projection system provides phasic changes in alertness. The frontal-thalamic gating system is responsible for selective and directed attention. The latter gating system appears to be under the influence not only of ascending fibers of the reticular activating system, but also of descending fibers from the frontal cortex. Hence afferent and efferent information can be integrated, interpreted, and used to control sensory pathways.

The specific effects of pathology in this tripartite system depend on the level of the lesion. With damage or dysfunction of the ARAS in the brainstem, the patient may be almost entirely unresponsive. This state is known as coma (Plum and Posner, 1980). With less severe pathology, there is a clouding of consciousness. The patient may respond and attend for brief periods of time, but will then return to a somnolent state. Benson and Geschwind (1975) characterized this state as "drifting attention."

When there is damage to the diffuse thalamic projection system, tonic alertness is intact and the patient may be responsive, but he will be easily distracted by external stimuli. The phasic component of alertness is impaired, and "attention wanders." According to Stuss and Benson, drifting and wandering attention represent poles in a continuum of attention: "in one attention cannot be sustained, in the other it cannot be directed."

Finally, damage to the frontal-thalamic gating system would produce disorders of complex behaviors that demand planning, selection, and monitoring of one's own performance. Stuss and Benson call this a deficit in conscious, directed, attentive behavior.

A Cortical Network for Spatial Selective Attention (Mesulam)

Mesulam (1981) described a cerebral system for spatial selective attention that accounts for the well-known attentional impairment in neurologic patients called hemi-inattention. This system or network has four components:

1. *Reticular*: provides the underlying level of arousal and vigilance
2. *Limbic*: in the cingulate gyrus, regulates the spatial distribution of motivational valence
3. *Frontal*: including the frontal eye fields, coordinates the motor programs for exploration, scanning, reaching, and fixating
4. Posterior *parietal*: provides an internal sensory map.

The latter two components are of paramount importance at the neocortical level. Important connections between the frontal eye fields and the superior colliculus have been noted in the parietal component. Experimental unilateral lesions in these structures in the macaque monkey result in deficits in saccadic eye movements. Thus, the frontal eye fields and superior colliculus appear to have parallel but complementary roles in modulating ocular movements. In the macaque, the cortical area known as PG is roughly comparable to the parietal cortex in humans. It is very probable that the output from PG to frontal eye fields and superior colliculus coordinates the motor sequences necessary for foveating, scanning, exploring, fixating, and manipulating relevant external events.

Although this four-component model is mainly based on experimental research with macaque monkeys, Mesulam believes that clinical literature supports the idea that a similar cerebral network may be responsible for the coordination of externally directed attention in humans. Data on *hemi-inattention* or *hemineglect*, a tendency to neglect one-half of the body, fits well with the Mesulam model. There appear to be four subtypes of hemineglect that can be related to the four components of the proposed network. For instance, neglect caused by lesions in the frontal component is characterized by a predominance of motor over sensory factors (Watson et al., 1978). This "frontal neglect" manifests itself as hypokinesia in exploration and manipulation of the area contralateral to the damaged hemisphere.

The Anterior, Posterior, and Vigilance Networks (Posner)

Posner and his coworkers have studied the relationship between cognitive processes and neuroanatomy for many years (Posner and Petersen, 1990). They have collected data from normal individuals, brain-injured patients and macaque monkeys. Their human studies have emphasized spatial attention, in particular, attention shifts in the visual field. Their basic paradigm included cues, mainly arrows pointing right or left, that caused the attentional focus to shift, even when the subject remained fixated on a central point. They demonstrated that there are three stages in shifting attention: disengage—move—engage. Disruption of the first two has been seen with focal brain lesions. Parietal lesions impair disengaging, and progressive supranuclear palsy, a neurologic condition that affects the midbrain selectively, impairs moving. The result of this many-faceted research was a model of attention based on three anatomical networks: posterior, anterior, and predominantly subcortical (Posner, 1992). These networks are highly interconnected and form part of a complex corticostriatothalamic neural circuit (Goldman-Rakic, 1988).

The *posterior network* involves orienting to visual locations. It has been demonstrated that if a subject is asked to move his eyes to a target, an improvement in efficiency at the target location begins well *before* the eyes move (covert orienting; see Chapter 2). The function of this covert shift appears to be a way of guiding the eye to the target area of the visual field (Posner and Cohen, 1984). Animal experiments suggest that three areas are involved in this: the posterior parietal lobe, the lateral pulvinar nucleus of the thalamus, and the superior colliculus (Petersen et al., 1987). Studies with normal individuals and neurologic patients confirm that injuries to any of these three areas will reduce the ability to shift attention covertly (Posner, 1988). However, each area produces a somewhat different type of deficit. Damage to the posterior parietal lobe affects the ability to disengage from an attentional focus in favor of a target located opposite the side of the lesion. Patients with progressive deterioration in the superior colliculus also show a deficit in shifting attention, but in this case the shift is slowed, whether or not attention is first engaged elsewhere. This deficit appears to be closely linked with mechanisms involved in saccadic eye movements. Finally, patients with lesions in the thalamus have difficulty attending to targets opposite the side of the lesion, and in avoiding distraction by events occurring at other locations. In other words, thalamic lesions appear to cause problems in engaging a target in a fully selective manner. In summary, the evidence from animal and human studies suggests a circuitry for covert attention shifts. The parietal lobe disengages attention from its present focus; then the midbrain area acts to shift attention to a new target; and, finally, the thalamic pulvinar reads out data from the new location.

The *anterior network* acts to detect sensory or semantic events, and appears to be related to awareness and voluntary control of attention. While the posterior system is involved in automatic or involuntary orienting (Luria, 1973), the anterior system is important for conscious, focused attention. These systems are related at both the psychological and the anatomical levels. Goldman-Rakic (1988) described a strong connection between the posterior parietal lobe and areas of the lateral and medial frontal cortex.

In Posner's theory, the anterior network has been charted to a lesser degree than the posterior network, and is more hypothetical. It implies a system involved in signal detection, regardless or source or sensory modality. The essential structure may be the anterior cingulate. Midline frontal areas, including this anterior cingulate gyrus and the supplementary motor area, are active during semantic processing (Petersen et al., 1988). Moreover, the degree of blood flow in the anterior cingulate increases with the number of targets to be detected (Posner et al., 1988). Anatomically, the anterior cingulate is closely linked with the posterior parietal lobe as well as with language areas of the lateral frontal lobe. Posner suggested a possible hierarchy of attention systems in which the anterior system can pass control to the posterior system when it is not occupied with processing other material.

Posner and Petersen (1990) also suggested the existence of a *vigilance network*. The ability to prepare and sustain alertness for processing high priority signals is an important function of attention. It seems that alertness does not affect the build-up of information in the sensory or memory systems. For example, letter identification appears to be possible at about the same rate, whether or not the subject has been alerted by a warning signal. In a state of high alertness, the selection of a response occurs faster, although the probability of errors increases.

Posner did not describe the vigilance network in great anatomical detail. He suggested that the right hemisphere is responsible for developing and maintaining an alert state, but as we shall see below, the data are contradictory. The assertion that lesions of the right hemisphere cause difficulty with alerting is based on psychophysiological studies in humans and monkeys (Heilman, Watson, and Valenstein, 1985; Yokoyama et al., 1987). Performance on vigilance tasks has also been found more impaired with right than with left lesions (Coslett et al., 1987; Wilkins et al., 1987). Moreover, blood flow and metabolic studies suggest a link between the right cerebral hemisphere and alerting (Cohen et al., 1988; Deutsch et al., 1988).

Posner and Petersen (1990) reviewed physiological studies that suggested a norepinephrine (NE) system in alerting. This system arises in the locus ceruleus, a brainstem nucleus at the level of the fourth ventricle. The NE pathways course through frontal areas, divide and trace backward toward posterior areas. Activation of NE works via the posterior attention system to increase the rate at which high-priority visual information can be selected for further processing. At high levels of alertness, this more rapid selection is often at the expense of lower quality information and higher error rate. The system is supposed to be more strongly lateralized in the right hemisphere. In the next section we will discuss the merits of various hypotheses with regard to functional asymmetries of attention.

FUNCTIONAL ASYMMETRIES

Macroscopically, the human brain is almost symmetrical in the coronal plane. Despite this anatomical symmetry, the brain develops during ontogenesis in such a way that the two hemispheres serve quite different functions in adults. The best-known example of this is dominance in dextrals of the left hemisphere for language. Thus, it is reasonable to consider the possibility of hemispheric specialization in attention. Since "attention" refers to a complex set of states, abilities, and processes, however, it would be naive to expect that one hemisphere would be dominant in all of these areas. It is conceivable that no hemispheric dominance exists for certain aspects of attention, while for others either the left or the right hemisphere may be most important.

Some publications on dominance for the *regulation of consciousness* have appeared. A graded scale of wakefulness and alertness may be distinguished, as described in the section on the mesencephalon in this chapter. Consciousness is distinguished from unconsciousness, and sleep from wakefulness at the lower end of this continuum. Serafetinides and colleagues (1965) observed that patients receiving intracarotid amobarbitol injections in the language-dominant hemisphere lost consciousness more often and for longer periods of time than patients receiving injections in the nondominant hemisphere. Albert and colleagues (1976) also found *left* hemisphere dominance for consciousness, after studying 47 patients with unilateral lesions following acute cerebrovascular injury. They measured the level of consciousness by means of a 5-point scale based on reflexes and behavioral indices: coma, semicoma, stupor, somnolence, and consciousness. Of the patients with left hemispheric lesions, 57 percent suffered initial impairment of consciousness, compared to 25 percent with right-sided damage.

Salazar and coworkers (1986) reported comparable findings after studying 342 Vietnam veterans who had survived penetrating brain wounds in combat, mainly caused by low-velocity fragments (shell splinters). These investigators studied the medical records of the survivors, focusing on what they called the "wakefulness" component of consciousness. Salazar and colleagues define wakefulness as the manifestation of a tonic activational component that maintains vigilance. The analysis of the relationship between site of injury and disturbance of consciousness was restricted to two subgroups for whom the acute state in the first few hours after injury had been reliably assessed as being either "alert on initial examination" or "unconscious at initial examination." Site and size of injury were accurately assessed by means of computed tomography scan. Salazar and colleagues found a preponderance of left hemisphere lesions in patients who had suffered prolonged unconsciousness, and right hemisphere lesions in those who had not. Structures much more commonly involved in patients with prolonged unconsciousness included the area of the posterior limb of the left internal capsule, the hypothalamus, the left basal forebrain, and the midbrain (mesencephalon). Involvement of the basal forebrain led to unconsciousness in 11 of 12 times.

Both Albert and colleagues (1976) and Salazar and colleagues (1986) speculated about a possible connection between left cerebral dominance for language and "dominance for consciousness." An interaction between wakefulness and language (Salazar et al., 1986) is conceivable in the light of Luria's theory (1973) that many psychological processes, including consciousness, are organized on a verbal basis and are linked to language processes. If one accepts the idea of an intimate working relationship between the left hemisphere and brainstem centers, a relatively superficial yet acute injury to that side could indirectly and transiently disrupt the ARAS and wakefulness, whereas a comparable injury in the right hemisphere would not. Although the link between language and the regulation of consciousness seems plausible, it must be noted that consciousness is regulated in all mammals except man without the help of language. In other words, while language is a relatively recent product of evolution, the regulation of consciousness is much older. If anything, one would expect that language would be most important for the finer regulations in the upper end of the continuum, that is, for gradations of alertness in awake subjects. We know that we can force ourselves to attend to a boring lecture—but it is less clear how language processes might move a patient from a comatose to a subcomatose state. Hence it should be kept in mind that even if the left hemisphere is dominant for the regulation of consciousness, this may be independent of its dominance for language.

In the previous section we referred to several studies reporting that performance in vigilance tasks was more impaired with right than with left hemisphere lesions. If poor vigilance performance is considered a sign of low (tonic) alertness, these findings seem to be at odds with the clinical evidence cited above.

The next topic is focused attention, in this case *attending to external events*, by subjects with a normal, waking level of alertness. There is strong evidence that functional asymmetries exist in this area as well. The anatomical symmetry of structures underlying the arousal reflex and orienting reaction suggests that each hemisphere monitors the area contralateral to itself, in well-balanced cooperation. This is indeed the case in lower animals, but in humans the phenomenon of hemi-inattention is proof of a functional asymmetry. Hemi-inattention, or unilateral neglect, is more frequent and more severe after damage to the *right* hemisphere than after damage to the left hemisphere (Heilman et al., 1985; Mesulam, 1985). Hemi-inattention is the phenomenon that animals and patients with unilateral cerebral lesions fail to report or respond to stimuli presented contralaterally. The phenomenon is not restricted to one modality, and not to the senses. Various theories have been proposed to explain unilateral neglect; some of these are attentional hypotheses. The term hemiakinesia was coined to

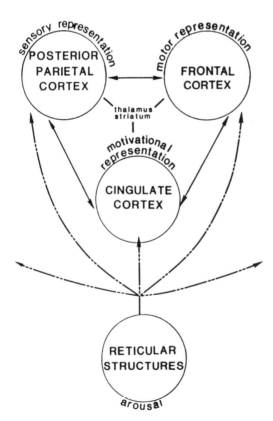

Figure 3-4   The network involved in the distribution of attention to extrapersonal targets, as proposed by Mesulam. (From Mesulam, 1985, with permission.)

describe the behavior of patients who do not use the extremity contralateral to a lesion, even in the absence of paresis. A spectacular manifestation of hemi-inattention is found in anosognosia, in which a patient fails to note that he has a hemiparesis (Babinski, 1914). As early as 1917, Poppelreuter introduced the term inattention, after studying the effects of penetrating brain injuries in World War I casualties.

Unilateral neglect can be induced by lesions in several brain regions: cortical areas such as the temporoparieto-occipital junction, limbic areas such as the cingulate gyrus, and subcortical areas such as the thalamus and the mesencephalic RF. See Figure 3-4. As described previously, these subcortical structures are important for mediating arousal and maintaining an adequate activation level, while the cortical component is involved in the analysis of the behavioral significance of stimuli. Heilman and colleagues therefore concluded that unilateral neglect was an attentional-arousal disorder, caused by dysfunction of a corticolimbic reticular formation loop. The Heilman model clearly resembles the Mesulam model in distinguishing between various types of unilateral neglect, depending on the component damaged in the corticosubcortical network.

Heilman and colleagues (1985) believe that the substantial asymmetry in hemispheric lesions causing unilateral neglect suggests that the brain mechanisms used for attending are asymmetrically distributed. The right hemisphere, in particular, is thought more important for this function than the left. Studies with both normal subjects and patients can be interpreted to suggest that the right

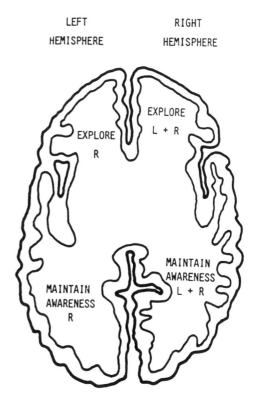

Figure 3-5 The functional asymmetry in the distribution of attention, according to Mesulam: while the left hemisphere is attending to and acting in the right hemispace only, the right hemisphere is attending to and acting in both halves of extrapersonal space. (From Mesulam, 1985, with permission.)

hemisphere is able to monitor both halves, while the left hemisphere merely monitors the space contralateral to it (Dorff et al., 1965; Heilman and Van den Abell, 1979). See Figure 3-5. There is also evidence that the right hemisphere is dominant for intention, or the preparation for action (Verfaellie et al., 1988). The right hemisphere is presumably capable of physiologically preparing *both* arms for action, whereas the left hemisphere can only prepare the right arm. Findings such as these imply that signs of hemineglect caused by lesions in the left hemisphere are usually less obvious, as the right hemisphere supplies compensatory mechanisms. On the other hand, if the right hemisphere is rendered inactive by a lesion somewhere in the corticolimbic reticular loop, the intact left hemisphere will only attend to and act in the right hemispace.

Kinsbourne's model of *imbalance of activation between hemispheres* (Kinsbourne, 1970, 1987) provides a very different view of hemineglect. In this model,

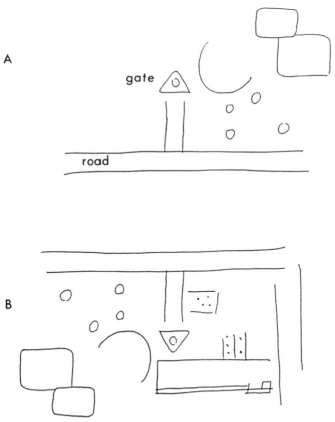

Figure 3-6 A case of hemineglect in visuospatial representation. When a farmer was asked to draw a map of his farm, he stopped drawing after putting in the elements to the right of the central drive and gate (A). The small circles represent trees, the rectangles represent the farmhouse. When the paper was turned 180 degrees, and the patient was asked to view his farm from the rear, he could activate the internal representation of the remaining elements and complete his drawing by adding stables and gardens (B). (Adapted from Tromp, 1993, with permission.)

unilateral neglect is seen as a bias in lateral attention (orientation and action), due to imbalance in a brainstem opponent processor control system for lateral orientation. Reuter-Lorenz and colleagues (1990) compare the model to the game tug-of-war in which the cerebral hemispheres are opponents. "The preponderance of left over right neglect syndromes is attributed to a more powerful rightward than leftward orienting tendency in normals, revealed in them by minor behavioral asymmetries, but resulting in major inequalities when these tendencies are disinhibited due to contralateral brain damage. It is thought that downward projections onto the ipsilateral colliculus superior influence lateral orienting strategies. Reciprocal inhibition between colliculi through the intercollicular commissure mediates the balance of attention. In the case of a hemispheric lesion producing neglect, the ipsilateral colliculus is chronically underactivated and therefore tends to be inhibited by the contralateral one." While the *right* hemisphere is seen as dominant for visual spatial attention in the theories of Mesulam (1981) and Heilman and coworkers (1985), Kinsbourne suggests that a stronger right orienting tendency in the *left* hemisphere is responsible for asymmetrical neglect. Disinhibition of the left hemisphere following damage to the right hemisphere leaves the strong rightward orienting tendency of the left hemisphere unopposed, resulting in left-sided neglect. The leftward bias of the right hemisphere that may predominate after left hemisphere damage is inherently weaker, leading to a directional bias of less severity (Reuter-Lorenz et al., 1990).

A strong point of Kinsbourne's theory is that it is able to explain why the leftmost stimuli are responded to less efficiently than stimuli presented more to the right, even within the not-neglected ipsilesional visual field. Failure to attend contralesionally is complemented by exaggerated attention in the preserved direction. "An ipsilesional stimulus is, as it were, a magnet for the patient." This theory is also used to explain neglect phenomena observed in mental representations of remembered scenes: "Representing may be a successive 'print out' process that is subject to the same directional biases as are submotor attentional shifts across an external field." See Figure 3-6. The implication from Kinsbourne's theory is that the left brain is dominant for spatial attention—although, strictly speaking, it might be the left superior colliculus rather than the left hemisphere.

At the beginning of this section we reviewed evidence suggesting that the left hemisphere might be dominant for the regulation of consciousness at the lower end of the alertness continuum. This could be considered tonic alertness as it refers to a change between global states of consciousness. The right hemisphere might be dominant in one aspect of *phasic alertness*, the short-term preparation for motoric action. This has been demonstrated in reaction time (RT) studies of normal subjects. Heilman and Van den Abell (1979) studied readiness to respond by presenting lateralized warning signals followed by central stimuli (a green light). Warning signals projected to the right hemisphere reduced RT of the right hand more than warning signals projected to the left hemisphere reduced left-hand RT. Warning signals projected to the right hemisphere reduced RT of the right hand *even more* than warning signals projected directly to the left hemisphere. The authors concluded that the right hemisphere appeared to dominate activation. Clinical studies in general confirm this hypothesis (Benton, 1986). A substantial number of studies found that patients with right hemisphere lesions had significantly longer simple RT than those with left hemisphere lesions (De Renzi and Faglioni, 1965; Howes and Boller, 1975). Moreover, simple RT is correlated with mass of lesion in the right hemisphere but not in the left (Tartaglione et al., 1986). In his review, Benton (1986) concluded that the right hemisphere played a special role in the mediation of basic high-speed responses.

Still, it cannot be said that the right hemisphere is dominant for speed of reaction in general. In the introduction to this section we hinted at the possibility that "dominance for attention" might be fractionated. That this can be the case, even in an apparently unitary paradigm, is illustrated by RT studies comparing simple and choice RT. Left hemisphere lesions lead to greater impairment in choice RT tasks, both in terms of speed and accuracy, compared to lesions of the right hemisphere (Benton and Joynt, 1958, Dee and Van Allen, 1973; Rey et al., 1983; Sturm et al., 1989). Studies with normal subjects also suggest that the left hemisphere is dominant in choice reaction tests (Jeeves and Dixon, 1970). Benton (1986) pointed out the distinction that is often made in RT between an arousal component and an information processing component. The level of alertness presumably determines response speed in all RT tasks while facility in information processing assumes progressively more importance in determining response speed as the complexity of task increases (Dee and Van Allen, 1973; Van Zomeren and Deelman, 1976; Van Zomeren, 1981).

The fact that different attentional components seem to play a role in simple versus choice reactions contains a warning that "dominance of attention" might be even more complex in more cognitive tasks. It may be assumed that attention becomes increasingly domain-specific when it is applied to higher order cognitive processes such as word identification or visual pattern matching. It will be even more difficult to extract the attentional component from the dominance dictated by hemispheric specialization in tasks such as these.

SUMMARY

For the present, any attempt to relate all aspects of attention to cerebral structures is bound to fail. This is partly due to the fact that psychological concepts and phenomena do not necessarily have a specific neural substrate; a concept that is psychologically valid may be misleading when transferred to the anatomical level. Even the omnipresent slowness of information processing in neurologic patients cannot be related to the anatomy and physiology of the brain with any certainty. Generally speaking, the connections between aspects of attention and anatomy are more or less understood with regard to basic phenomena such as regulation of the level of alertness, the orienting reflex and habituation. These *intensity* aspects of attention depend largely on subcortical structures that form the ARAS, or "the first functional unit of the brain," according to Luria's theory.

The basal ganglia and the limbic system, particularly the afferent part of the basal ganglia, which consists of the caudate nucleus and putamen, are probably involved in the *selectivity* component of attention. These structures, which seem to be integrated in the diffuse reticulothalamic projection system, have a gating function; a stimulus will neither be consciously perceived nor attended to if its diffuse projection component is suppressed by the gating system. The basal ganglia are closely connected with the limbic system via the hippocampus and amygdala. It is likely that these anatomic connections allow for the integration of emotional value and learning effects (memory) in attentive behavior.

The *cerebral cortex* has three functions in attention: activation, localization, and analysis. The first occurs in the prefrontal cortex where extensive downward projections influence the ARAS. This implies that the cortex is able to regulate the level of alertness in a subtler way than would be possible through more elementary mechanisms such as arousal and habituation only. This finely tuned regulation may be superimposed on the basic regulatory mechanisms, particularly in alert subjects engaged in a task. The cortex, as activator, is concerned mainly with the intensity component of attention.

The two remaining roles of the cortex are more important for selectivity. When it acts as a locater, the cortex is integrated in the system responsible for attending to the outside world. The parietal cortex and the frontal eyefields are essential for visual orienting and focused attention. Next, the cortex acts to analyze and to determine which stimuli will be attended to and which will not. This analysis may vary greatly in its psychological complexity. At one extreme, a preattentive system with a local cortical substrate seems to monitor continuous background stimulation, triggering an attention response when a mismatch occurs. At the other extreme, selective attending may be based on elaborate cortical processes typical of controlled processing and awareness. Language, either in the form of instructions or thought processes, may direct attention at this level.

The question of *cerebral dominance for attention* cannot be answered, but it is too simplistic to assume that attention is a unitary concept which can be related to one hemisphere. Functional asymmetries have been noted for several aspects of attention. On a very basic level, the left hemisphere seems to be more important for the regulation of consciousness since lesions in this hemisphere more frequently lead to loss of consciousness than do lesions in the right hemisphere. In awake subjects, the right hemisphere seems to be dominant for phasic changes in alertness, orienting, and preparation for action. It is not known whether the right hemisphere is dominant for attending to external space in alert subjects. Although the phenomenon of hemi-inattention is far more severe and more frequent after right hemisphere damage than after left hemisphere damage, this does not prove that the right hemisphere is dominant. An alternative explanation for these findings could be imbalance in a brain stem opponent processor system for lateral orientation.

The matter of dominance becomes even less clear at a higher cognitive level. No straightforward dominance can be discerned even with a comparatively simple paradigm such as a reaction time task. The evidence seems to suggest that the right hemisphere is most important in simple RT; basic timed responses are particularly impaired by damage to the right hemisphere. On the other hand, lesions in the left hemisphere seem to have a greater effect on choice RT. This dissociation has been linked to the distinction between an arousal component, essential in simple RT, and an information processing component, more important in choice RT.

Two developments in theories of attention and the brain are worth noting here. First, there is a strong tendency to view attentional mechanisms in terms of *anatomical networks*, or combinations of structures. Several investigators have proposed an anatomical circuitry based on experimental work in humans and animals. This is a welcome development in our view as it does justice to the fact that the brain is a highly integrated system in which various parts are "in concerted action," to use one of Luria's favorite expressions. If one thing has become clear in this chapter, it is that "we attend with our whole brain." This statement is not meant to suggest an extreme holistic point of view, but rather to avoid a phrenology of attention.

Second, increasing emphasis is being placed on the *frontal lobes* as the regulators of attention, particularly in nonroutine situations requiring deliberate planning and regulation. The fields of behavioral neurology and neuropsychology seem to be converging in their views on this part of the brain. In neuropsychology, concepts such as the supervisory attentional system and the central executive have been associated with the frontal lobes, particularly the prefrontal area. Although the idea that the frontal lobes have a role in regulating attention is not new, modern psychological concepts and advanced neurophysiological techniques such as positron emission tomography scanning have opened new possibilities in the study of the frontal component in attention.

4

Closed Head Injury

When one interviews head-injured patients about their cognitive problems, two complaints are almost invariably mentioned: forgetfulness and poor concentration. When asked to describe the latter, patients often say that concentrating on mental activities, such as reading, is unusually tiring for them. Some patients also report difficulty in performing two tasks simultaneously, which suggests that they cannot divide their attention adequately (Van Zomeren and Van den Burg, 1985; Hinkeldey and Corrigan, 1990). In 1987, Gronwall reviewed the quantitative evidence of posttraumatic attentional complaints. In her conclusion, data from self-reports of attentional problems after head injury suggest that although these usually may abate within three months of minor head injury, a significant proportion of more severely injured patients still may have problems two years posttrauma. Following her review, several further reports were published, particularly on surveys done in rehabilitation settings (Burke et al., 1990). Ponsford and Kinsella (1991) studied attention problems in a sample of 50 severely head-injured patients in a rehabilitation facility, using ratings made by speech pathologists and occupational therapists working with the patients. Of the 14 items in their Attention Rating Scale, the following five were most frequently reported:

Performed slowly on mental tasks
Was unable to pay attention to more than one thing at a time
Made mistakes because he/she wasn't paying attention properly
Missed important details in what he/she was doing
Had difficulty concentrating

In this chapter we will review studies of attentional impairments after head injury, which are based on a task-level typology of focused, divided, and sustained attention and supervisory control. Unless otherwise stated, all clinical studies discussed below concern attentional deficits in patients who were no longer in a state of posttraumatic amnesia (PTA). PTA is characterized by an obvious lack of continuous memory, its duration is often considered the best index of severity for closed head injury (Russell, 1971; Schacter and Crovitz, 1977; Brooks, 1984). We will use the terms subacute and chronic to describe the patient's stage after severe head injury. Admitting that such distinctions are more or less arbitrary, we will call the first month after injury the *acute* stage.

The period from 1 to 6 months after injury we will call *subacute*, and thereafter a patient is considered to be a *chronic* case of head injury. This chapter deals with the effects of closed head injury (CHI) only, as penetrating injuries can have quite different effects at the behavioral level.

FOCUSED ATTENTION

The object of focused attention studies is to measure task performance in the presence of distraction. Clinical interest in this aspect of attention stems from the complaints of many CHI patients, both mild and severe, about poor concentration, oversensitivity to noise and bustle, and irritability (Van Zomeren and Van den Burg, 1985). Early psychological investigators (Conkey 1938; Ruesch 1944a, 1944b) had some doubts about their subjects' ability to focus attention on a given task. However, in these papers remarks about selectivity seemed to be based mainly on observation of patients during assessment. Dencker and Löfving (1958) were the first investigators to test specifically for attentional deficits. They tested a group of patients, two-thirds of whom had experienced a PTA duration of 1 hour or less, making them cases of "mild concussion" in terms of the W. R. Russell classification of severity (1934). As they were tested at an average interval of 10 years postinjury, it must be assumed that many of the mild injury cases had recovered more or less completely.

Dencker and Löfving presented two texts to their subjects, reading them aloud. During the presentation of one of the texts, a recording of about a dozen persons talking simultaneously was played. Immediately after the presentation of each text, questions were asked about the content. Judging by the number of correct answers, it appeared that the irrelevant stimulation had no effect at all on the performance of either group. They therefore concluded that this experimental group showed no deficit in focusing.

Gronwall and Sampson (1974) tested focused attention in five mildly concussed patients (duration of PTA of less than 1 hour). Within 24 hours of admission to the hospital these subjects were tested with dichotic stimulation. Two texts were presented simultaneously through headphones, and the subjects were instructed to shadow (repeat word by word) the text presented to their left ear while ignoring the other ear. Halfway through the session the texts were switched between ears. In neither group were intrusions from the irrelevant message found, but in the control group the switch between ears caused a greater increase in omissions than in the patient group. The authors concluded that their patients were not abnormally sensitive to distraction, that is, showed no deficit in focused attention.

Kewman and colleagues (1988) presented tape-recorded paragraphs of a text read by a male voice to a head-injured group predominantly consisting of chronic cases, and to a hospital control group. Comprehension was assessed immediately afterward by means of questions on each paragraph. Half of the recordings had been dubbed over with a female voice reading a different text at the same volume as the male voice. In the double recordings, both texts were presented simultaneously through earphones, both ears receiving the same mixture of male and female voices. Head-injured patients made more errors in both the standard and distraction conditions. When error scores were compared between single-voice and double-voice conditions, it was found that the number of errors had doubled for both groups in the distraction condition. Kewman and colleagues interpreted their findings as an indication of enhanced distractibility after head injury, but stated that the poor performance in the distraction condition "may not entirely be due to a selective attention deficit but may be better explained by a general breakdown in a number of cognitive processes under conditions of greater informational loads."

Miller and Cruzat (1980) studied the effect of distracting stimuli on speed of card sorting in head injured subjects. The test was presented to a "mild" group with a median PTA duration of 20 minutes, and to a "severe" group with a median duration of 9 days. Piles of cards were sorted according to the occurrence of the letters A or B. The cards also contained a variable number of distracting letters (in conditions with 0, 1, 4, or 8 irrelevant letters). It appeared that only the severely injured group was significantly slower than the control group, but there was no interaction between severity and task difficulty. In other words, an increase in the number of irrelevant letters on the cards had no specific effect on the sorting speed of these patients.

Stuss and coworkers (1989) investigated the effect of irrelevant information during a choice RT task. Three groups of head-injured patients (mild concussions, severe concussions within one year after injury, and chronic severe cases) were tested with a series of RT tasks in which colored stimuli were presented on a personal computer. The stimuli had three dimensions: shape, color, and line orientation within the shapes. In the so-called Redundant Multiple Choice RT Test, subjects could detect the target stimulus in an array of four stimuli by attending to one dimension only; for example, by focusing on color the task became relatively easy, as none of the distractors were the color of the target. Stuss and coworkers found some evidence of unnecessary processing of redundant information: the Redundant Condition had a significant effect on choice RT in the chronic group. However, the authors themselves considered the effect "somewhat elusive," as it had not been found in the same group of patients one week before.

Most of the studies reviewed above made use of very obvious cues to determine choice: experimenter versus recording, left ear versus right ear, male versus female voice. In other words, selection in these experiments was possible on the basis of physical dimensions and did not demand much of the selective strategy. Moray (1969) pointed out that ear of presentation is a very potent cue for selective attention. Also, there were no conflicting response tendencies attached to the distracting stimuli: the results reflected the use of relatively weak distractors. The next experiments we will discuss were also concerned with focused attention but differed from those reviewed above by introducing distracting stimuli having *strong response tendencies* attached to them which conflicted with the task requirements presented. Thus, they are good techniques for assessing abnormal "focused attention deficits" (FAD) as described by Shiffrin and Schneider (see Chapter 2).

Dencker and Löfving (1958) included a test of *mirror-drawing* in their study. This test requires suppression of habitual visuomotor responses in order to deal with the mirror image visual feedback. This is clearly an example of interference by overtrained responses, or a FAD in terms of Shiffrin and Schneider's model. The task is usually experienced by any subject as difficult, but the chronic head-injured group in the Swedish study took significantly longer to complete the task than the control group. Still, this cannot be explained conclusively as a sign of pathological response interference in the patients. As no comparison was made of drawing speed without the hindrance of mirror feedback in either group, it could be that the experimental group was performing slower than the control group, but without a qualitative difference.

A classic case of response interference is found in the *Stroop paradigm*, where stimuli have two dimensions: a color, and a word meaning conflicting with the color (for example, the word "yellow" printed in blue letters). The Stroop Color Word Test has been presented to head-injury patients in several studies. This test consists of three subtests: reading color names, naming the colors of printed blocks, and naming the colors of words that are themselves color names. The latter condition creates response interference, as the subject must suppress the overtrained reading response. Chadwick and colleagues (1981) compared head-injured children with orthopaedic controls, testing them 1 and 4 months after injury. They found a difference between groups. The head-injured children were slower on all three subtests, however there was no specific response interference effect in the last subtest. Thomas (1977) reported similar results in a group of adult patients with mild concussions. Stuss (1985) and Ponsford and Kinsella (1992) reported that moderate and severe head injuries did not result in a specific interference effect.

To further increase response interference in the Stroop Test, we tried to distract subjects by means of delayed feedback of their own voice. While performing the test, a group of subacute CHI patients and controls heard their voices through earphones, after a delay of 180 or 350 ms. This is a very disturbing echo that has a clear effect on speed of performance. However, this delayed auditory effect had no special effect on the patients' reading and color naming. Only in the most difficult condition of the Stroop Test, where the color of the ambiguous words must be named, was the effect of distraction significantly greater in the patient group than in the control group, both absolutely and relatively (Elting et al., 1988, 1989).

Bohnen (1991) described another variation of the Stroop paradigm in which twenty percent of the ambiguous stimuli (colored words) were marked by boxes, that is, small rectangles around the stimulus words. Subjects were instructed to *read* these words, rather than to name their colors. Hence the unfamiliar task of color naming was interrupted repeatedly by stimuli that forced the subjects to switch back to reading. When testing mildly head-injured subjects with PTA durations not exceeding 60 minutes, in the first 2 weeks after injury (subacute stage), it was found that the classical Stroop paradigm had no specific effect on the patients. However, the modified Stroop condition had a slight but significant additional effect on the patient group, as compared to controls. Whereas patients and controls needed, respectively, 88 and 83 seconds to name the colors of the words in the standard condition, the respective values for the modified version were 106 and 97 seconds.

Van Zomeren and Brouwer (1987) studied the effect of response interference using *visual choice reaction times* (RT). Patients with injuries ranging from moderate to very severe on the Russell scale were tested between 3 and 6 months postinjury. RT was recorded in a four-choice task with a very high stimulus-response compatibility: the stimuli were buttons that had to be pressed as quickly as possible when they were lighted. This four-choice task was then repeated in a so-called "distraction condition." This time an irrelevant stimulus appeared simultaneously with each relevant one (Van Zomeren, 1981). The panel contained additional identical lights in close proximity to the stimulus lights. The presentation of these twin lights evoked conflicting response tendencies in the subjects. The patients' performance was compared in an analysis of variance with that of a group of healthy controls, matched for age and sex. See Figure 4-1.

The patients had significantly longer RTs than the controls, and both groups had significantly longer RTs on the distraction task than on the original four-choice task. Moreover, there was a significant interaction between groups and tasks: the irrelevant stimuli had a much stronger distracting effect on the head-injured group than on the control group.

The outcome of this experiment was statistically very clear: distraction had a greater effect on the patients than on the controls. A theoretical explanation is nevertheless difficult. Because of their close proximity and resemblance, and the high S-R compatibility in the task, the distractors may have evoked response tendencies requiring inhibition. If this is the case, the results suggest that sub-acute CHI patients are more susceptible to response interference. The question remains why this effect does not appear in the standard Stroop Test. As stated above, healthy controls and CHI patients are equally impaired by the distraction in the latter task.

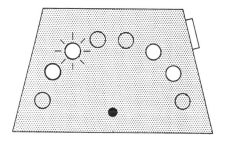 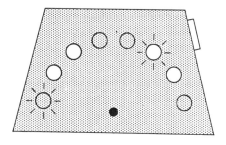

BASIC TASK   R-4   DISTRACTION   TASK

Figure 4-1   The apparatus used for recording RT in a basic four-choice task and in a distraction condition. In the latter condition, an extra stimulus appears along with the target stimulus and has to be ignored by the subject. On the actual panel all lights are physically identical, but in this illustration the positive stimuli are depicted unshaded. The black dot is the central button on which the subject keeps his index finger until he starts his movement toward a stimulus. The lights in the semicircular array are themselves push buttons.

An alternative explanation for the distraction effect in our RT task may lie in controlled processing. Both patients and controls experience response conflict in the distraction task, resulting in longer RTs than those registered in the basic four-choice task. The extra time is necessary for dealing with the conflict, that is, for making a final choice of where to go. As with every other mental process, head-injured patients need *more time* than controls to deal with response interference. Thus, the experiment demonstrated that patients show a slowing of controlled processing, but it produced no evidence for a focused attention deficit. This explanation was also considered by Deland and associates (1992) who found, in a comparable experiment, that distraction effects were proportional to the reaction times observed in the basic task condition without distraction. They considered the possibility that patients are not impaired in inhibiting automatic processes, but that the controlled discarding of irrelevant stimuli in a task with relatively new requirements costs them significantly more time.

Later studies have suggested that susceptibility to response interference may be typical of the acute and subacute stages following head injury, but that it wears off as patients recover. A group of patients was tested in our laboratory at 3 months and 6 months postinjury. On the first occasion, RT scores on the basic four-choice task and the distraction task contributed independently to the discrimination between control subjects and patients. At 6 months postinjury this independent contribution of the distraction task had disappeared. Other evidence supporting a temporary susceptibility to interference was found by Brouwer (1985) in a short-term memory comparison task and in a word learning task. The memory comparison task was administered to head-injured patients within a few weeks after the end of PTA, and again in the chronic stage (more than 6 months postinjury). On the first occasion, patients appeared to be particularly slowed in their reactions to items that did *not* match with the positive memory set, that is, in their NO responses. This could suggest that subacute patients have difficulty inhibiting the dominant tendency to give positive responses. In the free recall word learning task, slight proactive interference was recorded on the first occasion, but this was no longer the case 6 months after injury.

Some doubt with regard to the relationship between the interference effect and the subacute stage is raised by the outcome of a study reported by Deland and colleagues (1992). These authors used the same four-choice RT tasks, with and without visual distractors, as described above (Van Zomeren, 1981; Van Zomeren and Brouwer, 1987). The tasks were presented to a representative group of 14 consecutively hospitalized CHI patients 3 and 12 months after injury. Deland and colleagues did not find a greater improvement of RT over time in the distraction task than in the standard four-choice reaction task (approximately 35 ms gain in both cases). Further research into the issue of increased susceptibility to response interference early in CHI is clearly needed.

Summary

In spite of the clinical reality of complaints about increased distractability, there is little empirical evidence for increased effects of distraction on task performance in individuals who have sustained head injuries. When auditory or visual distractors are presented in a task, head-injured patients can ignore these as well as controls. Even when irrelevant stimuli are presented that provoke conflicting response tendencies, and thereby create response interference, the effects are often comparable to those in healthy controls. Although there are some inconsistent findings, the overall conclusion seems to be that chronic patients have a normal ability to focus attention. There is some evidence for increased sensitivity in *subacute* patients to interference from dominant response tendencies observed in modified Stroop tasks, a visual reaction time task and two memory tasks. This issue requires further study.

DIVIDED ATTENTION

As mentioned in the introduction to this chapter, complaints about dividing attention and mental slowness are frequent and persistent, particularly in patients with severe brain damage (Van Zomeren and Van den Burg, 1985; Ponsford and Kinsella, 1991). Individual performance in a divided attention task consisting of two or more subtasks that have to be performed simultaneously is determined by a number of components:

Allocation strategy: The individual attention allocation strategy (between subtasks), with greater emphasis on some tasks and less on others
Processing strategies: Within subtasks, and the level of skill obtained performing the subtasks
Speed: The duration and accuracy of the elementary cognitive processes required by the strategies for the subtasks
Switching: The time it takes to switch attention between subtasks that cannot be executed simultaneously
Time-sharing: The separability of processing systems required by the subtasks. Subtasks may require completely different perceptual, cognitive, and motor processes or there can be overlap. This separability may be determined both by task and subject characteristics, including the level of skill.

It may be argued that the latter three components are especially important for the clinical evaluation of divided attention in a general sense. These are not task-specific and are assumed to indicate general constraints on processing efficiency for unfamiliar tasks under time-pressure. The time-sharing factor, of course, must be corrected for skill level. Limitations in the speed of elementary cognitive processes and in switching attention are clinically interesting phenomena because of their general character. Individual abilities to time-share may be of interest as well. Theoretically, these could influence performance on a wide range of tasks and therefore provide a parsimoneous explanation for patients' problems in many everyday situations requiring divided attention. One could expect such general areas such as speed, switching, and time-sharing to be influenced by traumatic brain injury.

Generalizations based on abnormalities observed in individual strategies for allocating attention between and within subtasks could also be considered. Individuals will differ with regard to the quality and efficiency of cognitive strategies in nonroutine cognitive tasks, even if skill, speed of processing, time-sharing, and flexibility do not play a limiting role. Where there is evidence that CHI patients are impaired in the formation or use of such strategies in divided attention tasks it will be noted, but its discussion will be deferred until the section on Supervisory Attentional Control, as the ability to form and use Supervisory Attentional Control strategies is considered a specific function (Shallice, 1982; Baddeley, 1986) with implications for a wider range of tasks than divided attention tasks only.

What is known about speed of (controlled) processing and speed and efficiency of switching attention and time-sharing between tasks in people who have sustained head injuries will be reviewed below. Strictly speaking, the investigation of these aspects of attention requires an experimental procedure in which controlled processing, switching, and time-sharing requirements are varied independent of (unconfounded with) sensory and motor factors. For example, if simple reaction time and complex reaction time in nonroutine tasks are compared, the time difference may not immediately be interpreted in terms of controlled processing as the tasks differ in terms of visual and motor requirements. As many studies on the speed of processing, particularly in older CHI studies, have not controlled for such confounding, strict adherence to this procedure would leave us with a very limited data set. We will therefore broaden the scope of this review, commenting from case to case on the degree to which controlled processing may have been involved in the difference between CHI patients and control subjects.

Impaired Speed of Processing

"Mental slowness" in individuals with head injuries has been frequently reported by clinical observers. This observation was confirmed when psychologists began to study the effects of head injury. In contrast to early statements about "attention," reports on slowness are less questionable. For example, Ruesch (1944a) reported that his patients were slow in color naming and in reading. In a second study (Ruesch 1944b) he demonstrated that head-injury patients, tested while still in hospital, showed significantly longer reaction times than control subjects. In 1961, Norrman and Svahn reported on the reaction times (RT) of patients who had suffered severe cerebral concussion at least 2 years earlier, and who had been in coma for at least 1 week after the injury. In this chronic group, a three-choice reaction to visual stimuli revealed a highly significant slowness compared with a control group of neurotics. Simple visual reaction showed no difference between the groups.

Van Zomeren and Deelman (1976) compared simple and four-choice visual RT in subjects with varying severity of injury and in controls matched for sex and age. They found a significant interaction between groups and tasks, that is, the choice reaction resulted in a significantly larger difference between groups than the simple reaction. In a second experiment they demonstrated that the slowing of information processing was proportional to the severity of injury as expressed by duration of coma. A follow-up study (Van Zomeren and Deelman, 1978) showed clearly that even after almost 2 years the most severe group, with a coma lasting over a week, performed significantly slower than less severely injured groups on the four-choice task.

Ponsford and Kinsella (1992) tested very severe CHI patients consecutively admitted to a rehabilitation program and orthopedic controls with a large battery of tests of attention, including a simple and a four-choice reaction time task. Patients were tested in the first year after injury, some in the subacute and some in the chronic stage of recovery. The tasks provided for separate assessments of decision-time (DT) and movement-time (MT), and the former was taken as the reaction time measure. It was found that the CHI patients were significantly slower than controls and that the difference was significantly larger in the choice reaction task.

Many investigators have observed that choice RT is generally more effective than simple RT in revealing residual impairments (Stuss et al., 1989; Ponsford and Kinsella, 1992). The disproportional effect of an increasing *number of stimulus alternatives* on patients has been termed a "complexity effect" (Van Zomeren and Deelman, 1978; Benton, 1986; Braun et al., 1989b). This factor has been investigated in more detail by a number of authors.

Miller (1970) studied visual RT in a small group of head-injury victims, comparing their performance with the behavior of a control group matched for sex and age. His subjects had been in PTA for more than 1 week and were tested between 3 and 12 months after injury, with some in the subacute and some in the chronic stage of recovery. The subjects stood before a horizontal panel containing a circular array of push buttons. The buttons were numbered from 1 to 8. As soon as a number appeared in a small visual display subjects were required to push the appropriate button in the array. RT was tested under four conditions, with increasing numbers of stimulus alternatives: 1, 2, 4, and 8 numbers.

The groups differed in reaction time, the head-injury group being slower in all conditions. Moreover, the difference between groups increased with the complexity of the task. Miller concluded that the effect of head injury was slowed decision-making and central information-processing. In addition to the number of stimulus alternatives, the apparatus used by Miller also differed from instruments used in the clinical studies described above by employing symbolic stimuli. This feature decreases the stimulus-response compatibility as the response is not directly indicated by the physical features of the stimulus.

In a study by Gronwall and Sampson (1974), the influence of *S-R compatibility* was specifically tested in a choice reaction time experiment, along with the effect of increasing the number of stimulus alternatives. Twelve mildly concussed males, (PTA duration of less than 1 hour) were tested within 24 hours of admission to hospital, with symbolic and nonsymbolic 2, 4, 6, 8, and 10-choice tasks. The stimulus was a table-tennis ball falling down the alleys of a pinball machine. In the symbolic condition, a button below an alley other than the one in which the ball had fallen had to be pushed (mirror-image position). As the concussed patients had significantly longer RTs in the most complex subtests of the symbolic version only, the authors concluded that central processing time was significantly increased following concussion.

The studies described above suggested that the RT of head-injured patients is influenced disproportionately by two variables: the number of stimulus alternatives and stimulus-response compatibility. Such observations have inspired a search for the *locus of the slowness* in terms of information processing stages. The additive factor model (Smith, 1968; Sternberg, 1969), in particular, has been applied. This model involves the following successive stages between S and R:

Stimulus encoding
Memory comparison
Decision-making
Response selection
Response execution

Number of stimulus alternatives and stimulus-response compatibility are thought to influence the cognitive stages of decision-making and response selection. In a more global sense, the RT data suggested a selective impairment (slowing) of controlled processing because it involved the central symbolic aspects of the reaction process (Van Zomeren et al., 1984). This hypothesis of impaired controlled processing after CHI has an additional attraction as, even in the PTA stage, patients often seem well able to apply thoroughly learned, automatized sequences of information processing. It is also consistent with the complaints of slow thinking and difficulty with doing two things at the same time, frequently expressed by very severe CHI patients, and significantly correlated with the severity of injury (Van Zomeren and Van den Burg, 1985).

Following the formulation of the *controlled processing hypothesis*, a number of relevant studies appeared. Brouwer (1985) varied the complexity of automatic and controlled memory search in a binary choice paradigm, controlling for perceptual and motor differences between task conditions.

Subjects sat behind a tilted response panel with both index fingers on response buttons marked YES and NO, and viewed a video monitor. After the presentation of a fixation mark, a set of digits appeared (1, 2, or 3 digits) on the monitor. These had to be memorized. Following a short visual mask, a simple addition problem (e.g., 4 + 3 =) was presented. An affirmative response had to be given if the answer to the sum was in the memorized set. The principal dependent variable was RT. The set of digits was varied from trial to trial (varied set). See Figure 4-2.

A sample of initially hospitalized CHI patients (predominantly very severe concussions according to the Russell scale) and a control group comparable for age and education were tested on two separate occasions at about a 5-month interval. Patients in the subacute stage were tested as soon as possible after the termination of PTA, and in the early chronic stage. It appeared that increasing the complexity of controlled processing slowed patients significantly more than controls. It also appeared that the patients had recovered significantly when subacute and early chronic scores were compared to overall RTs and to the effects of increased complexity of controlled processing. Further, it was observed that while patients were significantly slower in the least complex task conditions,

STIMULI

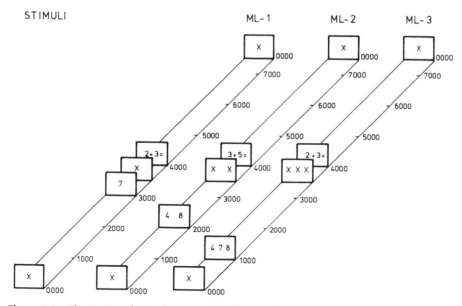

Figure 4-2   The timing of stimulus events (milliseconds) in each of the experimental blocks of a controlled memory search task. ML, memory load. At first, 1, 2, or 3 digits are shown that have to be kept in memory. Then a simple addition problem is presented, and the subjects have to indicate, as fast and accurately as possible, whether the answer to the problem matches with a digit in the memory set. Numbers along the oblique strips are milliseconds. Boxes with X's are either fixation points or visual masks to suppress the afterimage of the memory set.

the *relative* increase in reaction time with increasing complexity was almost identical for patients and controls.

Task variables used to vary the difficulty of controlled processing were the number of elements in the memory set and the binary variable indicating a match or a mismatch between the memory set and the answer to a simple addition problem. It appeared that the mismatches, in particular, took the patients much longer: the interaction of the match/mismatch variable and groups was significant. However, this specific effect was found only at the initial testing (subacute stage). See Figure 4-3.

Stokx and Gaillard (1986) varied memory set size in a fixed set memory search task (Sternberg task) presented to chronic, very severe head-injured patients more than 2 years postinjury, who were currently active car drivers. "While RTs increased with increasing set size, and were longer with nontargets than with targets, these effects were not larger in the patient group than in the control group" (p. 428). This result contradicts the controlled processing hypothesis. With regard to testing procedure, it should be noted that the same positive set was used (fixed set) in the whole experimental block and may have led to some degree of automatization in memory comparison. Another possible criticism of the study is that the choice of subjects was not representative as only patients who were judged to be fit to drive had been selected.

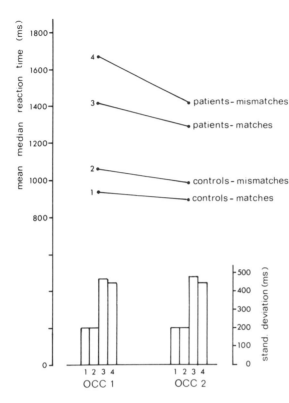

Figure 4-3 Mean median RT and its standard deviation as a function of occasion, required response, and group membership. Lines 3 and 4 clearly reflect recovery in the patient group. Patients improved their RT particularly in the case of mismatches (4). (From Brouwer, 1985, with permission.)

In the latter study, other task variables were included in the framework of the method of additive factors (Sternberg, 1969). The authors used a four-stage information processing model (Sanders, 1983): stimulus encoding, memory comparison, response selection, and motor preparation. Task variables believed to influence each of these stages were varied to determine whether CHI interacted with any of these variables. Although some individual patients were very sensitive to specific task variables, the general effect of slowness in any task was a much more robust phenomenon than these specific effects. For the total group, the results of the reaction time task provided no conclusive evidence that severe concussion of the brain affects particular stages of information processing.

Shum and colleagues (1990) also used the additive factor method in a study on visual RT in subacute and chronic CHI patients. Unfortunately, the nature of the patient selection was not mentioned. It appeared that *subacute* very severe patients were considerably slower than controls, both in decision-time (DT) and movement-time (MT). They also made a high number of errors. In addition to these main effects, significant interactions on DT were found between CHI and the task-variables, "signal similarity" and "S-R compatibility." The latter variables are thought to influence the stages of stimulus identification and response selection. In *chronic* very severe CHI patients, slowness was less excessive and apart from significantly slowed MT, only a significant interaction between CHI and S-R compatibility was found in the DT data. No significant effects of CHI whatsoever were found, either on errors, DT or MT in *mild* subacute patients'

DT or MT. However, this group consisted of only seven patients, three of whom were tested more than a month after injury, which is too long to expect marked impairments after such mild injuries.

Finally, Schmitter-Edgecombe and coworkers (1992) studied the effect of CHI on three stages of information processing: stimulus encoding, memory comparison, and decision-making/response-selection. Patients were chronic cases tested more than 18 months postinjury. Their injuries had been very severe, with durations of PTA ranging from 8 to 360 days and reported duration of unconsciousness always more than 48 hours. The stimulus encoding stage was tapped by varying the quality of target stimuli (unmasked, slightly masked, and strongly masked words). These target stimuli were the words RITE and LEFT. Stimulus-response compatibility was varied by directing subjects to react to the target word RITE with either their "right or left hand," and to the word LEFT with either their "left or right hand." This manipulation should have had an effect on the stages of decision-making and response selection. The stages of memory comparison and response selection were tested by means of the Sternberg (1969) memory scanning paradigm: subjects were presented with a memory set of one, two, or four digits, and had to respond YES or NO to a probe digit presented immediately afterward, depending on whether the probe had been included in the memory set.

Stimulus quality had a much stronger effect on patients' RT than on the RT of controls. Schmitter-Edgecombe and colleagues (1992) concluded that very severe CHI may affect the stimulus-encoding stage. This seems to be consistent with electrophysiological evidence, which shows an increased latency of P-300 after head injury (Papanicolaou et al., 1984; Campbell et al., 1986; Papanicolaou, 1987; Rugg et al., 1988). Heinze and colleagues (1992) studied EPs and ERPs in 11 chronic, very severe CHI patients with a visual selective attention task. They found abnormalities in early and intermediate ERP components: "The results were interpreted as an index of CHI dysfunctions in perceptual processes such as simple feature registration and early target discrimination."

The difference between compatible and incompatible responses was somewhat greater for the CHI patients, suggesting that they were impaired in decision-making and response-selection processes. In the memory scanning task, head injured subjects' RTs were *not* slowed more than controls' as memory set size increased. On the other hand, the effect of the match/mismatch variable was much stronger in the CHI group. This is similar to the pattern of results Brouwer (1985) found in subacute patients performing a comparable task (see above). The investigators conclude that their findings do not support a late-specificity hypothesis, as the patients' deficits were not restricted to the decision-making and response-selection stages. On the other hand, they do not feel that their results support a *global slowness hypothesis* (according to which all stages of information processing should be affected by CHI). They point out that some processes, such as the ability to scan items in short-term memory, may be more resilient than others to the effects of severe head injury. Still, in their study, as in those described previously, the main effect of head injury appears to be much more impressive than specific effects. In this regard, these authors' results tend to support the global slowness hypothesis rather than a more specific hypothesis.

To summarize, the controlled processing, or late-specificity, hypothesis is not supported in severe CHI patients. Nonspecific slowing is the most conspicuous phenomenon; it is very easy to demonstrate a slowing of information processing after severe CHI, but attempts to identify the slowness with specific stages have either failed or have revealed specific effects that were small in comparison to the general slowness.

The mental slowness of CHI patients has been studied extensively with the *Paced Auditory Serial Addition Task* (PASAT), a popular clinical test of information processing after head injury. Gronwall and Sampson (1974) devised this test, a task that is clearly aimed at divided attention deficits (DAD), in which tape recorded one-digit numbers are presented in different blocks at different rates. Subjects are required to add every pair of successive numbers and to give the answer immediately, as follows:

Stimulus   7   1   3   5   2   4   etc.
Response   8   4   8   7   6   etc.

This infers dividing attention between stimuli, stored memory elements, mental transformations, and responding. The dependent variable is the percentage of correct answers. Gronwall and Sampson presented this task to hospital controls and concussed patients classified in two degrees of severity, according to duration of PTA. Patients were significantly more influenced by rate of presentation, and within the patient group there was an interaction of severity and rate of presentation. It was thought unlikely that patients used a qualitatively different control strategy as the nature of errors did not discriminate patients from controls. Both patients and controls could do the task almost perfectly without time pressure, and early processing up to the level of meaning of individual verbal stimuli was found to be normal in these patients.

No decreased PASAT performance was found by Thomas (1977) when testing a head-injured group with comparable mild injury. However, as she used a lower rate of presentation, her results may well indicate that processing speed is indeed the critical factor. Later studies have generally confirmed the clinical usefulness of the PASAT in group studies of CHI patients (Gronwall, 1977; O'Shaughnessy et al., 1984; Ponsford and Kinsella, 1992), as well as for studying the recovery of processing capacity (Gronwall, 1987; Stuss et al., 1988).

Reaction Time After Head Injury: A Meta-analysis

It would seem that while there is convincing evidence for slowed information processing after head injury, until now this slowing has not consistently yielded to componential analysis, either in terms of the automatic-controlled distinction, or of stage analysis of reaction time. In fact, slowed information processing has been described in many different tasks: simple and complex, automatic and controlled, perceptual, cognitive, and motor. To illustrate this and to get an overview of the general pattern of results with regard to reaction time data, the reaction times of CHI patients and control subjects were plotted on a linear scale over a wide range of RT experiments (Figure 4-4). Only studies involving patients in the first year after injury were used as patient selection from subacute

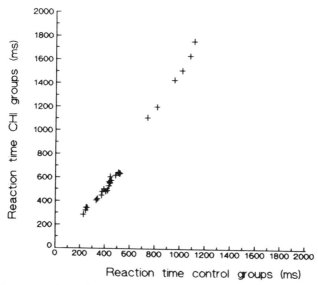

Figure 4-4 A meta-analysis of seven reaction time studies in head-injured subjects. Mean RT scores of patient groups are plotted as a function of mean RT in the corresponding control groups. [Data from Van Zomeren and Deelman (1976), Van Zomeren (1981), Brouwer (1985, p. 99), Brouwer (1985, p. 131), Stuss et al. (1989), Ponsford and Kinsella (1992), and Veltman et al., (1990).]

groups has generally been more uniform and a number of studies have used fairly large representative samples of (initially) hospitalized patients. [Data from the small, very severe subacute group ($n = 10$) of Shum and coworkers (1990) are not plotted in Figure 4-4 as the nature of patient selection was not specified and because the high error percentages and extreme movement times suggest that they may have had an atypical patient sample. Had they been included in the figure, they would have shown a far steeper regression line than the other results. Even on the simplest version of their reaction time tasks, these patients were much slower than would be expected from Figure 4-4.]

The general impression from studies on representative groups of subacute (and early chronic) patients is that the data from all classical RT methods reveal a remarkably constant relationship between the CHI and control groups. For example, if the CHI patients' and controls' reaction time scores are computed for clinical tests, for example, the Trailmaking Test or Symbol-Digits Substitution Tests, comparable ratios are found. In the group of subacute patients represented in Figure 4-4 JC Veltman and colleagues (1990) recorded 31 and 67 seconds for Trailmaking A and B, respectively, in the control group, and 44 and 91 seconds for the subacute patients. The ratios between patient and control scores are 1.42 and 1.36, respectively, which is close to the average ratios for reaction time data. This suggests that an explanation in terms of global slowing suffices and that the choice of tasks for assessing this robust phenomenon can be based on purely practical grounds. A small qualification is that the ratio between patient and control reaction times appears to be slightly larger in very complex tasks

(Brouwer, 1985, p. 99) than in more straightforward choice reaction time tasks. In the above section on focused attention, the possibility was considered that increased difficulty in inhibiting dominant responses may have contributed to this. An alternative explanation is considered below.

Until now, poor divided attention performance was explained by slow processing alone. No psychological mechanisms or structures specific to multiple-tasks or rapid switching between tasks were considered. In the following sections, aspects of divided attention and switching between tasks which are theoretically independent of processing speed within (sub)tasks are investigated.

Time Sharing

An interesting method for testing the ability to divide attention in this restricted sense was described by Somberg and Salthouse (1982) in a study on aging. It has two important features. The first is that individual differences in processing speed on the level of single task subroutines are controlled for by the use of adaptive tasks. Prior to the dual task situations, the difficulty of each separate task is individually adjusted so that all subjects reach a comparable accuracy. The second attractive feature of this method is the use of a performance-operating-characteristic (POC), which enables measuring divided attention independent of the allocation strategy of each subject (Wickens, 1984). This could be considered a control for individual differences in supervisory attentional control. In order to be able to construct the POC, subjects are instructed to vary their emphasis on each of the tasks in several dual-task conditions. Performance in one task is plotted as a function of performance in the other. Differences between individual POCs can be considered as differences in ability to divide attention.

Brouwer and coworkers (1989) applied this method to study the ability to divide attention in *chronic* CHI patients. Fifteen very severe patients tested 5 to 10 years postinjury and 34 control subjects performed two continuous visuomotor tasks in a driving simulator, in single- and dual-task conditions. Both the patient group and the control group consisted of active licensed drivers at the time of the study. One task was a compensatory tracking task requiring lane-tracking, a basic car driving skill. The subjects had to compensate for course deviations resulting from an unpredictable "sidewind." The other task, dot counting, was a self-paced visual choice reaction time task requiring analysis of dot configuration in a small area of the road display (Figure 4-5).

Before beginning the dual-task, single-task difficulty was individually adjusted for by adaptive task procedures. This was done to equalize the difficulty of the two tasks in the dual task condition for both groups so that any differences in dual-task performance could not be explained by impairments in processing speed. Adaptation to the lane-tracking task prior to the dual task conditions, consisted of the individual calibration of a factor multiplying the response of the steering wheel to the sidewind (see Figure 4-5). This factor was increased step-wise until a stable level of steering quality was obtained. As a result of individual calibration, the size of the steering movements was the same for subjects with low and high sidewind scores. The only difference between subjects was in the

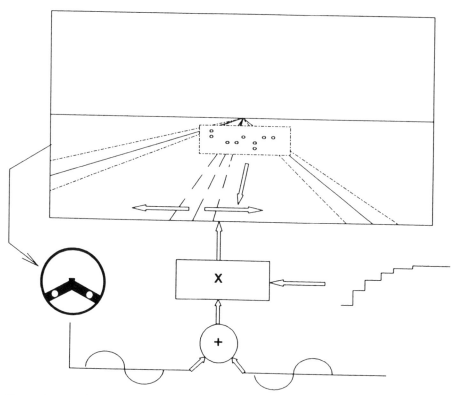

Figure 4-5 A schematic representation of the dual-task simulator as used by Brouwer and colleagues. In the central box on the screen, the groups of 8, 9, or 10 dots are presented. The subject is reacting to these signals by means of the YES and NO buttons on the steering wheel (which is shown here on the lower left side, but which is situated centrally below and before the screen in the real simulator). The sinuses at the bottom symbolize the artificial electronic "sidewind" for which X is the multiplication factor. (From Brouwer et al., 1989, with permission.)

number of compensatory movements made per unit time. The dot-counting task was adaptive by its self-paced character. Individual adaptation of tasks implied that for each subject a force of sidewind was determined that resulted in 90 percent of time "on target," and a 90 percent correct score in the dot counting. An attempt was made to control for individual differences in attention allocation strategies by making all subjects perform the dual-tasks under three different emphasis conditions: emphasis on tracking, emphasis on dot-counting, equal weight for both tasks.

As expected (from decreased speed of information processing), CHI patients reached significantly lower levels of performance in the single-task conditions of the adaptive tasks. They could handle less sidewind and reacted slower in the dot counting than control subjects. However, with individual differences in processing speed and task allocation strategies controlled for, the ability to divide attention was found to be approximately equal in the chronic CHI patients and the control group. An unexpected finding, however, was a significant positive correlation between severity of injury (PTA duration) and divided attention impairment in the patient group. The possibility was considered, post hoc, that the patient sample was too selective as it consisted of active drivers only. Maybe this group had superior divided attention abilities prior to having sustained the head injuries, which would have the effect of shifting the distribution of their abilities into the normal range.

In a subsequent study, a sample of *subacute* very severe CHI patients (Veltman et al., in preparation) was tested with this task within a larger battery of tests. Eighteen CHI patients, consecutively hospitalized at the Neurology Department of the Academic Hospital in Groningen, were tested on average 118 days after injury (SD 44.7 days). The average PTA duration was 20.8 days (SD 22.3 days) and all patients were out of PTA when tested. A questionnaire on mental complaints was administered at the time of testing (Van Zomeren and Van den Burg, 1985). The majority of patients mentioned concentration difficulties, mental slowness and difficulty in doing two things simultaneously.

Basically the same results were found in the divided attention task as in the chronic group. Again, the performance level on the adaptive single tasks was significantly lower in the head-injured patients than in a healthy control group, although the subacute patients were more impaired, on average, than the chronic group. The dot-counting task appeared to be especially sensitive to the effects of CHI with a correlation between PTA duration and reaction-time of $+.60$. The CHI group and the healthy control group did not differ at all in ability to divide attention in the restricted sense used here. Once more, a significant positive correlation (.49) between PTA duration and divided attention impairment was found. As patients were not selected in this case, the post hoc explanation given for the chronic group is considered less likely. It is possible that some of the very severe patients used a more sequential control strategy, switching attention between tasks instead of time-sharing. Future research should focus particularly on divided attention performance in subgroups of very severe patients. At present, the most important conclusion to be drawn is that experimental control for slow information processing removes most of the differences between CHI patients and control subjects in divided attention performance. It should be noted that this concerns attention divided between two visual motor tasks. Whether it holds for other task areas remains to be demonstrated, for as stated in Chapter 2, a general time-sharing ability does not exist.

Switching Attention

In the simulator studies mentioned above, two tasks had to be performed simultaneously. In an earlier study we used a task version in which only one task, lane-tracking, was performed, but under variable environmental conditions. The multiplying factor of the artificial "sidewind" was doubled or halved at unexpected moments. When such a change was discovered, the subject had to change his behavior radically, in this case with driving speed, either slowing or increasing, to maintain accuracy (course deviation) within the required limits. The goal of the study was to determine whether chronic CHI patients are less *flexible* than healthy control subjects (Van Wolffelaar et al., 1990) in adapting to such

environmental changes. Twenty very severe chronic CHI patients (PTAs between 11 and 124 days) were tested 5 to 10 years after injury. All patients were
active car drivers at the time of testing. The complete task consisted of three
main stages and took more than an hour to perform. Because the study has not
yet been separately published, the task will be described in somewhat more
detail than the previous items. The basic task is compensatory lane-tracking as
described above.

1. In the first, adaptive stage of the test the subject's lane-tracking performance at fixed speeds of driving is assessed, resulting in individual *sidewind
   factors* (see above) separately assessed for a fixed driving speed of 50 km/
   h (factor A) and for a fixed speed of 100 km/h (factor B).
2. In the second stage the subject has to learn to maintain a fixed level of
   tracking error by keeping speed and steering within certain limits, in the
   two global sidewind conditions: sidewind factor fixed at A and B, respectively. Separate blocks for each of the two sidewind conditions consist
   of 20 trials of 15 seconds duration. Feedback on speed, deviation and
   credit points earned is given on the screen after each trial. A *short-term
   flexibility factor* can be derived from performance in this stage which
   reflects the efficiency of finely tuning speed and course deviation to a
   constant norm in a situation with knowledge of results. In an earlier
   publication, this factor was called a learning factor (Van Wolffelaar et
   al., 1990).
3. In the third and final stage the sidewind conditions (at forces A and B,
   respectively) are intermittently administered in an unpredictable mix without any knowledge of results about speed or course deviation given. The
   task is to detect shifts rapidly and adjust for the required combination of
   speed and deviation, keeping the course stable and the loss of credit points
   minimal. A *long-term flexibility factor* can be derived from performance
   in this stage. In earlier publications, this factor was called a flexibility, or
   adaptivity, factor (Brouwer et al., 1988; Van Wolffelaar et al., 1990).

As in the divided attention task, the chronic CHI group performed worse
than the control group at the adaptive task stages. This resulted in significantly
lower sidewind factors, with the patients reaching approximately 80 percent of
the normal control group level. When this was controlled for, the chronic CHI
patients' flexibility scores in the subsequent stages of the experiment were surprisingly good, and in fact did not differ appreciably from the scores in the
control group.

In all three studies described above, CHI patients were found to be unimpaired in the higher order aspects of attention measured. In addition to these
studies, there are a number of results from *clinical tests* which are consistent
with this finding. The well known Trailmaking Test (Reitan, 1958) has been
presented to subacute, very severe (Veltman et al., in preparation) and to chronic,
very severe patients (Brouwer et al., 1989). This paper and pencil test consists
of two versions, A and B. In version A, lines have to be drawn between randomly
distributed numbered circles in ascending order from 1 to 25. In version B, the
numbers 1 and 13 and the letters A and L are used and the task is to proceed

from a number to a letter to a number etc., also in ascending order (1–A–2–B–3–C, etc.). The important dependent variable is time to complete the test. The principle difference between versions is that version B requires rapid switching between sets of stimuli to be selected.

Brouwer and coworkers (1989) found that CHI patients were significantly slower than controls on both versions of the test. When B was compared with A, the proportional increase was approximately the same in both groups, however (CHI: 41.5 and 86.7 seconds for A and B, respectively; controls: 31.0 and 66.9 seconds, respectively). Veltman and colleagues (in preparation) recorded 44 and 91 seconds for the subacute patients. For the patients, the mean proportional increase in the time score is approximately 110 percent, which is similar to the 116 percent in the young/middle-aged control group from Brouwer and colleagues (1989). In neither study was the significance level of the difference between B-scores of patients and controls larger than for the A scores.

Finally, Elting and colleagues (1989) and Veltman and colleagues (in preparation), in their studies on subacute CHI patients, recorded visual/manual four-choice RT both with and without a simultaneous auditory/pedal reaction time task. Auditory and visual stimuli never appeared at the same time, thus the task is better described as a flexibility task than a dual-task. A comparable task was described by Benton and colleagues (1962), who reported that patients with diffuse brain damage resulting from degenerative diseases showed a larger "crossmodal retardation" in RT than controls. However, in both samples of head-injured patients the proportional increase in reaction time, when CHI patients were compared with controls, appeared to be larger in the single-task condition than in the dual-task condition. Hence in two independent samples of severely head-injured patients, the flexibility demands on the combined RT task and Trailmaking B had no specific effect.

The results from *divided attention and flexibility* tasks can be summarized as follows: When adaptive tasks were used to control for the patients' slower information processing, no additional impairments were seen. When tasks were used which were not adaptive, the proportional performance decrement for dual-tasks and tasks requiring shifting attention was no greater in the patients than in normal controls. The tentative conclusion to be drawn from this is that the ability to divide and shift attention—where impairments in single task performance are controlled for—is not impaired in chronic severe CHI patients. This suggests that it is not necessary to infer the existence of any impairment other than slow information processing in order to understand the problems that severe CHI patients complain of in everyday, divided attention situations.

ALERTNESS AND SUSTAINED ATTENTION

Phasic Alertness

Phasic alertness refers to the process taking place in the brain of a person who is expecting a relevant stimulus in the immediate future. According to Posner (1975), alertness is a hypothetical state of the nervous system that affects general receptivity to stimulation. This could involve both orientation to a stimulus and readiness to make a motor reaction. A psychophysiological operational definition of phasic alertness is "contingent negative variation" (CNV). In a CNV paradigm a warning signal precedes an imperative stimulus that requires a fast motor response. The slow negative shifts in EEG between the warning signal and the imperative stimulus are called the CNV, or expectancy wave (Walter et al., 1964). Further study has revealed that the CNV has at least two components (Gaillard, 1978; Curry, 1984): an early one related to the information present in the warning signal and later components, which are a sign of preparation for action. A psychological operational definition of phasic alertness is the gain in RT when task performance with and without warning signal is compared.

A number of studies have been published on the "expectancy wave" in head-injured patients. Rizzo and coworkers (1978) studied the central CNV in patients with chronic, very severe head injuries and an average duration of coma of 15 days. A significant decrease in CNV amplitude (unspecified in terms of early and late components) was found when the head-injured patients were compared with normal subjects.

Curry (1981) studied CNV in a group of subacute patients with degrees of injury ranging from mild to severe (PTA longer than one week). Testing was carried out as soon as possible after the PTA ceased. In accordance with the findings by Rizzo and colleagues, Curry noted a decreased CNV amplitude when comparing his patients with a control group. In the severely injured group even absence of a measurable CNV was observed frequently.

Rugg and coworkers (1989) also found a decreased CNV amplitude in a group of 20 severely head-injured patients who were tested with a GO/NO-GO paradigm more than six months after injury. An attractive feature of the study by Rugg and colleagues was that it allowed for the separate study of early and late CNV components. They summarized their findings as follows:

> In the control group both the early, frontal maximum, and the later, vertex-maximum, components of the CNV were larger on GO and NO-GO trials. In the patients the early frontal CNV wave did not differentiate GO and NO-GO trials, and the late CNV showed a smaller separation between these trial types than did the late CNV of the control group.

The clinical significance of these CNV findings is difficult to evaluate because the relationships between CNV parameters and reaction time in the GO/NO-GO task, neuropsychological tests, severity of injury and localization of damage are low. Segalowitz and colleagues (1992) published a study on CNV, using a simple paradigm (GO only) administered to 20 chronic CHI patients recruited through local chapters of the Head Injury Association. They computed correlations between CNV amplitudes for 5 consecutive time periods, from 600–930 ms to 1960–2290 ms after the onset of the visual warning signal (the imperative stimulus was presented 2300 ms after the onset of the 500 ms warning) and a number of neuropsychological test scores. A significant correlation for the WISC-Mazes test was found for the late CNV-amplitude only. On the other hand, they did find significant correlations between the amplitude of earlier CNV components and performance on the Trailmaking Test (A and B), the Wisconsin Card

Sorting Test and the WISC-Mazes Test. They related this finding to frontal-lobe functioning in the patients, but in our opinion this is not a necessary conclusion. What can be concluded from their study is that CHI patients with relatively poor neuropsychological task performance tend to show relatively small CNV amplitude in the middle period of the CNV wave. It is hard to tell which processes are responsible for this part of the CNV wave (and for the poor neuropsychological task performance). In any case, the early CNV components are not necessarily related to phasic alertness since, as Segalowitz and colleagues (1992) stated, the early CNV probably indicates processing of the first stimulus (warning signal) and not preparation for the subsequent stimulus.

We now turn to *behavioral data* relevant to phasic alertness. Ponsford and Kinsella (1992) studied the effect of a warning signal on RT in head-injured patients and controls. These investigators tested severely injured patients in a rehabilitation setting, most of whom were in the subacute stage. The introduction of a warning signal reduced RT in both groups nearly equally on both simple and choice RT tasks. Thus, in this group of head-injured subjects, there was no evidence to support the presence of abnormal phasic alertness responses. This finding is similar to a number of earlier findings reviewed by Van Zomeren and colleagues (1984, 1987).

Thus, there seems to be a discrepancy between electrophysiological and behavioral indices of phasic alertness after severe CHI. While CNV data indicate a weakened alertness response, the behavioral data suggest that this does not influence RT. This apparent contradiction is partly resolved by more recent CNV studies which suggest that the most important differences between CHI patients and controls occur in the early CNV processes. These are probably not important for motor preparation and most likely do not contribute to the shortening of RT after the warning signal. It has been argued that the early CNV does not necessarily indicate phasic alertness. We may conclude that the issue of phasic alertness after CHI is still open.

Sustained Attention

Tonic alertness may be described as a continuous receptivity to stimulation, lasting from minutes to hours. Tonic alertness after CHI has been discussed at length in our earlier reviews (Van Zomeren et al., 1984, 1987) and the conclusions have not changed. Therefore we will discuss it only briefly here. As is the case with phasic alertness, tonic alertness may be operationally defined both in psychophysiological and psychological terms. With regard to the latter, tonic alertness is more or less synonymous with sustained attention, or the stability of task performance over relatively long periods of time. Sustained attention after head injury has mainly been tested with an emphasis on *time-on-task effects*. In our 1984 review we concluded:

> Tonic alertness was studied with continuous RT tasks and with a low-event rate vigilance task; in both studies head-injured patients performed worse than controls, but their performance was remarkably stable over time.

Since that time, a number of new studies have appeared which support and extend this conclusion. In our own research on driving skills in head-injured subjects (Brouwer, 1985; Van Zomeren et al., 1988), lateral position control, that is, tracking ability in an instrumented car on a highway, was significantly poorer in a patient group consisting of very severe chronic CHI patients than in matched controls. However, there was no specific time-on-task effect in the head-injured subjects during a 1-hour ride on a quiet straight highway. In a dot-cancellation test (a modified Bourdon task) requiring self-paced visual search we found that subacute patients worked somewhat slower, but maintained their initial level of performance just as well as controls (see Figure 4-6).

Performance curves of patients and controls were more or less parallel in all these studies, indicating that sustained attention was normal even though the absolute level of performance was usually somewhat lower in the patient groups. In the Bourdon study it was likely that patients found their speed-accuracy trade-off in the same way as normal subjects: for both groups the number of missed targets was somewhat higher in the first block of 3 minutes, while time-per-line was somewhat shorter than in the next four blocks, when both groups improved. In addition, it is noteworthy that patients were working at the same level of accuracy as controls. This latter point was also noted recently by Ponsford and Kinsella (1992), who report that their head-injured patients were no less accurate than controls in a continuous choice RT task lasting 45 minutes. This conclusion must be qualified insofar as it is based on a situation where the subjects have

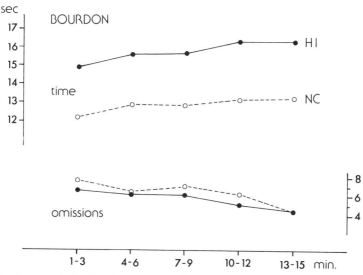

Figure 4-6 Sustained attention in a prolonged visual search task, the 15-minute Bourdon test. Although head-injured patients are working much slower than controls in this self-paced task, in their accuracy they are comparable to their noninjured counterparts. Note that performance curves are identical, both for time per line and number of omissions. HI = head-injured patients, NC = normal control subjects. (From Elting et al., 1988, with permission.)

enough time to inspect the stimuli. Both in the Ponsford and Kinsella study and our Bourdon study, the patients took significantly more time for the detections.

An extensive study of sustained attention in subacute mild CHI patients was reported by Parasuraman and colleagues (1991). They were able to produce significant time-on-task effects on detection in difficult visual vigilance tasks, both in CHI patients and controls, but these effects were no greater in the patient group than in the control group. As in an earlier vigilance study (Brouwer and Van Wolffelaar, 1985), patients performed worse than controls on a signal detection measure of perceptual sensitivity, but this effect was present at the beginning of the experiment.

Other operational definitions of sustained attention are *lapses of attention* and increased *intraindividual variability* of performance. It is a question of choice whether these should be treated under phasic or tonic alertness. The similarity with time-on-task effects is that it concerns spontaneous changes over time, independent of specific stimuli or warning signals. The similarity with preparation effects is the relatively short time frame. In our 1987 review we concluded that "there is no evidence for the occurrence of lapses in attention after head injury. Likewise there seem to be no specific increases in intraindividual variability in RT studies, as variability measures show increases that are proportional to the increases in mean or median RT."

In summary, the evidence on sustained attention and alertness is described both in terms of phasic and tonic aspects. With regard to phasic alertness there seems to be a discrepancy between electrophysiological (CNV) and behavioral indices after severe CHI. CNV data suggest a weakened alertness response seen as less good, or less specific, preparation for a subsequent response. However, behavioral data show normal effects of warning signals on RT. Tonic aspects of sustained attention, as indicated by time-on-task effects on performance in long continuous vigilance and reaction time tasks, are unimpaired.

SUPERVISORY ATTENTIONAL CONTROL

As we noted in Chapter 2, neuropsychological research on attention has taken on a new dimension over the last 15 years. There has been increasing interest in strategies guiding the focusing, dividing, switching, and sustaining of attention.

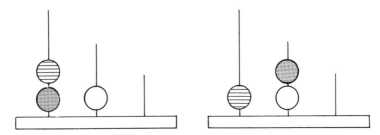

Figure 4-7 The Tower of London as used by Shallice (1982). Starting with the arrangement on the left, the beads must be moved one by one until the arrangement shown on the right is duplicated. This particular problem can be solved in three moves.

In particular, the question arose which agent or system is employed to overcome the subject's automatic response when he or she is faced with a non-routine situation or a disturbance of routine in a well-trained task. Shallice (1982, 1988) presented an information processing model with two modes: contention scheduling and supervisory attentional control. The first mode refers to the automatic execution of routine schemata, the second to the suppression of routine reactions by a higher-order agent. Shallice devised a test called the Tower of London to test his hypothesis (see Figure 4-7). This is a look-ahead puzzle or planning task, derived from the Tower of Hanoi, that has frequently been used in the study of artificial intelligence. Three colored beads must be arranged on three vertical sticks of decreasing length, in a limited number of moves, in order to form a certain pattern. The solution requires intermediate steps in which a particular bead must be placed temporarily in a side position, i.e. on a stick that is not its final destination. Shallice demonstrated that patients with focal left-frontal lesions did poorly on this test, and he argued that the supervisory attentional system is part of the executive functions of the frontal lobes (Luria, 1966; Lezak, 1982). Although both the theoretical model and the test were received enthusiastically in clinical neuropsychology, it must be noted that the relationship between them is not a close one. In particular, it is not clear which routine schemata are suppressed by subjects who have never before seen the Tower of London Test. Only if a very broad interpretation is given to the term "routine schemata" will the test serve the model.

Ponsford and Kinsella (1992) presented the Tower of London Test to subacute head-injured patients consecutively assigned to a rehabilitation hospital. The time after injury ranged from one to seven months. They found that the patient group needed more time than a control group to solve the problems, but that the groups made the same number of errors. These authors stated that: "Once again the pattern of reduced speed of information processing, but comparable accuracy, was apparent in the head-injured subjects." We had the same experience in our own department with a group of 20 very severe patients who were at a chronic stage (time since injury between 5 and 10 years). In this group too, patients required more time, particularly from the presentation of the task until the first move, but they did not differ from controls in the number of items solved correctly (Van Wolffelaar et al., 1990; Rosenboom and Brouwer, 1989). Like the patients in Ponsford and Kinsella's study, they even were significantly better than the control group in the number of problems correctly solved in one attempt. In this respect they seemed to be less impulsive than the normal control group.

Another approach of the Supervisory Attentional System makes use of the *dual task methodology*, in which subjects have to divide their processing capacity between two tasks. Although this approach is clearly related to divided attention research, the emphasis here is more on strategies for allocating attention. A task was designed in which chronic and subacute CHI patients had to divide attention between a lane-tracking task and a visual analysis task (dot-counting). Subjects were instructed to give priority to either task 1, both tasks, or task 2. Very strong and significant effects of instruction were found in both studies in the analyses of variance on performance of the subtasks. In the chronic CHI study the interaction of groups and instructions was negligible, both for the tracking and dot-counting task. In the subacute group there was a small but significant interaction between groups and instruction on the relative performance in the tracking task. Patients were influenced less strongly by the priority instructions than controls. However, no corresponding effects were found in the dot-counting task. Therefore, a tentative conclusion is that CHI patients are as able as controls to allocate attention to subtasks, according to instruction.

RELATIONSHIPS WITH SEVERITY AND RECOVERY

Severity of Injury

There are two kinds of evidence for indicating a relationship between severity of injury and attentional deficits. First, systematic studies of patients' *complaints* suggest that problems of concentration and mental slowness are reported more frequently by more severely injured groups. Gronwall (1987) presented a table summarizing the findings of 10 studies in which the percentages illustrate the relationship. For example, McLean and colleagues (1984) expressed severity of injury as "Time to obey commands," or TOC, this being the interval between injury and the moment when a patient responds to spoken commands. When questioned one month after injury, 47 percent of a group of patients with TOC less than 24 hours reported attentional problems. In a more severely injured group, with TOC exceeding one day, the percentage was 75. The use of PTA as an index of severity reflects the same effect. Wrightson and Gronwall (1981) interviewed patients 2 years postinjury who had been in PTA for less than 36 hours. Six percent of the patients still reported attentional problems. Van Zomeren and Van den Burg (1985) also interviewed patients two years after injury and found that 17 percent reported complaints when PTA had ranged from 1 to 7 days, and 40 percent when PTA had been longer than 1 week.

Objective *tests* also indicate a significant relationship between severity and attentional impairments. Van Zomeren and Deelman (1978) demonstrated that mental slowness as revealed by choice RT, was proportional to severity of injury as expressed by duration of PTA and coma. RT at 5 months postinjury correlated .66 with PTA and .62 with coma duration. Gronwall and Sampson (1974) found a relationship between severity and PASAT performance: patients with PTA exceeding 24 hours performed worse than subjects with mild concussions.

Recovery

Attentional deficits after head injury tend to show some recovery. Once more, there is both subjective and objective evidence for this statement. The percentages of attentional complaints in Gronwall's review (1987) show a general decline in reported complaints in longitudinal studies. For example, Wrightson and Gronwall (1981), studying 66 patients with PTA of less than 36 hours, recorded that 16 percent reported complaints at 3 months postinjury, and 6 percent 2 years postinjury. Objective longitudinal studies of recovery have made use of choice RT (Van Zomeren and Deelman, 1978; MacFlynn et al., 1984; Saan, 1994), PASAT (Gronwall and Sampson, 1974; Stuss et al., 1989), and Trailmaking (Stuss et al., 1989). These investigations have shown clearly that recovery can be complete after minor to moderately severe head injury. Recovery of PASAT performance to a normal level takes from 20 to 40 days in cases of mild head injury (Gronwall and Sampson, 1974; Gronwall, 1977). In a review of the literature on cognitive deficits after minor head injury, with PTA less than one hour, Gronwall (1991) concluded: "Most group studies show that recovery of cognitive function after MHI occurs within 1 to 3 months after injury (Dikmen et al., 1986; Gronwall and Sampson, 1974; Levin et al., 1987c)." Stuss et al. (1989) also conclude that there is complete recovery or minimal problems by 1 to 3 months after mild head injury.

In more severely injured patients recovery clearly takes more time. O'Shaughnessy and colleagues (1984) studied a group of patients with a mean duration of PTA of 5.65 days, severity ranging from mild to very severe. Within the first week after injury, 89 percent of the sample showed impaired PASAT performance. Six months after injury, this number had decreased to 56 percent. RT studies have revealed lasting problems in severely head-injured subjects (Norrman and Svahn, 1961; Van Zomeren and Deelman, 1978; Saan, 1994). In this group of patients prolonged choice RT can be found as long as 2 or more years after injury (Figure 4-8).

The overall pattern seems to indicate that mild head injury causes some attentional problems, which tend to disappear in a matter of weeks or months. More severe injuries result in impairments that last longer. In very severe cases, with PTA duration exceeding one week, a certain mental slowness usually remains, with resulting divided attention deficits. The recovery curves of severely injured patients indicate that most of the recovery takes place early, that is, in the first half-year after injury (van Zomeren and Deelman, 1978; Saan, 1994).

The longitudinal studies quoted above are burdened by a variety of specific methodological problems, such as patient dropout and the confounding of test-retest effects with recovery. Useful papers on these topics have been published by D. N. Brooks (Brooks et al., 1984; Brooks, 1987), Dikmen and Temkin (1987), Strauss and Allred (1987), and Stuss et al. (1989).

It was noted above that both subjective complaints and objective test performance indicate partial or complete recovery. However, the *correlations between complaints and performance* are not impressive. Generally speaking, complaints may persist even when performance has recovered to a normal level (Minderhoud et al., 1980; Dikmen et al., 1986; Gronwall, 1991). As Gronwall points out, the ability of a patient to obtain a normal score on a given test in a quiet and well-structured testing situation does not guarantee that his cognition will likewise be normal in a noisy social gathering. In our own experience (Van Zomeren and Van den Burg, 1985), we have observed a special group of very severely injured patients who disrupt the statistical relationship between complaints and performance. Some patients who have severe cognitive impairments may fail to report these through lack of insight. Thus, the absence of complaints does not guarantee the absence of deficits.

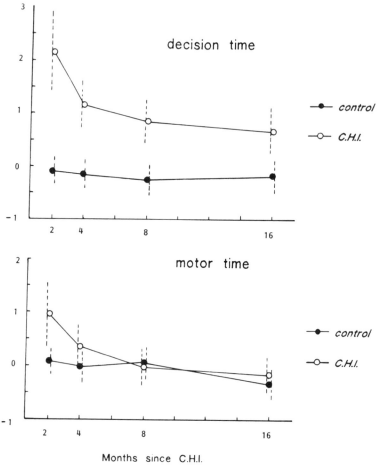

Figure 4-8   Recovery curves of decision time and movement time in a group of 40 severely head-injured subjects who were tested on four occasions in a period covering 16 months after injury. A control group of 53 subjects was likewise tested four times. For decision times, group differences are statistically significant on all occasions. For movement time, the group difference was significant on the first occasion only. Note that decision time remains prolonged, while movement time normalizes completely. However, both patient curves show that recovery mainly occurs in the first half year after injury (Saan, in preparation). RT had been recorded with the apparatus shown in Figure 4-1. Individual RTs have been converted into z-scores.

CONCLUSIONS

From the evidence presented in this chapter, it can be concluded that slower information processing is a very important attentional deficit following CHI. Taking this into account, surprisingly little evidence may be found for impairments in tasks of focused, divided and sustained attention. This conclusion, based on many experimental studies, is in line with patients' complaints and with systematic observations and ratings of their behavior in rehabilitation settings. We will try here to give a theoretical explanation for the origin and nature of this symptom, using factors related to normal aging as a guideline. Although studies of CHI have been limited compared to research on normal aging, a number of parallels come to light. In the case of aging as well, the phenomenon of slowing has not yielded to componential analysis and remains largely unexplained, although it has been described (Salthouse, 1982) as "the most pronounced, the most striking, the most pervasive and most reliable phenomenon in the psychology of aging."

Myerson and coworkers (1990) claim that: "Older adults' latencies can be predicted from younger adults' latencies without regard to any specific information about the experimental condition or the component process involved." For this prediction they use a mathematical model that generates a mildly positively accelerated relationship between the reaction times of young adults and older adults that appears to be quite similar to the relationship outlined in Figure 4-4. The theory behind this mathematical model is a variation of the *neural noise theory* of aging (Welford, 1962, 1981), which assumes that neural pattern recognizers suffer from a worse signal-to-noise ratio because of proportionally more irrelevant activity, either from residual neural activity from previous processing, from increased spontaneous noise levels or from weaker input signals.

Myerson and associates (1990, p. 485) argue that it is possible to distinguish between two alternative concepts of the neural noise theory, one of which, the information loss model, appears to be supported by the reaction time data on aging and head injury:

> It is possible to further distinguish between two alternative conceptions of random noise that lead to clearly different, testable predictions concerning the relationship between the performances of older and younger adults. Both conceptions assume that at each step in the neural processing of information a degraded pattern of inputs may still be detected, although it will take longer. Thus, neurons are able to compensate to some degree for age-related decreases in signal-to-noise ratio by accumulating information longer. One possibility, a noncumulative noise hypothesis, is that the compensation is complete in the sense that there is no progressive decrease in signal-to-noise ratio through successive processing steps. The other possibility, and this the position of the information loss model, is that the loss of information or decrease in the reliability of messages sent between neural ensembles is likely to be cumulative as processing proceeds. That is, longer step durations cannot compensate completely for decreased information. Although there is some compensation for information loss at each processing step, there will be a residual that cannot be compensated for and to which additional loss is added. With this cumulative information loss, more and more compensation is required, and successive processing steps become progressively slower.

The general pattern of the results of reaction time experiments with CHI patients suggests that these results may be explained using a *cumulative noise hypothesis*. However, much more data are needed, particularly for experiments requiring relatively long reaction times, to make a precise assessment. An attempt has been made to explain the global effect of head injury on the speed of information processing, using a theory which states that the signal-to-noise ratio in central neural pattern recognizers has decreased (Van Zomeren, 1981;

Stokx, 1984; Brouwer, 1985; Korteling, 1990). Increased noise levels could be caused by residual neural activity from previous mental operations (Korteling, 1990) or just be random noise. To investigate the possibility of *residual neural activity*, Korteling varied the difference between consecutive compound stimuli and the duration of the response stimulus interval in a complex choice reaction task administered to chronic young adult CHI patients, healthy aged adults and young adult controls. He found no interactions of these variables with groups. Stokx and Gaillard (1986) had previously varied response stimulus interval duration in CHI patients and had obtained inconsistent results. Therefore, it is not considered likely that residual neural activity from previous processing plays a role in the slow information processing of CHI patients, at least not in chronic CHI patients. On the other hand, in subacute CHI patients tested early after injury, Cant and colleagues (1975) demonstrated a longer recovery time for a slow auditory evoked potential response, which might be taken as evidence for longer lasting residual neural activity. So, in subacute patients, it may be a factor of some importance.

Residual neural activity as described above is a source of systematic noise, as it can be related to a discrete stimulus and is not random activity. Interfering neural activity resulting from the processing of irrelevant stimuli presented in parallel with relevant stimuli, could also be described as a form of systematic noise. As argued in the preceding section on focused attention, the evidence with regard to this is generally weak; with a few exceptions in subacute patients, most studies showed no negative effect of CHI on focusing. In any case, it is not considered likely that neural activity resulting from "overprocessing" of irrelevant stimuli plays an important role in the slow information processing of chronic CHI patients.

This leaves us with the concept of an information processing system with relatively increased random noise levels. The theory of Myerson and associates (1990) described above gives a more precise and quantifiable character to this concept. Whether the relatively increased noise levels are the result of increased noise or decreased signal cannot be answered on the basis of reaction time data. Brouwer (1985, p. 139), on the basis of a pathoanatomical argument, stated that *decreased signal strength* with normal noise levels is a more plausible cause of the decreased signal-to-noise ratio for neural pattern recognizers in CHI than increased noise levels at the pattern recognizers:

> Consequently, the basic deficit after concussion must be in the longer access time of the data base and not in the application of procedures as such. If the data base is viewed as an associative network consisting of a large set of interconnected nodes, the author views the effects of concussion as a global decrease in strength of associations between nodes, possibly as a result of diffuse functional (in the acute and subacute stage) and structural loss of axonal tissue.

Neuroanatomical studies (Strich, 1961; Adams et al., 1982; Snoek, 1990) have shown that CHI damage occurs at the long axonal connections between neurons and between parts of the brain and not in the gray matter itself, which is presumably the location of the pattern recognizers. Of course, this is as yet speculative, as "connection" and "pattern analyzers" at the conceptual/meta-

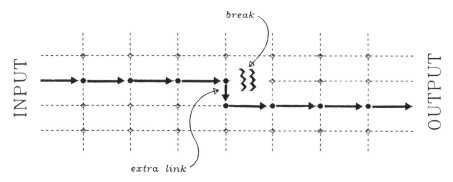

Figure 4-9 Damage in a schematic neural network, as described by Cerella. Nodes represent neurons and dotted lines axon connections between neurons. The illustrated network performs no computation, merely transmits signals from top to bottom. Latency is determined by the number of links, in this case 8 in the intact network. However, one link on the optimal route is broken, forcing the signal to detour and adding one more link to the path for a total of 9. According to Cerella, progressive loss of connectivity in a schematic network matches quantitatively the increase in information-processing latencies observed in elderly subjects. (From Cerella, 1990, with permission.)

phorical level of the neural noise theory are more or less equaled here to connections and neural structures at the anatomical level. Whether such speculations will actually help in understanding the effects of CHI on cognitive tasks can only be effectively studied with dynamic computer simulations of human information processing. Ideally in such dynamic models, impairments mimicking CHI patients' task performance should emerge when basic parameters of the model are changed from normal to abnormal, according to neuropathological assessment of these patients. See Figure 4-9.

SUMMARY

In this chapter evidence about impairments of attention in CHI patients in the subacute and chronic stage of recovery was reviewed. With regard to *focused attention*, there is little empirical evidence for increased effects of distraction on task performance despite the clinical reality of complaints about increased distractability. When irrelevant auditory or visual distractors are presented in a task, head-injured patients can ignore them as well as control subjects. Even when irrelevant stimuli are presented that provoke conflicting response tendencies, and thereby create response interference, the patients' responses, at least those of chronic patients, are often comparable to those of healthy controls. In subacute patients, the picture may be different as there is some evidence for increased sensitivity to interference from dominant response tendencies. This issue requires further study. Concerning *divided attention*, a nonspecific slowing of perceptual-motor and cognitive processes, approximately proportional to task difficulty, is the most conspicuous phenomenon. When adaptive tasks are used to control for the patients' slower information processing, no additional impairments are demonstrated in dividing and switching attention between tasks. Concerning *phasic alertness*, there seems to be a discrepancy between electro-physiological (CNV) and behavioral indices of preparation for a subsequent stimulus or response. CNV data suggest a less good or less specific preparation. Behavioral data show normal effects of warning signals on reaction time, however. This issue, too, requires more study. Tonic aspects of *sustained attention*, as indicated by time-on-task effects on performance in long-continued vigilance and reaction time tasks, are unimpaired by CHI. The chapter concludes with a theoretical speculation about the nature and origin of slow information processing, the most pervasive limitation of attention after CHI.

5

Dementia of the Alzheimer Type

Alzheimer's disease is the most common degenerative neurologic disease. In the Netherlands it has been estimated (Muskens, 1993) that between 5 and 10 percent of the population over 65 years is demented as a result of this condition. However, even between the ages of 50 and 65 the disease is not uncommon, and every neurologist and neuropsychologist is familiar with the tragic course of the condition when it befalls middle-aged people. After a healthy and productive life, the disease begins insidiously, and subtle changes in the behavior of the patient may be noted by friends, family, or co-workers long before the person is finally classified as suffering from Alzheimer's disease. The following case from our outpatient clinic is illustrative:

Our patient, T.B., was a 66-year-old retired businessman who had led a very active social life. In World War II he had flown a fighter plane as a Dutch volunteer in the U.S. Air Force. After the war he had a successful career in publishing. He came to the Department of Neurology outpatient clinic because of forgetfulness that had been noted by his wife and had developed over the past few years. A neurological examination revealed no convincing pathological signs, but the neurologist noted that the patient was bradyphrenic and disoriented in time. It also struck the neurologist that T.B. underwent the examination passively, leaving the talking to his wife.

A CT scan showed no abnormalities. EEG was somewhat slow and irregular, but seemed to remain within normal limits. When the patient was tested neuropsychologically, the IQ (Groninger Intelligence Test) was 96, definitely below his estimated premorbid level. Memory functions were clearly affected, as the patient scored beneath the normal range for his age group on verbal and nonverbal tests of learning, recall, and recognition. Motor functions, however, were perfectly normal when assessed with a finger-tapping test and a blockboard task requiring manipulation and goal-directed movements. T.B. was also agile in walking and bicycling; according to his wife, he was considered swifter and more stable than she.

In an interview with his wife she stressed that forgetfulness was the first sign that started her worrying. Later, she also noticed that her husband was often disoriented in time and sometimes in place. For example, in the car he might stop at intersections, not knowing whether to turn left or right. He had stopped playing bridge, with the comment that his play demanded "too much thinking." She noticed that he talked less in social situations and had a decreased interest in others. She also judged his general behavior to be slow, as he seemed to have trouble switching from one activity to another or interrupting the daily routine. Somewhat surprisingly, she reported that her husband still liked to drive and that the couple had even made a trip by car to Morocco 4 months before the neuropsychological examination. On further questioning, these feats turned out to be somewhat less impressive than they seemed at first. The wife actively coached her husband as he drove, particularly with regard to route planning and route finding. Moreover, the trip to Morocco with their caravan had been made in a convoy, as the couple were members of a caravan club that had organized and guided the journey.

T.B. was diagnosed as suffering from Alzheimer's disease (AD). While his severe memory problems and disorientation fit this diagnosis well, impairments of attention were just as remarkable. These contrasted sharply with his very good preservation of sensory and motor functions. There appeared to be a striking discrepancy between performance elicited by well-known or obvious environmental stimuli and performance requiring active mental control. T.B.'s visual reaction times were within the normal range on the basic four-choice reaction task, but he was completely unable to handle two more complex conditions. When distracted by irrelevant additional lights, and when a dual-task demanded divided attention between visual and auditory stimuli, he became confused and made so many errors that the testing had to be discontinued.

Descriptions of the clinical features of AD, the major dementing disease, seldom mention attentional impairments (Lishman, 1978; Kolb and Wishaw, 1990). Nevertheless, problems with regard to simultaneous activities were observed during the initial application of information processing methods to the study of dementia (Inglis, 1965, 1970). Results obtained with dichotic listening tasks at that time were interpreted in terms of impaired memory processes.

The first stage of the disease, which may last from 2 to 3 years, is characterized at the behavioral level by deficits in memory, language, and perception, by decreased efficiency in everyday tasks, spatial disorientation, and disturbances of mood. Although attentional deficits may play a role in most of these areas, investigators rarely refer to this aspect. Loss of memory has generated by far the most research interest, and theoretical memory models have been tested for usefulness in the study of AD (Miller, 1977). In retrospect, it must be admitted that neuropsychology tended to reduce the disease, at the behavioral level, to an amnesic syndrome. This is probably due to the fact that psychology, as an objectifying and quantitative discipline, was then best equipped to study this conspicuous aspect.

A similar reduction has occurred in neurology. AD has traditionally been viewed anatomically as a degeneration of certain parts of the cerebral cortex. The main histological features are extensive degeneration and loss of nerve cells with senile plaques and neurofibrillary tangles, resulting in cortical atrophy, particularly in the temporal and parietal lobes. See Figure 5-1. The neuronal degeneration especially affects the outer three layers of the cortex, and is often concentrated within the hippocampus and amygdaloid nuclei (Lishman, 1978). Hyman and coworkers (1984) reported that the medial temporal lobes, specifically the entorhinal cortex, are selectively affected early in the course of the disease. Senile plaques appear particularly in the amygdala and hippocampus (Corsellis, 1970). Tangles are likewise found in the cortex, amygdala, and hippocampus, as well as in the subcortical nuclei that serve as the genesis for various

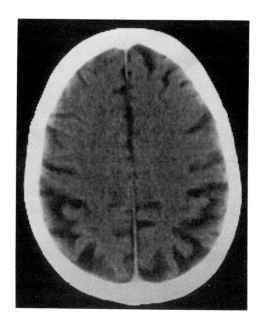

Figure 5-1 Computed tomography scan of a 59-year-old woman with Alzheimer's Disease showing marked cortical atrophy, particularly in temporoparietal areas.

neurotransmitter systems: the locus ceruleus for norepinephrine, Meynert's nucleus basalis for acetylcholine, the raphe nuclei for serotonin, and the ventrotegmentum for dopamine. This implies the reduction by AD of the input of these neurotransmitter systems into the cerebral cortex (Price, 1986; Saper, 1988).

From such findings, students of AD tended to adopt the view that temporoparietal degeneration is the main locus of neuropathology and memory loss the main clinical feature. However, the scene changed after 1980. Several investigators were able to show that there are subgroups of AD patients in whom language or visuoconstructive problems are the first or most severe impairments (Martin et al. 1986). Schwartz (1987) propagated a multiple component concept of cognitive deterioration in AD that included frontal symptoms. The latter have recently become the focus of interest for several investigators (Longley et al., 1990; Bhutani et al., 1992). Hence the neuropsychological view of Alzheimer's disease seems to be broadening, and studies of impairments in the area of attention have been undertaken. A longitudinal study of a small group of patients suggested that the first nonamnestic neuropsychological consequence of AD is a loss of attentional capacity (Grady et al., 1988).

Neurologists have also changed their views on the disease. Positron emission tomography studies have revealed that AD patients constitute a heterogeneous group, some of whom show clear focal damage outside the traditional temporoparietal area (Martin et al., 1986). Furthermore, there is growing evidence from blood flow studies that AD may have a frontal component (Grady et al., 1988, Montaldi et al., 1990).

The fact that AD patients do not represent a homogeneous group presents a methodological problem in research. In early studies of the neuropsychological effects of dementia, patients from various etiologies were lumped together as "seniles" or "demented patients." Such samples must have been very hetero-geneous, containing AD, multiinfarct dementias, and so on. Research efforts have been gradually homing in on purer cases of AD. The criteria supplied by DSM-III and the National Institute for Neurology, Communicative Disorders and Stroke/Alzheimer's Disease and Related Disorders Association have been very important in this development (NINCDS/ADRDA; McKhanu et al., 1984). The use of these strict nosological systems guarantees that AD research is cur-rently indeed dealing with AD patients, but, as mentioned above, it is now recognized that even in this seemingly homogeneous group there may be quite a variability in patterns of degeneration and cognitive impairment.

The fact that AD is a *progressive* disease, with a pattern of deficits that may change in an individual patient over the years, presents another methodological problem. For research purposes it is therefore important to control for disease stage as indicated by its duration. If this variable is neglected, another source of heterogeneity remains uncontrolled. In present AD research, there is a ten-dency to classify and describe patients not according to duration of illness, but on the basis of quantifying assessment methods such as the Mini Mental State (MMS) Examination (Folstein et al., 1975). The selection of patients according to MMS score is basically classification by quantified symptomatology. Although the duration of the disease will have an important influence on MMS score, premorbid factors, and localization of lesions may also play a part.

Finally, the progressive character of AD confronts us with the question of *when* to study patients. Investigators tend to select patients with a well-estab-lished diagnosis of AD to ensure that their sample does not contain patients with pseudodementia, depression, and so on. If this caution is stretched too far, subjects may be selected who already have a multitude of aspecific symptoms such as bradyphrenia, reduced tolerance for stress, impoverished speech, and understanding of complex instructions. Although it is easy to find significant differences between such patients and control subjects, the aspecific symptoms make it difficult to single out specific impairments. In our view, the real challenge of neuropsychological research lies with the patient in a very early stage of the disease, when the diagnosis is still doubtful. Ideally, AD research should be carried out with a longitudinal design in which patients can be classified afterward as definite cases of AD, after having been tested when symptoms were still subtle and the diagnosis uncertain. Such studies are beginning to appear, with inter-esting results (Jones et al., 1992). This shift to the milder end of the severity dimension would have a great practical advantage as psychologists in clinical practice are often confronted with doubtful cases, that is, people who may or may not be progressing toward dementia.

FOCUSED ATTENTION

One of the first studies of focused attention in senile dementia (Alexander, 1973a) made use of the Continuous Performance Task (Rosvold et al., 1956). It consists of a random series of letters, presented singly in a visual display facing the subject. In the simple condition, subjects are required to press a button whenever the letter X appears. Alexander tested 14 patients with a psychiatric diagnosis of senile dementia. He found that these patients did almost as well as elderly control subjects: hit rate was 97 percent in the control group, and 93 percent in the patient group. In the next condition, subjects were instructed to react to the X if, and only if, it was preceded by the letter A. This instruction means that A becomes a warning signal, sometimes followed by X and sometimes not. In addition, this condition requires response inhibition, as subjects are now supposed *not* to react when the X appears without a preceding A. This X − A condition was still easy for the control group, whose hit rate decreased only slightly, to 95 percent. However, the condition had a strong effect on the patients, for whom the hit rate decreased to 80 percent. The latter's many errors consisted for the main part of commission errors, that is, reacting to nontarget letters, presumably X's not preceded by A's.

Alexander concluded that his patients demonstrated a disturbance in selective attention. In our view, this conclusion needs some qualification, as the patients showed normal selectivity in the first, simple letter detection task. Selectivity broke down in the second condition only, when selection was based on a more complex decision rule. Before turning to a deeper analysis of this effect, we will continue the description of studies aimed at focused attention on the basis of simple stimulus characteristics.

Nebes and Brady (1989) studied a basic form of selective attention in which the color of stimuli was the essential cue. Healthy elderly subjects and Alzheimer patients were presented with arrays of six black letters, presented in a tachistoscope in two rows, for example:

L E S

D V A

Subjects were instructed to indicate with a YES or NO answer whether a particular target letter was present. The patients could do this quite well, although their reaction times were significantly longer than those of the control subjects (969 ms versus 725 ms, in the YES condition). The experiment also contained a condition in which the target letter and one other letter in the array were black, while the remaining four letters were red. This color cue reduced reaction times considerably, both in the Alzheimer and the control group (887 ms versus 671 ms, in the YES condition). The significant condition effect in ANOVA indicated that the color cue had a general facilitory effect on both groups, but the lack of interaction between group and condition meant that the cue facilitated letter search in the demented patients just as much as it did in the normals.

Nebes and Brady analyzed the selectivity of their subjects once more by comparing search times for arrays of two or six letters. In a separate condition, subjects had to search for targets in arrays of black letters only, the size of the array being, 2, 4, or 6 letters. The investigators could therefore compare search times with two black letters to search time with two black letters plus four irrelevant red letters. They found that the presence of the irrelevant red letters slowed search time somewhat, indicating that the subjects could not totally ignore the red letters. Hence merely segregating the letters by color does not lead to as great a reduction in search time as that produced by reducing the actual number of letters in the array. However, the distracting effect of the red letters was not greater in the Alzheimer group than in the control group.

The above experiment demonstrated that AD patients are not particularly hindered by irrelevant visual distractors, at least when these can be discriminated on the basis of a clear physical distinction. It may be noted that the distractors used in this case were "meaningless," that is, no response tendency was attached to them. A different situation occurs in the familiar Stroop task (see Chapter 2). In the distracting "Color-Word" (CW) condition selection is based on the color of the words, while at the same time the response tendency attached to their meaning causes a strong interference, even in normals.

Koss and coworkers (1984) presented the Stroop Color-Word Test to 9 mild and 5 moderate cases of AD. Slowing on the control conditions of reading and color naming was observed, and was greater in moderate than in mild dementia subjects. The Stroop interference effect was high in individuals with mild AD, but the more severely impaired AD subjects showed less interference effect than the mild AD patients when reaction time was adjusted for color naming performance. The mild AD group needed 40.7 seconds for simple color naming of 20 stimuli, and 186.1 seconds for the ambiguous CW. For the more severely demented patients these scores were 109.2 and 227.8 seconds, respectively. Hence the absolute interference effect was smaller in the patients with moderate AD. Koss and coworkers assume that this unexpected finding must be attributed to variation in speed-accuracy trade-off—differences in linguistic impairment and attitudes to errors. Both the mild and the moderately demented patients made many errors during the interference condition, but perhaps only the mild patients had enough preservation of cognitive abilities to appreciate their deficient performance. Their unsuccessful concentrated effort to master the interference task, and awareness of their errors, may have been a source of significant slowing down. In contrast, in moderate AD patients a lack of self-criticism combined with significant impairment on color naming may have accounted for adjusted reaction times closer to those observed in controls. Nestor and colleagues (1991a) also reported that the Stroop paradigm was able to demonstrate a breakdown of selective attention in patients with mild AD.

Grady and coworkers (1988) used the Stroop Color-Word Test in a *longitudinal* study of cognitive impairments in 11 AD patients. All of them were mildly demented, and they were followed up over 3 years, most of them being assessed three times in this period. At the initial evaluation, all patients had a significant memory impairment but five had a score on the Interference subtest of the Stroop CW Test within the normal range. On successive occasions, almost all patients developed impairment on the test; only one patient had a perfectly normal interference score, even 3 years after the initial assessment. Generally speaking, deterioration in performance on the CW part increased regularly with duration of illness.

Summarizing the evidence reviewed so far, it can be stated that focused attention in AD is unimpaired where selection can be made on the basis of a clear physical dimension and where there are no conflicting response tendencies attached to the distractors. When such conflicting response tendencies are present, as in the CW condition of the Stroop test, selectivity suffers. However, the magnitude of this effect is relatively small compared to the slow reading and color naming seen in the reading and color naming condition of the task.

Several investigators have studied the effect of *cues* on focused attention in AD patients. In particular, position cues in visual attention have been manipulated. Freed and colleagues (1989) used the "endogenous" covert orienting paradigm, in which a warning signal in the shape of an arrow directed the subject's attention to either the right or the left half of a video screen (Posner et al., 1978; see also Chapter 2). On one-third of the trials an arrow pointed right; on one-third an arrow pointed left; and on one-third a double-headed arrow pointed both left and right (these trials were called neutral, as the warning signal gave no information about the location of the imperative stimulus). A few seconds after the cue, an X appeared to the right or the left of the arrow. The subject's task was to press a single response key as quickly as possible after the appearance of the target. Subjects were told that when the warning cue was a single arrow, the X would probably appear in the direction of the arrow, and when the warning signal was a double-headed arrow, the two locations were equally likely. The single-arrow cues were valid 80 percent of the time (valid cue trials). On the remaining 20 percent of the single-arrow trials, the X appeared on the side opposite the direction indicated by the arrow (invalid trials). Subjects were reminded verbally throughout the session to press the response key as soon as they saw the target. The performance of normal subjects is typified by the occurrence of a positive value for the mean difference in RT between valid and invalid trials. Freed and coworkers tested 17 AD patients with this paradigm. Six of them obtained a negative value, meaning that on average they reacted faster on invalid cue trials than on valid cue trials. All effects of cueing were positive in control subjects, ranging from 14 to 165 ms gain, while the six AD patients obtained values ranging from 26 to 153. In a second experiment, 11 of 17 AD patients obtained negative values on the valid/invalid index. This sign of impaired focusing was significantly related to unusual performance on a picture recognition task, inspiring the authors to consider the patients with combined impairments as a cognitive subgroup in the Alzheimer population.

A second report from the same institute (Dolgushkin et al., 1989) once more presented evidence indicating that AD is a heterogeneous syndrome. This time 23 AD patients were tested with the covert orienting task, and 10 of them had longer latencies on valid cue trials than on invalid cue trials. In this paper too, the data were interpreted as indicating that selective attention tests can distinguish behavioral subgroups of AD patients. The question may be raised, however, whether this is the most parsimonious explanation. Inspection of individual scores shows that the valid/invalid index results in scores that seem randomly scattered around zero, which could mean that the AD group simply does not profit at all from the endogenous covert orienting technique. If one looks at the data for all control subjects, it appears that 57 percent of them had their shortest RT with valid cues, as expected. However, 9 percent reacted fastest on invalid cues, and 34 percent reacted fastest with neutral cues. For the Alzheimer group, these percentages are, respectively, 39, 26, and 35 percent. It would appear that AD patients, as a group, act as if there were no cues at all. Thus, about half are bound to get a negative valid/invalid index by chance. If all samples are combined, it appears that 27 of 57 patients obtained negative scores on the valid/invalid index.

Another method of cueing in the covert orienting paradigm is to precue the *exact location* of the stimulus to be detected, for example, by a short flash (the exogenous covert orienting paradigm, see Chapter 2). This would presumably cause attention to be drawn more automatically. It is therefore possible that AD patients would do better here than on the endogenous version with a central arrow pointing left or right. To our knowledge, no study using this paradigm has been published. However, a study by Cossa and colleagues (1989) contains a corresponding condition. Cossa and colleagues studied visual selective attention in 24 mildly deteriorated Alzheimer patients, using a letter detection task. Subjects faced a monitor on which a circle of capital letters was presented for 5 seconds. Subjects had to react by pressing a button when they found a letter T in the display. In the first condition of the experiment, the target was presented in randomly varied positions. It was found that Alzheimer patients reacted much more slowly than healthy elderly controls: the histogram in the publication indicates that the patients needed about 1400 ms to react, while the controls reacted in about 600 ms.

In the next condition, the target letter T appeared in a selected position (lower center) for 70 percent of the trials, and scattered elsewhere for the remaining trials. This condition, which corresponds somewhat with an endogenous covert orienting task, was called *memory-driven* as the procedure gives the subject an internal cue facilitating reactions in 70 percent of trials. In the final condition, called *data-driven*, two T's were displayed in the same location, one immediately after the other, and RT was measured on the second T. In this condition the precue can be considered exogenous.

In both groups, the memory-driven and data-driven conditions resulted in shorter reaction times than the uncued condition. Thus, no strong evidence was provided that AD patients have difficulty in focusing on the basis of a simple precue. However, Newman-Keuls multiple comparisons across the groups were not similar: in the control group comparisons there were significant differences between both facilitatory conditions against the random condition. The RT profile of the Alzheimer group was different: all differences between conditions were insignificant. In particular, the memory-driven and the data-driven condition produced about the same RT in the Alzheimer group, while in normals the data-driven condition was obviously easier, resulting in shorter RTs than the memory-driven condition. These results are inconsistent with the notion that memory driven (endogenous) attention is more impaired than data-driven (exogenous) attention. As the authors themselves noted, there are a number of peculiarities in their data which limit the generalization of results. For example, the patients seem to apply a different strategy in terms of speed-accuracy trade-off, reacting very slowly, but making hardly any errors. Cossa and colleagues stated that the Alzheimer patients behaved as if accuracy of performance was almost their only concern, and the stimulus-context of only marginal relevance.

Both this and the extreme baseline differences in RT between groups make the lack of interactions of groups and conditions on RT difficult to interpret.

Summary

It can be stated that focused attention in AD is spared only when selection can be based on a clear physical dimension of stimuli and when there are no conflicting response tendencies elicited by distractors. Focused attention, as tested with the Stroop paradigm, is impaired. With regard to exogenous position cues, the evidence is currently less clear, but selection on the basis of endogenous covert orienting (Posner paradigm) is severely impaired. The strongest effects of AD have been found with the Continuous Performance Test A-X condition and the Posner paradigm. Common factors in tasks that are difficult for AD patients seem to include an endogenous selection principle and a relatively frequent change of that principle.

DIVIDED ATTENTION

Divided attention performance is determined by the availability of processing mechanisms, their capacities and the strategies for utilizing those capacities. In the first part of this section, we will deal primarily with processing capacity. For the moment we will define this as the temporal rate of processing information (see Chapter 2). If mental operations are performed slowly, the processing capacity will be limited and divided attention deficits may occur. This will be the case when the rate of external information to be handled by a processing mechanism exceeds its capacity.

In the preceding sections mental slowness as a feature of AD was invoked frequently, either implicitly or explicitly. Recently, Nebes and Brady (1992) performed a meta-analysis of all RT studies carried out with AD patients, comprising 61 different experimental conditions. See Figure 5-2. Regression of the RTs of Alzheimer patients against those of normals yielded a linear function with a constant proportion describing the delay. The authors state that the linearity of this function suggests that AD produces a *generalized* slowing of cognitive processing, rather than a slowing of specific stages. This interpretation is supported by findings of Nestor and colleagues (1991a) from letter- and pattern-matching tasks. AD patients performed these tasks while an auditory probe signal was presented at various stages of their processing and responding. RT to the tone provided a "probe" of the attentional demands or costs of the component mental operations underlying the matchings tasks. It was found that the difference in RT to the probes between patients and controls was practically constant, that is, not influenced by the temporal relationship between probe and matching. The authors report: "A more detailed chronometric analysis indicated that the slowing of choice RT (in the matching task) was not associated with increased attentional cost of any particular component mental operation underlying performance."

An interesting additional finding in Nebes and Brady's (1992) meta-analysis was a relationship between degree of RT slowing and dementia severity. This was analyzed by restricting the number of studies to those that made use of the

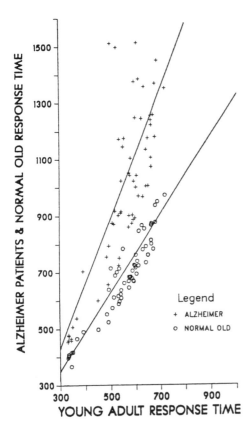

Figure 5-2 A meta-analysis of RT data from Alzheimer patients. Response times (in milliseconds) of Alzheimer patients and normal old adults are plotted as a function of the response times of young adults, on 61 different experimental conditions. (From Nebes and Brady, 1992, with permission.)

Dementia Rating Scale (DRS) as proposed by Mattis (1976). Patients from these investigations were divided into two subgroups: those with scores of 119 or more were considered mildly demented, those with lower scores, as moderately demented. Cognitive slowing was significantly greater in the more severely afflicted AD patients, or, as the authors put it: "It appears that the magnitude of the slowing rises with increasing dementia severity."

As noted in Chapter 2, a general slowness in information processing will result in divided attention deficits. If we look at studies of divided attention in AD patients, the visual search task with a letter array as described by Nebes and Brady (1989) is a prime example: rate of search was used by these authors as an index of processing capacity. Subjects were presented with arrays of letters in a tachistoscope. In the first part of the study, only black letters were presented in groups of either 2, 4, or 6. The investigators were interested in the relationship between array size and response time. They found that an increase in array size was associated with a slowing in response time, both in the elderly normals and in the AD patients. However, the slowing seen in demented patients was significantly greater than that in the elderly normals, disproportionate to the array size. The group difference was evident not only in absolute response time, but also in percent change. Between the two-letter and six-letter arrays (positive and negative trials combined), decision time rose by 17 percent in the elderly normals and by 26 percent in the demented patients.

Divided attention has also been studied with *dichotic listening* tasks, in which subjects have to attend to two different digit strings presented simultaneously to the right and left ear. Inglis (Inglis, 1965, 1970) was the first investigator to apply this method to the study of AD. He demonstrated that demented subjects have a specific loss of information presented to the second ear in comparison with healthy elderly controls. Several more recent reports also describe the performance of AD patients in situations where they have to divide their attention between two sources of information. Grady and colleagues (1989) studied dichotic listening in 32 patients in whom severity of dementia ranged from mild to moderate. Control subjects were 33 age-matched healthy volunteers. Stimuli were spondaic words: two-syllable words in which each syllable is stressed (e.g., toothbrush). These stimuli are presented so that the first syllable of the first spondee is presented monotonically to either the right or left ear. The second syllable of the first word, and the first syllable of the second spondee are presented dichotically (i.e., one syllable to the right ear and one to the left, simultaneously). Finally, the second syllable of the second word is presented to the ear not stimulated initially. Hence two spondaic words would be presented like this:

tooth L . . . brush L/grass R . . . snake R

The score on this Staggered Spondaic Words Test (SSW) was the percentage of words correctly identified.

DAT patients were significantly impaired in their recognition of these stimuli. Percentages of correct recognition varied from 15 to 93 percent in the patient group, while in the control group all subjects scored between 80 and 100 percent correct. This effect could not be explained by primary perceptual problems, as the patients had also been tested with time-compressed and filtered speech. Although a minority of the AD patients were also deficient on these speech perception tasks, performance of the AD group on SSW was only minimally correlated with performance on time-compressed and filtered speech tests. An interesting feature of this investigation was the assessment of cerebral glucose metabolism by means of PET scanning and of cerebral atrophy with CT scanning. Statistically significant correlations were found between rCMRglc and SSW performance. The correlation was .58 between the right SSW and rCMRglc in the left anterior superior temporal region and it was .57 between the right SSW and rCMRglc in the left posterior superior temporal area. Regarding CT data, SSW scores were significantly related to atrophy in both hemispheres, such that those patients with more severe atrophy in the anterior temporal regions showed poorer SSW performance than those with less.

Divided Attention in AD has also been studied with *dual-task* techniques. Parasuraman and colleagues (1985) found that patients with early, mild AD had difficulty time-sharing a letter classification task with a simple reaction time task, although each task could be performed reasonably on its own. About 30 percent of the subjects could not perform the dual task at all. Two later reports from the same institute (Nestor et al., 1991a, 1991b) confirmed this finding, again using samples of patients with mild AD. The main tasks in the dual-task condition consisted of letter matching or pattern-matching. Subjects reacted vocally by saying "same" or "different." The second task was a simple auditory reaction, the auditory signals functioning as probes that hindered the processing of letters and figures at fixed points in the stimulation program. Slowing of RT in the dual task correlated with local reductions in brain metabolism in right premotor and right parietal association areas in the patient group, but not in the healthy control group. Nestor and coworkers concluded that this finding points to a reduced capacity of association cortices to time-share activities in mild AD patients.

Additional evidence for a specific impairment of divided attention comes from our ongoing research on driving in AD patients. As described earlier (see Chapter 4), we use a paradigm in which task difficulty in single tasks conditions is individually adjusted on the basis of performance. These individually adjusted tasks are subsequently combined in a dual-task condition. Our experience shows that in AD patients performance breaks down in the dual task condition, in spite of this adjustment. For example, the patient described at the beginning of this chapter became so involved in the visual analysis task presented during driving that he forgot to steer (see Brouwer et al., 1991, 1992 for details of the task). This is fairly typical of moderately severe AD patients. In mild patients, performance may only break down in more complex dual-task conditions in which monitoring of peripheral information must be combined with driving and visual analysis. See Figure 5-3.

Summary

Mental slowness in AD is well-documented, but attempts to localize it in specific stages of information processing have failed. Rather, it seems to be a general and global phenomenon. Taken by itself, extreme slowness of information processing can explain many problems of divided attention in AD patients. However, apart from the slowness, there appears to be an additional problem in combining two different tasks or two different task elements. This has been demonstrated in AD patients with methods such as dichotic listening and dual tasks.

SUSTAINED ATTENTION

Very few reports have been published on sustained attention in AD. Interest has seldom focused on changes in performance over time. For example, although Alexander (1973a) used the Continuous Performance Test in a study of patients with senile dementia, time-on-task effects are not mentioned or discussed in his paper. Nissen and colleagues (1981) reported that AD patients had difficulties maintaining focused attention in a visual detection task, although their phasic levels of arousal were normal (quoted in Parasuraman and Nestor, 1986). Lines and colleagues (1991) studied sustained attention in a small group of AD patients: 8 subjects had a Mini Mental State (MMS) (Folstein et al., 1975) score of 20 or more and were considered mild cases, 8 had a MMS score between 11 and 19, and were considered moderate-severe cases. Two attention tests were applied, the first being the Wilkins Auditory Sustained Attention Task (SAT). In this test the subject is required to listen to trains of bleeps and to count their number

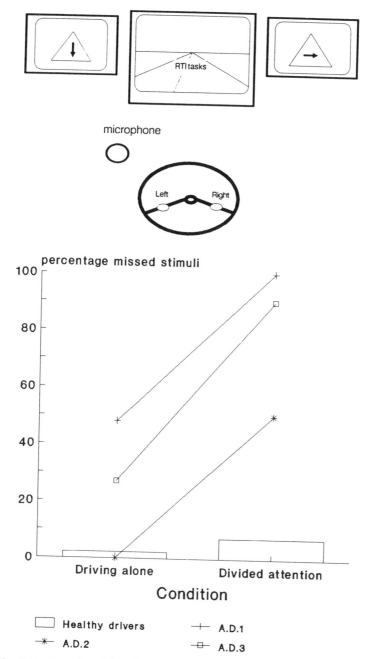

Figure 5-3 Detection of peripheral stimuli by Alzheimer patients in a divided attention task in a car simulator. Arrows were presented on small video screens 30 degrees outside the point of fixation for driving, and subjects had to react to these signals by pressing buttons on the steering wheel. In the basic condition "driving only" detection is optimal in elderly control subjects, and in one Alzheimer patient. Two more AD patients miss many peripheral signals. In the "divided attention" condition, subjects have to react vocally to the presentation of dot groups in the center of the main screen while driving. In this condition, healthy elderly subjects miss a few peripheral signals, while detection decreases dramatically in the AD patients.

(Wilkins et al., 1987). Train lengths from 5 to 14 were presented, and as the average interstimulus interval was 4 seconds, train length varied from about 20 to about 56 seconds. This short time scale is unusual in sustained attention research. However, there are no theoretical or methodological objections to considering this counting test as a test of sustained attention. The second task lasted 5 minutes and employed visual stimuli. Digits were presented briefly on a computer screen against a background of visual noise. The digits were presented at a rate of one per second, and subjects were instructed to push a button whenever they saw the target digit, "7." Performance of AD patients was compared to that of age-matched controls.

No significant differences between *mildly afflicted* patients and controls were found. Both elderly normals and mild AD patients made few errors in the bleep counting task. Both normals and patients responded to nearly all the target stimuli and made very few errors of commission in the visual vigilance task. Time-on-task effects were analyzed by comparing errors and false alarms over five successive 1-minute blocks in the visual task. No significant group × block interactions were found, indicating that the AD patients sustained their attention just as well as the normals.

Patients comprising the *moderate* group varied greatly with respect to performance in both tasks. In the bleep counting task, four patients made a large number of errors, and four made none. Similarly, in the visual vigilance task (presented to 7 patients) four patients had relatively high hit rates and low false alarm rates, while three performed very poorly.

All patients had also been tested with verbal memory tasks such as free recall, delayed recall, and fluency. Both AD groups showed the expected memory deficits. Hence for the mild group there was a clear dissociation of memory and sustained attention performance. The authors suggested from this that the memory deficit in early dementia does not involve a failure of sustained attention. The difference between mild and moderate AD patients could mean that this aspect of attention is preserved until late in the course of the disease.

Sheer and Shrock (1986) published a series of studies on a state of consciousness called *focused arousal*. This somewhat ambiguous term refers to a state of consciousness assumed to be important for cognitive processing in humans. The word "focused" is probably used here either to indicate that the phenomenon is task-related, or that it is a focal cortical phenomenon. In animals, a state of visual attending, without motor activity, has been related to certain frequencies in the EEG spectrum. The same approach has been applied to human subjects attending to a visual task. Alertness in humans is related to a desynchronized EEG. It has been demonstrated that a number of different electrical patterns can be found in this desynchronization. The 40-Hz EEG, with a frequency window between 36 and 44 Hz represents one such distinct pattern. The pattern can be both increased and suppressed with operant conditioning. The subjective state consistently reported by subjects in 40-Hz conditioning included, in a Q-sort procedure, such words as attentive, concentrating, vigilant and effortful (as contrasted with such words as active, energetic, excited, and restless associated with the general EEG desynchronization pattern). Hence "focused arousal" must be seen as a task-specific alertness within the range of normal wakefulness. As such, it can be considered as an aspect of sustained attention.

Sheer and Shrock were able to manipulate focused arousal, as revealed in 40-Hz EEG, by presenting subjects with verbal versus spatial tasks. The verbal task consisted of sentence repetition, while the spatial task consisted of same/different judgments of pairs of three-dimensional geometric figures. In normal elderly subjects, presentation of the verbal task causes a shift in focused arousal to the posterior cortex of the left hemisphere, while presentation of the spatial task produces a preponderance of 40-Hz EEG in the right hemisphere. EEG analysis used a laterality ratio $(L - R)/(L + R)$, which resulted in a .44 value for the verbal task, and $-.24$ for the spatial task. In a group of early Alzheimer patients, this index of focused arousal did not show a task-dependent lateralization, and for all conditions (baseline, verbal, spatial) the absolute levels of 40-Hz EEG activity was markedly lower and significantly different from the levels in geriatric controls. In a replication study (Loring, 1982) Alzheimer patients were compared with both normal geriatric controls and multiinfarct groups. The two patient groups performed worse than the control subjects on both the verbal and the spatial tasks. Test performance, however, did not discriminate between Alzheimer and multiinfarct patients. On the contrary, the 40-Hz EEG revealed significant differences between the two patient groups: the mean absolute levels of 40-Hz EEG under all conditions were significantly lower for the Alzheimer group than for the multiinfarct group and the control group. Once more there was no task-dependent lateralization in the Alzheimer patients. Sheer emphasized that the more molar, multidetermined neuropsychological measures discriminated poorly between Alzheimer and multiinfarct groups, while the electrophysiological index of focused arousal differed in a highly significant manner between patient groups.

Summary

Evidence on sustained attention in AD is so scarce that a general conclusion is as yet not warranted. One study indicated that sustained attention as measured by two tests is normal in mild cases of AD. Sheer and Shrock demonstrated that a task-specific alertness as reflected by 40-Hz EEG is disturbed at an early stage of the disease.

SUPERVISORY ATTENTIONAL CONTROL

In the previous sections impairments of attention in AD have been described at task level, and it appeared that few aspects of attention escape the deleterious effects of the disease. The question now arises whether explanations for the impairments can be found on a more theoretical level. The explanatory value of the Supervisory Attentional System in particular should be examined here. Many implicit suggestions of decreased supervisory attentional control (SAC) in Alzheimer patients can be found in studies on task level. One important function of SAC is the suppression of task-irrelevant responses or *response inhibition*. As early as 1973, Alexander reported that his senile patients made far more commission errors in the Continuous Performance Test than elderly controls, particularly in the A-X condition that required suppression of the response trained in the preceding part of the experiment. Studies using the ambiguous Stroop stimuli (Koss et al., 1984, Grady et al., 1988) have also demonstrated a marked weakening of response inhibition.

Furthermore, several investigations have clearly shown that AD patients do not profit from *cueing* as much as control subjects. Freed and his coworkers (Freed et al., 1989) found that a directional cue in the shape of an arrow had no facilitating effect at all in many of their subjects. Cossa and associates (1989) reported that their patients were apparently unable to use a probability cue (memory-driven) in a letter searching task. Neither were they helped by repetition of the target letter in the same position on two successive trials (data-driven). In all three experiments, the patients responded to the stimuli presented, albeit significantly slower than control subjects, but made no use of additional cueing information presented in the same tasks. It would seem then that simply reacting to an imperative stimulus is one thing, but optimizing that reaction on the basis of the temporal or spatial pattern of stimulation is another, obviously requiring the supervision of a higher-order system. The failure of AD patients to profit from cues cannot be explained as a result of reduced processing capacity, as there was ample time to process the information supplied by the cues. Within the Posner paradigm, for example, the arrow cues were followed by an interval of about 2 seconds before the imperative stimulus appeared. Hence, the fact that information from cues was not used seems to indicate that AD patients simply do not attend to all information available in the task situation. An inability to maintain an internal representation of all stimuli recognizable to an external observer might be assumed on the basis of this deficient performance.

The performance of AD patients can also be considered in terms of *flexibility*, that is, the ability to change a response set. A lack of flexibility, or conversely, behavioral rigidity, is certainly observed in the daily behavior of patients, and reported by their caretakers. The Trailmaking-B test is considered a test of mental flexibility because of its continuously changing response set. The clear failure of AD patients in this task can once more be interpreted as an impairment in supervisory control (Grady et al., 1988). Reduced flexibility in AD was also reported by Hart (1985) who presented a reaction-time task with cross-modal shifts (visual and auditory stimuli). Shifting the imperative stimulus from one modality to the other had a markedly greater retardation effect on AD patients than on controls.

Koss and coworkers (1984), doubted that patients with advanced AD were aware of their errors in the Stroop task. This *deficient monitoring* of their own performance can also be interpreted as an impairment of supervisory control. Monitoring the quality of one's own production is another form of attention to a task situation. Finally, the qualitatively different pattern of behavior of AD patients in dual tasks can also be explained by impaired SAC.

The available empirical evidence thus suggests that the Supervisory Attentional System breaks down with AD. A related conclusion was reached by Jorm (1986) in a review of *controlled processing* in AD patients. Although Jorm's conclusion was mainly based on data from experiments on memory and language, it appears to be directly related to the problem of supervisory control in attention tasks. Jorm points out that the bulk of evidence on cognitive decline in senile dementia can be interpreted as evidence of a breakdown of controlled processing which begins in an early stage of the disease. The review indeed presents an impressive number of studies bearing on the problem of automatic versus controlled processing in dementia. The main point is that cognitive performance based on well learned skills and automatic processing (i.e., automatic schema selection based on contention scheduling) remains unaffected in dementia. For example, in the area of *language* it has been demonstrated that the highly automatized aspects of language production, such as syntax, remain intact long after semantic knowledge has begun declining (Bayles and Boone, 1982). In the area of *intelligence* Performance IQ in the WAIS declines more and at an earlier stage than Verbal IQ (Alexander, 1973b). Again, this is explained by stating that the verbal part of the WAIS tends to test skills which are reasonably automated, while the performance part involves largely unfamiliar tasks demanding controlled processing. In the area of *memory*, dementia causes problems in learning tasks that require controlled processing, particularly with conscious effort. Retrieval of information from long-term memory remains intact as long as the process is based on well-trained schemata that automatically evoke and organize recall. But retrieval fails when it demands an active memory search of the subject. Weingartner and colleagues (1981) and Miller (1984) demonstrated this effect with verbal fluency tasks: even at an early stage of AD, patients recall far fewer words beginning with a given letter, or words belonging to a certain semantic category, than control subjects.

It is clear from the example above that controlled processing implies the use of attentional strategies. In the case of word fluency in a given category, search is effective only if the subject is flexible enough to switch between subcategories, such as from "animals around the house" to "animals in the zoo," when the experimenter uses animals as the semantic category in the fluency task. As such, the conclusions in Jorm's review support the idea that AD results in an impairment in strategies of attention, that is in SAC.

The distinction between intact automatic processes and impaired controlled processes can also be found in some of the studies of attentional deficits in AD reviewed above. It is striking that Nebes and Brady (1989) found two automatic processes intact in their AD patients: in addition to normal discrimination on the basis of a simple color cue, they also found a gradual development of automatic search in the letter recognition task. Neither process demands conscious effort on the part of the subject, and he may even be unaware of the development of automatic search. The fact that controlled search was disproportionately slow in the same sample of patients convincingly demonstrates dissociation of impairment in controlled versus automatic processing in AD.

Still, the hypothesis in terms of impaired SAC can be criticized as being very global and aspecific. Hart and Semple (1990) pointed out that a similar pattern of automatic versus controlled functioning may be found in other patient groups such as schizophrenics and depressed patients, and in normal elderly. This aspecific character of the hypothesis seems to reduce its explanatory power somewhat. Furthermore, the distinction between automatic and controlled processing might be confounded with the dimension of task difficulty.

It must be stressed that the impairment in supervisory control does not mean that the demented patient is left completely without any strategy. In mild cases, particularly, one can sometimes observe strong efforts to concentrate, but often directed at only one aspect of the task which seems to command all of the patient's attention. In the study by Alexander (1973a), patients were obviously unable to suppress irrelevant responses, and made many commission errors in the Continuous Performance Test. Nevertheless, they apparently applied a deliberate strategy for identifying the letters presented successively in the display. In contrast to normal subjects, patients tended to name each letter aloud. Possibly they were trying a kind of rehearsal strategy with regard to successive letters in the hope of remembering an X when an A appeared. This is certainly a strategy, but apparently not an effective one. An alternative interpretation could be that the senile subjects simply could not suppress the letter name, each time a stimulus was presented. However, this is in contradiction with clinical experience: demented individuals have never been conspicuous for displaying a tendency to name everything they see. A second indication of remaining supervisory control stems from the report by Koss and coworkers (1984). Mildly demented patients still noted their errors and slowed their performance, as if aware of their problem. Hence the decline of supervisory control should not be seen as an absolute phenomenon, but rather as a deterioration that proceeds with increasing duration of disease.

IN SEARCH OF AN EXPLANATION

Although studies of attentional impairments in AD are not abundant, the available evidence allows for the conclusion that attention is impaired in most of its aspects. The most conspicuous effects are in the areas of divided attention and supervisory attentional control. Relatively speaking, focused and sustained attention are less impaired. In a qualitative sense, impairments of attention are less striking than memory impairments. In this respect, studies confirm the traditional view that AD manifests itself initially as a memory impairment. When focused attention was assessed together with memory at the beginning of a longitudinal study, it was found that AD patients with memory deficits performed normally in the Stroop paradigm (Grady et al., 1988). Lines and colleagues (1991) found normal sustained attention in patients exhibiting memory deficits associated with mild AD. If we consider Digit Span as a test of attentional capacity, another longitudinal study supports the idea that attentional deficits appear later than memory impairments. Jones and coworkers (1992) reported that Digit Span did not differentiate between dementia and pseudodementia on a first test occasion, although a Temporal Orientation Questionnaire and the Benton Visual Retention Test revealed significant differences between groups. When patients were retested at least 6 months later, Digit Span performance had clearly deteriorated in the dementia group.

There has been speculation on the relationship between the *cortical pattern of degeneration* in AD and the sequence of the appearance of behavioral deficits. A sequential appearance has even been suggested within the class of attention deficits. Lines and colleagues (1991) point out that studies of regional cerebral blood flow using PET and SPECT scans suggest that temporoparietal abnormalities are most common in the early stages of the disease (Grady et al., 1988) with frontal abnormalities occurring later. This picture of differential regional involvement might have implications for attention. There is evidence (Wilkins et al., 1987) that the frontal lobes are involved in sustained attention as tested by Lines et al. (bleep counting, and digit detection over 5 minutes). One might predict, according to Lines et al., that sustained attention would be preserved until later on in the disease. One might also predict that other aspects of attention, such as divided attention and attentional shifting, which are more susceptible to parietal damage (Posner et al., 1988), could be impaired early on in the disease. However, two caveats should be added: First, as stated in the introduction to this chapter, AD is far more heterogeneous in its pattern of cortical degeneration than was previously assumed. It therefore seems unwarranted to assume a fixed sequence of early temporoparietal and late frontal degeneration. Next, at the behavioral level there is some evidence that frontal symptoms may be present from the beginning. Bhutani and coworkers (1992), using a delayed alternation task and a subject-ordered pointing task, concluded that their results strongly suggested that some degree of frontal involvement does occur during the earliest stages of AD. In a closing remark, they state that "AD should no longer be defined as a posterior dementia."

In the area of *electrophysiology*, studies of AD seem to reveal one general feature: a decreased functional differentiation. This is suggested by the disturbed topography of event-related potentials such as P-300 and CNV (Goodin et al., 1978; O'Connor 1980a, 1980b; Remond and Bouhours, 1988; Maurer and Dierks, 1988; Rugg, 1992). O'Connor (1980b) observed less differentiation between central and frontal recordings of CNV in patients than controls and suggested that increased overlapping of neuronal generators may exist in demented subjects. Sheer and Shrock (1986), studying "focused arousal" by means of the 40-Hz frequency in EEG, noted decreased task-dependent lateralization of this phenomenon. These electrophysiological changes seem to suggest that the AD patient's brain loses the normal pattern of functional differentiation to a certain degree. This conclusion is in line with a remark by Parasuraman and Nestor (1986): "Neuronal degeneration in the corticocortical network results in a loss of functional distance in the cortex, such that mental operations begin to compete for the same neural processing units."

AD is increasingly viewed as resulting from deficiencies in *neurotransmitter systems*. Both the noradrenergic and the cholinergic neurotransmitter systems appear to be affected in AD, although it is not yet known how extensively these two patterns of neuropathology overlap in individual patients (Freed et al., 1988). Several investigations have reported pathology of the locus ceruleus (LC), a brainstem nucleus that is the origin of noradrenergic projection to the cerebral cortex (Bondareff et al., 1982). Neuropathology in the locus ceruleus causes a reduction in cortical levels of norepinephrine. Freed and colleagues (1988) reported that reduced levels of MHPG, a metabolite of norepinephrine, were related to deficits in attentional focusing as tested with the Posner paradigm (arrow cues). Tariot and colleagues (1987) reported improved cognition in AD patients after treatment with a monoamineoxidase (MAO) inhibitor in a double-blind serial treatment design (MAO inhibitors increase noradrenergic activity by suppressing one mechanism for the neurotransmitter's metabolic destruction.)

The cholinergic system plays an important role in the active control of attention and AD has been described as a disorder of marked cholinergic deficiency (Davies, 1979; Buchwald et al., 1989). Midbrain cholinergic cells may be dysfunctional in AD, and it is known that a cholinergic component of ARAS generates P-1, an evoked potential that has been described as abnormal in AD (Pollock et al., 1989; Buchwald et al., 1989). Finally, cortical levels of serotonin and dopamine can also be reduced in AD by degeneration in the raphe nuclei and the ventrotegmentum.

The well-established fact that neurotransmitter systems are deficient in AD might have implications for a recently developed view on the cognitive deterioration in these patients. It has been postulated (Parasuraman and Nestor, 1986) that *energetic factors* in information processing are impaired in AD. The interest in these factors resulted from an important development in cognitive psychology. As described in Chapter 2, the computer metaphor has long dominated the scene in this field, and one of its drawbacks is the implicit assumption that information processing systems are in a stable state. Indeed a computer will never be tired, bored, or depressed, and computation will proceed according to fixed rules as long as the computer is plugged in, receiving its energy from the electric mains. The shortcomings of the computer metaphor became manifest in the 1970s, and in the 1980s cognitive psychology turned to connectionism with its network models as a more promising approach (Schneider, 1987). As part of this development, energetic factors were discovered as relevant for information processing (Hockey et al., 1986). On the basis of his own research on visual masking Bachman (1984) concluded:

> Classical works in the physiology of arousal and nonspecific systems have proved convincingly that the neurophysiological substrate necessary for energising the brain and providing sufficient activity for the manifestations of consciousness is located subcortically and consists of the brain stem reticular formation and non-specific thalamic activating system. The importance of energetic, rather than purely structural or algoristic, processes in visual masking and information processing is rarely stressed. . . . In visual masking, the interaction of specific sensory systems with nonspecific 'energising' pathways is crucial.

Two criticisms should be made here. First, energetic factors are vague concepts. Parasuraman and Nestor (1986), who elaborated the energetic viewpoint as an explanation for cognitive decline in AD, formulated this problem. They pointed out that energetic concepts as they had been used so far were less well defined than information-processing concepts. Terms such as arousal, alertness, effort, capacity and resources have been used, but not always defined. Moreover, the use of the terms may vary: resources are sometimes looked upon as subjects' abilities, and sometimes as a kind of energy that can be allocated to various mental processes. Effort has likewise both the meaning of subjective experience and an energetic factor.

Second, the importance of energetic factors for information processing in AD should be demonstrated by manipulating them. Only if the state of the system can be varied, and only if this variation influences the quality of cognitive processes, can an important role of energetic factors be assumed. Manipulation of energetic factors might take two approaches; a pharmaceutical one and a psychological one. In the latter case it should be demonstrated that AD patients perform better on cognitive tasks when they are alerted, or when their motivation is increased. We tend to be rather pessimistic, at least about the motivational approach, as it is hard to conceive that, for example, retrieval from long-term memory in AD patients will improve if they try harder. It is very probable that AD is marked by severe structural impairments in the neural substrates of cognition, impairments that cannot be ameliorated or overcome by manipulating the state of the information-processing system.

SUMMARY

AD has traditionally been viewed as a progressive cerebral disease with mainly temporoparietal cortical degeneration, and memory loss as the main behavioral feature. Since 1980, the neuropsychological view of AD has broadened and investigators have shown that impairments of attention, although they are less conspicuous than memory impairments, can even exist in mild cases of AD.

Focused attention is normal as long as selection can be based on clear physical characteristics of stimuli, and if no conflicting response tendencies are elicited by distractors. Selectivity breaks down if it depends on an endogenous selection principle, or a principle that is frequently changing. This more or less boils down to the conclusion that automatic attention responses are preserved, while controlled selection is impaired.

Serious impairments of divided attention are present in AD. They are mainly the result of a general slowing of cognitive processes, a deficit that has not yielded to attempts to localize it in particular stages of information processing. It appears that the magnitude of the slowing rises with increasing dementia severity. In addition, AD patients have difficulties in switching and demonstrate impairments in dual-tasks which cannot be explained on the basis of mental slowness only. Sustained attention has been studied insufficiently to warrant a conclusion. The scant evidence currently available seems to suggest that sustained attention remains normal in early stages of the disease.

Supervisory attentional control is also deficient in AD patients. Response inhibition is weakened, flexibility is decreased and self-monitoring of one's performance is poor. There is some evidence suggesting that strategies can still be developed by patients with mild AD, although they are not always effective.

The overall picture then is dominated by deficits in divided attention and supervisory control. In recent years there has been speculation about a temporal pattern of attentional impairments, with problems in sustained attention appearing last. Although such a pattern analysis could be rewarding from an academic and a practical point of view, it should not be forgotten that AD is a

far more heterogeneous condition, both on the neuroanatomical and the behavioral level, than was assumed in the past.

In electrophysiology the disturbed topography of event-related potentials
and the decreased task-dependent lateralization of 40-Hz EEG have suggested
that a decreased functional differentiation may exist in the brains of AD patients.
AD is increasingly viewed as resulting from deficiencies in neurotransmitter
systems, particularly the noradrenergic and cholinergic systems. Two broad neuropsychological hypotheses were postulated in the 1980s. It was suggested that
AD mainly affects the controlled processing of information, while automatic
processing remains spared until the later stages of the disease. Further, attempts
were made to explain the cognitive decline in AD as a result of a deficiency in
energetic factors in information processing.

6

Attention in Parkinson's Disease

Parkinson's disease (PD) is a progressive neurodegenerative disease with a relatively high prevalence, estimated to be between 1.1 and 1.2%. The great majority of patients are over 50 years old. In this disease, a progressive degeneration of the dopaminergic cells of the substantia nigra affects the nigrostriatal input to the basal ganglia. It has been estimated that striatal dopamine content must fall to 20 percent of the normal value before PD becomes manifest. Above this threshold, compensatory physiological reactions such as augmented activity of the remaining dopaminergic neurons are able to maintain function (Wolters and Calne, 1989).

Despite much research, the cause of the selective degeneration is still unknown. One possibility is that a long-latency toxin, presumably contained in one or more agents to which the patient has been exposed during a period of susceptibility, initiates the process of neuronal degeneration (Langston et al., 1989).

Clinically, the disease is characterized by the *motor symptom triad* of rigidity, tremor, and akinesia. The first two are rather conspicuous "positive symptoms," manifested by an excess of muscle activity, which is presumably caused by a release of the basal ganglia's normal inhibitory control on other brain structures (Marsden, 1982). Akinesia is a so-called "negative symptom," which may take many different forms and is initially much less conspicuous. Nevertheless, it is thought to be the cardinal symptom of the disease (Hallett and Khoshbin, 1980; Marsden, 1982).

James Parkinson defined "the shaking palsy" in 1817 and concluded that it "leaves the senses and the intellect intact." Nevertheless, although motor disturbances are the obvious features of the disease, subtle mental impairments have also been described. Many neuropsychological studies have focused on these mental impairments over the last decades, both in the areas of affect and cognition (attention, perception, memory).

A general methodological problem in evaluating neuropsychological studies of mental function in Parkinson's disease concerns the selection of patients. A random selection of Parkinson patients contains a much greater proportion who are clinically demented than the same age group in the general population (Brown and Marsden, 1984, 1987; Raskin et al., 1990). Two explanations are given for this: 1) there is a tendency for simultaneous occurrence of Alzheimer-type disease with PD (Boller, 1979), and 2) cognitive impairments peculiar to

PD are themselves a form of dementia, a subcortical dementia, when they occur in a very severe form (Cummings, 1988).

This methodological problem is usually handled by testing only those patients who are not clinically suffering from dementia and are at a relatively early stage of Parkinson's disease. The necessity for such selection would be obvious if the first explanation given above is correct. It would still be quite acceptable and practical, but theoretically unnecessary if the second one is correct. Patients in that case would differ only in the severity of their affliction rather than comprise two different nosological categories.

Although dementia is substantially more prevalent in Parkinson patients than in healthy control subjects, "the overwhelming clinical impression is of a group of patients devastated by motor incapacity, but with preserved cognitive (in the clinical sense) function" (Marsden, 1982). Nonetheless, much of the evidence gathered in the last 15 years or so indicates that nondemented Parkinson patients as a group perform significantly worse on certain mental tasks, including tasks of focused and divided attention, than healthy controls matched for age and background. According to Marsden (1982), one of the initial reasons for studying attention in Parkinson patients had to do with findings from animal studies which suggested that the basal ganglia played a role in corticosubcortical control loops that modulate the state of preparation of the cortex. For example, a small lesion in the striatum (the "input" area of the basal ganglia) would produce the same deficits as a lesion in the cortical zone projecting onto that area (Rosvold and Schwarcbart, 1964). Such findings suggest that the basal ganglia play a role in brain activity not restricted to motor control. This line of reasoning led to an unusual development: on the basis of animal models of cognition, investigators began to look for attentional impairments in patients who had not previously expressed such problems. This contrasts starkly with the approach taken in other fields, for example, head injury, where patients' complaints of poor concentration lead clinicians to note their mental slowness. Likewise, lapses of attention had been observed in epileptics. As a result, investigators began to study these clinical phenomena and explained them in reference to theoretical models of cognition. The starting point in the field of PD was quite different; a model was available, and impairments had to be found. It also seems likely that the motor problems of Parkinson patients, particularly with starting and alternating motor responses, inspired investigators to look for similar problems in cognition, that is, decreased ability in switching or decreased flexibility in attention. Consequently, the literature on attentional impairments in PD is mainly concerned with these topics and related issues such as divided attention and supervisory control.

THE BASAL GANGLIA AND THE NONSPECIFIC
THALAMOCORTICAL PROJECTION

Important names in the early study of nonmotor functions of the basal ganglia are Rosvold (Rosvold et al., 1958; Rosvold and Schwarcbart, 1964), Denny-Brown (1962; Denny-Brown and Yanagisawa, 1976) and Hassler (Jung and

Hassler, 1960; Hassler, 1978). Rosvold and his colleagues described the similarities of the effects of basal ganglia lesions and prefrontal lesions in rats and monkeys performing tasks which required a delayed selective response. This was followed by a number of publications on neuropsychological indicators of frontal dysfunction in PD. However, in the 1960s there was as yet no anatomical explanation for the more conspicuous effects of basal ganglia lesions on prefrontal functions than on other brain functions.

It was known that a nonmotor part of the output of the basal ganglia projected onto the centrum medianum of the thalamus. It is the origin of the nonspecific thalamocortical projection which diffusely projects onto all secondary and tertiary cortical areas. Thus, it was thought that the nonmotor effects of basal ganglia lesions were the result of interference with this system and that the areas affected should include all secondary and tertiary cortex. Based on the then current neuroanatomy, Hassler (1978) made a detailed model showing the role of the basal ganglia in selective attention (Figure 6-1).

Although the model is elegant, it has been refuted because it predicts too many attentional problems in Parkinson patients. According to Marsden (1982), PD is the clinical testing ground on which all theories of basal ganglia function must be measured. His clinical arguments against Hassler's theory and related views are characterized by the following passage on attention in Parkinson's disease (p. 517):

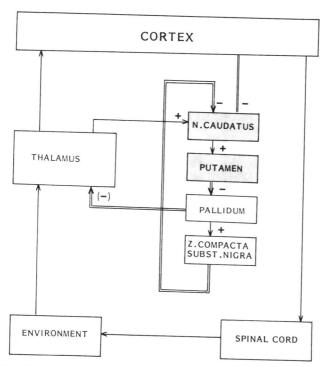

Figure 6-1 The Hassler model of basal ganglia function. (Adapted from Van Vreden, 1986, with permission.)

. . . Nor is a deficit of attention evident in this illness. Patients do not complain of a flood of sensory information swamping their processes of thought, as would be expected if the function of the basal ganglia normally is to suppress unwanted input. Nor do those with hemiparkinsonism complain of unilateral inattention or difficulties in perception in one half of space. Matched against Parkinson disease, it is hard to believe that the basal ganglia are primarily concerned with general inhibitory actions to focus the attention of the conscious mind on single events.

Although the passage seems convincing, it doesn't do justice to Hassler's theory by suggesting that it would predict a flooding of sensory information in Parkinson's disease. Figure 6-1 shows that the effect of the failing dopaminergic input to the striatum is to enhance the putamen reaction, with overfocusing, arrest and fixation of attention as a likely outcome. Moreover, there is some evidence of neglect phenomena in basal ganglia disease. Damasio and colleagues (1980) reported two cases of unilateral vascular lesions of the striatum, with left-sided hemineglect as indicated in a line cancellation task. Villardita and co-workers (1983) also demonstrated subclinical neglect in Parkinson patients performing a cancellation task. So on closer examination, there is some evidence for impairments of focused attention in perception, just as predicted by Hassler's model. Still, the fact that attentional impairments appear much less pronounced than motor impairments, both qualitatively and quantitatively, does not agree with Hassler's theory (Rafal et al., 1984; Stelmach et al., 1989).

Greater understanding of the nature and causes of attentional impairment in PD is needed to explain its apparent similarities with that arising from prefrontal lobe lesions. The two types may be related since "the intimate functional association between prefrontal cortex and the head of the caudate has been shown in studies which found equivalent impairments following lesions to either region" (Gotham et al., 1988, p. 301). A number of reciprocal connections between the basal ganglia and the frontal and prefrontal cortex have been described in recent years (Nauta, 1979; Alexander et al., 1986). It seems neuroanatomically plausible to seek a common explanation for the similar effects of basal ganglia and prefrontal lesions on aspects of attention (see also Chapter 3).

> Anatomical studies thus provide ample evidence that a selective impairment of frontal lobe function may be possible in PD. They do not however, prove that it is the case, nor can they prove that the specific pattern of cognitive impairment observed in PD stems from a selective dysfunction of prefrontal areas. (Goldenberg et al., 1990, p. 142).

In this chapter we discuss the evidence obtained from tests of attention in Parkinson patients. We will try to structure the evidence under the headings Focused Attention, Divided Attention, and Supervisory Attentional Control as in other chapters, although it must be said that the literature does not easily permit this distinction. Flexibility in attention, or the ability of PD patients to shift attention, has been studied in such a way that it becomes intertwined with supervisory control. PD patients have frequently been studied using tests found sensitive to frontal damage because of the similarity of symptoms in frontal and basal ganglia lesions. Findings obtained with such methods fit best under the heading Supervisory Attentional Control. The section on sustained attention is omitted in this chapter for lack of evidence.

FOCUSED ATTENTION

The level of difficulty in focused attention tests can be varied according to the nature of the distraction and the salience and consistency of the object of focus. A very elementary manipulation of the object of focus concerns the *spatial location of the stimulus*. As we mentioned above, subclinical neglect phenomena have been reported in Parkinson patients with right-sided and bilateral symptoms (Villardita et al., 1983).

Rafal and coworkers (1984) carried out a more refined test of the hypothesis that Parkinson patients have a central deficit in the spatial orientation of attention. Covert orientation of attention in the visual field was tested in 10 Parkinson patients of varying severity both on and off levadopa medication. Throughout this experiment, subjects had to fixate on a central cross. A cue-box, either 10 degrees to the left or right, was brightened at random intervals between 50 and 1000 ms, indicating the high probability (80 percent) of the appearance of an asterisk at that position. The subjects responded by pressing a key. Trials in which the stimulus appeared at the indicated position were called "valid," and those in which it did not were "invalid." Controlling for the effects of PD on motor speed, the effects of interval duration and validity were the same with and without levodopa, and the same for healthy subjects. The authors concluded: "This experiment gave no indication that Parkinsonian patients are slow in shifting attention in the visual field" (p. 1090). Sharpe (1990) reported similar findings in patients with early PD.

Rafal and coworkers did not distinguish in their data analysis between cues to the right and left visual fields or for patients with unilateral and bilateral involvement. Because of the overall integrity of their patients' spatial orientation, it is probably safe to assume that neglect played no role in determining the results. This seems to contradict the results of Villardita and colleagues (1983) showing the occurrence of subclinical neglect in similar patients. One possible cause for the discrepancy could have been Rafal and colleagues' use of a discrete external cue prior to each imperative stimulus (exogenous covert orienting, see Chapter 2). This was not the case in the other study, which required an internally directed search in a cancellation task.

Cossa and colleagues (1989) tested bilateral Parkinson patients and age-matched controls under conditions similar to Rafal and colleagues' covert orienting task, but this time with an internal cue (memory driven). Their patients appeared to be helped by this information as much as the control subjects.

Several investigators have used the classic Stroop Test to assess PD patients' ability to restrict their attention to information presented in one *stimulus dimension* while overcoming the effect of interference by that presented simultaneously in another (Portin and Rinne, 1980; Cools et al., 1984; Heitanen and Teräväinen, 1986). Patients were found to be significantly slower in responding to color-word cards than healthy controls in the two Scandinavian studies. In neither study, however, were the data analyzed to separate interference from basic psychomotor slowing. In the study of Cools and colleagues (1984) the difference in performance between patients and controls on the Color-Word test was quite small and not statistically significant. They concluded that set-maintenance was no problem for their patients.

A further indication that *set-maintenance*, at least at the perceptual level, is not a problem comes from a study by Bradley and associates (1989) on visuospatial working memory in Parkinson's disease. They compared medicated, mildly to moderately impaired patients who had been screened for global cognitive deterioration, with a matched control group. They found no abnormal interference effects of irrelevant auditory and visual information on performance in tasks of verbal and visual working memory. However, the interference must have been very mild as it had no negative effect on performance in either group.

The studies described above were concerned with visual selective attention. Sharpe (1992) investigated auditory focused attention in early PD using a dichotic monitoring task requiring a push-button response to target words. She found some evidence for poorer focusing in the patients on one of her dependent variables, but the effect is hard to interpret as a description of experimental details was lacking.

To summarize, aspects of focused attention which have been shown to be unimpaired are: inhibiting a dominant response tendency, as seen in the Stroop Test, and covert orienting of visual attention (both with internal and external cues).

SPEED OF PROCESSING AND DIVIDED ATTENTION

Akinesia, the delayed initiation of a movement, and bradykinesia, its slow execution, are prominent symptoms of Parkinson disease which can be easily observed in almost any isolated motor activity (Marsden, 1982). In addition, "it has been repeatedly demonstrated that Parkinsonian patients are impaired in performance of simultaneous and sequential movements beyond and above the impairment shown in performing isolated movements" (Goldenberg et al., 1990, p. 139) (see also Schwab et al., 1954; Benecke et al., 1986; Horstink et al., 1990). Various explanations have been given for this, both at the level of motor control (Hallett and Khoshbin, 1980; Marsden, 1982), and more generally by postulating "an additional deficit of a general supervisor" (Goldenberg et al., 1990, p. 139). One reason for the latter notion is the observation that Parkinson patients tend to interrupt motor activity when a concurrent nonmotor task attracts their attention. A simple explanation for this is that previously automatic components of the motor activity have degenerated and now need to be replaced by components controlled by the supervisory attentional system. If the concurrent nonmotor tasks also requires supervisory attentional control, a divided attention deficit may occur, even if the capacity for controlled processing is itself normal. Further explanations have been offered, for example, that controlled processing capacity has declined and/or that higher order planning and regulating functions of the supervisory attentional system have declined in a qualitative way, over and above the capacity limitations. Karyandis (1989), for example, argued that the poorer performance of PD patients on tests of concept formation, planning, learning, memory and spatial organization can all be explained by a capacity limitation, namely, the reduced speed of information processing. On the other hand, specific impairments with regard to higher order cognitive functions have also been suggested as an explanation for the performance differences between PD patients and healthy controls. The merits of the latter possibility and the evidence with regard to mental slowness and capacity limitations will be assessed in the following section.

Capacity Limitations

The earliest mental chronometry studies usually involved the complexity factor, *simple versus choice RT*. In a pioneering study, before the introduction of levodopa, Talland (1963) tested 25 patients of varying severity and an age-matched control group using simple and choice visual RT tests involving a traffic light (right-hand response to green only in the simple condition; respectively, right and left hand response to green and red in the choice condition). The interstimulus intervals were short and variable and the stimulus light remained on until a response was made. The Parkinson patients as a group were not significantly slower, on either RT task, nor did they make more errors. No analysis of variance was done for interaction of complexity and groups, but the difference between simple and choice reaction was somewhat larger in the patient group (130 ms vs 96 ms). A subgroup of severely disabled patients were significantly slower than the rest of the patients and the control group, on both simple and choice RT tests.

Goodrich and colleagues (1989) reviewed subsequent studies comparing simple and choice reactions. None of them reported a significantly larger effect of Parkinson disease in the choice reaction time (CRT) than in the simple one. In fact, simple reaction time (SRT) was found to be more sensitive: "Such studies have either revealed a selective deficit, with significant impairment of SRT even when CRT cannot reliably be distinguished from that of age-matched controls . . . , or they found a dissociable deficit, in that while CRT was substantially improved by dopaminergic replacement therapy, SRT was scarcely affected" (Goodrich et al., 1989, p. 311).

Still, this differential effect on simple and choice RT may be partly dependent on the progression of the disease. In a recent study, Zimmermann and coworkers (1992) found that SRT (visual) is not impaired in untreated early PD patients, at least not in the decision time component. In advanced, medically treated PD patients, they again saw a greater effect of PD on SRT than on CRT. A peculiar result was that early PD patients' movement times were more influenced than advanced cases', relative to normal controls, by task complexity (i.e., simple versus choice RT and compatible versus incompatible responding). They tentatively attribute this to an alleviating effect of the L-dopa replacement therapy, which all of the advanced patients were receiving, on cognitive slowing. Alternative explanations in terms of qualitative differences in task control are possible as well. For example, it might be that normal controls are able to perform the movement almost without controlled processing but that in early PD patients it requires a certain amount of such control, at least in the CRT situation. If controlled processing has been completely committed to the decision process, it may cost additional time to shift control for the movement execution. The difference between advanced and early PD cases is explained by assuming that in advanced cases, movement execution always requires full controlled processing for SRT as well as CRT.

We will return to the possibility of qualitative differences in movement control, but for the present it suffices to conclude that the evidence from combined simple and choice RT studies does not support the idea of a capacity limitation with regard to controlled processing.

Of course, it could be argued that choice in a visual or tactual RT task does not depend upon controlled processing, and therefore no real distinction exists between SRT and CRT demands. In reply, we will now turn to studies in which the effects of a "more cognitive" symbolic manipulation were investigated. Wilson and colleagues (1980) administered the well-known *Sternberg Memory Scanning Task* to a group of nondemented Parkinson patients and an age-matched control group. Subjects were given a list of digits to memorize. They were then immediately shown a single digit and required to make a RT response indicating whether or not the number was a member of the previously memorized set. Memory scanning speed, which may be considered as the reciprocal of the rate of controlled processing, was derived from the slope of linear function relating reaction time (RT) to the number of digits in the memorized set. The results only revealed a slowing of memory scanning in the older Parkinson patients. Rafal and colleagues (1984) also used this paradigm in a study of Parkinson patients of varying severity, testing them both on and off levodopa medication. According to them: "The slope relating RT to set size in the range from 2 to 6 items is about 40 ms per item, which is well within the normal range for this age." In addition, Rafal and colleagues found no correlation between the rate of memory scanning and bradykinesia and dopaminergic dysfunction.

The *Paced Auditory Serial Addition Task* (PASAT) is another test presumed to load heavily on controlled processing (Gronwall and Sampson, 1974; see also Chapter 4). Gotham and colleagues (1988) and Brown and Marsden (1988) administered it to nondemented Parkinson patients, using both a fast and a slow rate of presentation (i.e., one digit per 2s and 4s, respectively). Patients made significantly more errors than healthy controls. However, the difference between the slow and fast condition was larger in the control group than in the patient group, in both studies. Also there was no interaction between on/off levodopa medication and the slow/fast variation of the PASAT. These consistent findings are an argument against an effect of capacity limitation on controlled processing in PD.

Perceptual Speed and Motor Preparation

The results reviewed above do not support the notion of general retardation of symbolic processing in PD. However, it cannot be denied that slower than normal reaction times are often found in this condition. If this is not the consequence of slower controlled processes, what other central components could be responsible? In very global terms, central components of reaction time may be divided into perception, decision, and motor preparation. The evidence with regard to the complexity effects discussed above is relevant to the speed of decision processes, but less so to the perceptual and preparatory motor components.

It is possible to estimate the speed of *central perceptual processes* in RT by recording P300, a long latency positive potential in the event-related EEG. It occurs when a subject detects an unexpected but relevant stimulus in the auditory, visual, or somatic modalities. Hansch and coworkers (1982) measured P300 latency in Parkinson patients and age-matched controls and found it significantly longer in the patients. Brouwer and Lakke (1983) and Bodis Wollner and colleagues (1984) also observed prolonged latencies in individual Parkinson patients. In the former study, 2 out of 5 patients had a P300 latency more than 2 sd's above the normal range. One of these patients was clinically demented. Goodin and Aminoff (1987) were also only able to find significantly delayed latencies in demented patients. Yet the relationship between dementia and P300 latency is a well-known phenomenon, and not specific to Parkinson's disease (see also Chapter 5).

In summary, these studies provide evidence for an effect of Parkinson's disease on the latency of P300 in demented PD patients only. There have also been a number of studies designed to show how P300 latencies vary with levodopa therapy in PD patients. A decreased P300 latency during the on levodopa phase compared to that during the off phase was described in two recent studies of nondemented Parkinson patients (Starkstein et al., 1989; Amabile et al., 1991). In the former, the mean latency decreased within the normal range from 336 to 324 ms. Amabile and colleagues stated that "preliminary data-analysis shows that in Parkinsonian patients, basal P300 latency is delayed in comparison with that of normal subjects of the same age. The P300 latency seems to be reduced by dopaminergic therapy . . . to the point that it does not significantly differ from the P300 of the control group" (p. 119). On the other hand, Prasher and Findley (1991) observed that P300 latency increased when newly diagnosed Parkinson patients were put on optimal levadopa treatment. Before treatment, their latencies were normal, but after treatment they were significantly longer than an untreated control group's. These results cannot be fully explained by progression of the disease over the treatment period. For the purpose of the present chapter, it may be concluded that perceptual impairments plays a minor role in the delayed reaction time of nondemented Parkinson patients.

We will now examine the role of impaired *preparatory motor processes* in prolonged RT of Parkinson patients. If a warning signal gives advance information about the subsequent response in a choice RT task (e.g., lifting the right or the left index finger), control subjects profit significantly more than mildly impaired Parkinson patients both at short and longer delays (Bloxham et al., 1984; see also Evarts et al., 1981). Interestingly, in this study Parkinson patients profited only from the warning signals preceding the imperative stimulus at short intervals (100 to 800 ms) and not at the long ones (3200 ms). Controls profited from the preparatory cue in both conditions. However, control subjects also lost the warning signal's advantage at the 3200 ms interval, while the advantage at the short intervals remained, in a divided attention condition where one hand was engaged in a simple rhythmic visual-motor task. The performance pattern of controls in the dual-task, which prevented them from sustaining the anticipated motor program, and Parkinson patients in the single task, were strikingly similar. Bloxham and colleagues (1987) suggested that performing the secondary task engenders "noise" and decreases the signal to noise ratio (S/N) of information processed within the basal ganglia. This mimicks the effect of Parkinson's disease which is thought to diminish S/N within information transmitted between the striatum and the adjacent prefrontal cortex.

Goodrich and colleagues (1989) also studied the ability to use advance information for controlling movement. They contrasted the simple and choice RT, both with and without a secondary task (reading aloud), in medicated Parkinson patients with mild to moderate affliction with that of healthy controls. The principal finding was mentioned earlier: after variable foreperiods, 1.5–3 seconds, patients' and controls' simple, tactual RTs differed more, absolutely and relatively, than they did with respect to CRT. However, the difference between patients' and controls' simple RTs disappeared in the dual-task condition, leading the authors to conclude that "These findings converge on the notion that the Parkinsonian deficit in simple RT is due to the impairment of an attention demanding process which facilitates RT performance when the required response is known in advance" (Goodrich et al., 1989, p. 309). These authors discussed various possible explanations for their results. They favored a description in terms of attentional resources, as described above, or of strategic adaptation: "In this view, the simple RT deficit is not the immediate and inevitable consequence of damage to some structure or resource required for efficient simple RT performance. Instead, it is an adaptation to the consequences of having a 'noisy' motor system, characterised by inaccurate execution of fast or forceful actions" (p. 328). As we have seen, the SRT effect is also partly dependent on the severity of the disease. The early patients are presumably still able to maintain a normal mode of movement programming and execution in a SRT situation.

Regarding speed of processing and divided attention it may be concluded that large differences exist between PD patients and controls in tasks requiring movement preparation and movement execution. When perceptual and cognitive processes are studied in conditions where motor impairment is controlled for, the effects are much smaller, at least in nondemented PD patients.

SUPERVISORY ATTENTIONAL CONTROL

It has often been noted that rapid shifting between target stimuli is particularly difficult for Parkinson patients (Talland and Schwab, 1964; Cools et al., 1984). Brown and Marsden (1988) incorporated an attention shifting requirement into the Stroop Test, using the Stroop paradigm with cued and noncued conditions. The cued condition is similar in concept to the classic Stroop Test except for the fact that the relevant dimension is more frequently alternated. They presented color words (RED or GREEN) singly, in conflicting colors (green or red) on a computer screen. After the presentation of a color word, the subject had to push an appropriate button, according to either the color or the meaning of the word. The relevant dimension, color or meaning, remained fixed for 10 trials. After 10 trials the command to "switch" was given on the screen, indicating that the relevant dimension had changed. The cue (Color or Meaning) was presented immediately prior to each word. The dependent variables measured were reaction time and number of errors. Appropriate control conditions with unconfounded words and colors were run.

Brown and Marsden presented this task to Parkinson patients and normals matched for age, sex, and education. Taking their basic psychomotor retardation (observed in the control task) into account, it appeared that the patients were *not* hindered more than the normals were in the interfering condition, in the cued part of the experiment. The first response after the "switch" command was significantly slower than the subsequent responses for both normals and patients. That this effect was not greater in the patients, suggests it is not the switch per sé which creates the problem: "This implies that the patients cannot be considered to have a generalized switching deficit, even in tasks when there are competing stimulus attributes. The theory of Cools and colleagues (1984) therefore seems untenable" (Brown and Marsden, 1988). However, something more should be said in defence of the "shifting hypothesis." As far as shifting tasks go, the one used in the cued condition was very simple. It could even be argued that the command to switch only provided redundant information in this experiment and that the lack of a specific effect in Parkinson's patients is irrelevant to the "switching hypothesis." We will return to this hypothesis following the discussion of the Brown and Marsden experiment.

A different pattern of results was seen in the noncued condition of the experiment. The command to switch relevant dimension was likewise given every tenth trial, but the stimuli were not preceded by external cues. Thus, subjects had to maintain internal control on the relevant dimension to avoid "switching" before the times indicated for them to do so. The patients were significantly impaired in this condition, both their errors and reaction time increased. This remained the case when their basic psychomotor retardation was taken into account. On the other hand, the control group's performance was almost identical in the cued and noncued conditions. Thus, Parkinson patients are impaired when forced to rely upon internal control for maintaining the relevant stimulus dimension.

Brown and Marsden adopted Baddeley's (1986) model of Working Memory for interpreting their results. Working memory (WM) was defined as the interface between current information and long-term memory. WM was divided into a central executive and a number of slave systems. The central executive functions as a supervisory attentional system (Shallice, 1982), applied to nonroutine cognitive tasks, where preprogrammed schemata are not available and/or suppression of some strong habitual response is required (see also Chapter 2). The supervisory attentional system was thought to be strongly capacity limited.

Brown and Marsden explained their results by suggesting that Parkinson patients have less supervisory attentional system capacity. Performance decreases when the difficulty of a cognitive task requires more capacity than is available. "Provided attentional resources are not overstretched, performance will be maintained despite increases in task demands" (p. 344). So, according to these authors, the qualitative difference between Parkinson patients and healthy controls with respect to ability for shifting attention can be explained by an underlying quantitative difference in their supervisory attentional system capacities. This explanation would be more convincing if no qualitative differences had existed between the tasks they applied and if some effect of switching had been seen in the control group. In fact, the control's performance hardly differed in the two conditions, despite the lack of obvious ceiling or floor limitations, as if the use of the internal cue was a very simple additional task for them.

Goldenberg and colleagues (1990, p. 140) proposed a hypothesis similar to Brown and Marsden's (1988), stating that "there is a weakness of the Supervisory Attentional System, which may cause a deficiency of dual task performance if it is required in a context where other demands on Supervisory Attentional Control are high." Remarkably, this statement follows a description of their own experiments on verbal and visual immediate memory (1989) in which they were unable to demonstrate any additional difficulties for Parkinson patients in dual tasks. However, they did find that Parkinson patients showed more intrusion from previous lists when four lists of six words had to be learned consecutively; but this effect was significant only in the single task condition.

Our opinion is that the evidence presented above does not strongly support an explanation for PD patients' difficulties in performing complex cognitive tasks as attributable to diminished WM capacity, or any other quantitative supervisory attentional system limitation. A further piece of evidence against this explanation was described in the section "Capacity Limitations" in Chapter 6: In nondemented PD patients' central capacity limitations in terms of speed of processing are small.

The next question is whether specific operations in the control of nonroutine cognitive tasks are impaired in PD patients. A global distinction with regard to supervisory attentional system control may be made between planning and regulation. For historical reasons, our discussion will address the regulation aspect first. Many studies with PD patients have been carried out using card-sorting tasks to assess concept-formation and concept-, or category-, shifting. Concept-shifting, particularly as it implies flexible inhibition of a previous selection set, may be seen as an important element of supervisory attentional system regulation. Of course, impaired performance in these tasks could be attributed to capacity limitations; but, it could also be due to an inability to carry out specific cognitive operations required for regulation, even when capacity is available. Such specific cognitive operations should be studied in situations involving a low demand on resources, or a limited set within almost any patient's capacity. Unfortunately, most studies, particularly the older ones making use of card sorting tests, did not meet this criterion.

Cognitive Flexibility and Concept-Shifting

Results from studies of animals with basal ganglia lesions suggested to Cools and coworkers (1984) that Parkinson patients might have a generally impaired ability for shifting between components of behavioral programs, manifested at the perceptual, cognitive, and motor levels. They tested nondemented Parkinson and control subjects, matched for age and intelligence, with

Two verbal fluency tasks

Two category-shifting tasks, one figural and one verbal, requiring shifts of the sorting dimension,

A finger-tapping test, requiring a shift between two different motor sequences

The authors considered the verbal fluency tasks as a specific test of set-shifting, that is, the subjects had to name as many animals, then occupations, as possible within successive 1-minute periods. In the two other task domains, category shifting and tapping, experimental conditions with and without switching were compared.

The patients performed significantly worse than controls in all three tasks with a switching requirement. However, only in the motor sequences differences remained significant, when correction was made for group differences when the tests were done without switching. Correlations between scores from the shift conditions were relatively low for both controls and patients, but slightly higher for the patients. In spite of this rather shaky evidence, the authors interpreted their results "as reflecting a central programming deficit that manifests itself in verbal, figural and motor modalities, that is a diminished 'shifting aptitude' characteristic of patients with dysfunctioning basal ganglia" (p. 443). In our opinion, their results might still be explained by a quantitative difference between PD patients and controls in processing resources, with the probable exception of the motor sequences.

Card Sorting Tasks

Following this and similar research, more detailed studies of shifting aptitude were carried out with category shifting (card sorting) tasks and tasks of verbal fluency. In this section we will only discuss category shifting as recent studies on verbal fluency have indicated that the slightly impaired performance of Parkinson patients in these tasks is neither dependent on switching requirements (Gurd and Ward, 1988) nor related to the disease process (Hanley et al., 1990).

Evidence for *impaired category shifting* in both medicated and non-medicated patients has been obtained with the Wisconsin Card Sorting Test (WCST) (Milner, 1963). A subject begins the WCST holding a deck of 64 cards. Each is imprinted with a unique combination that can vary in three dimensions—color, shape, and number. He is instructed which dimension is relevant for sorting the cards into four separate piles. Locations for these are indicated by (1) one red triangle, (2) two green stars, (3) three yellow crosses, and (4) four blue circles. Given the instruction to sort for the color blue, the subject should place every card bearing symbols of that color, irrespective of their shape or number, on pile 4; the same for cards bearing yellow symbols on pile 3, green on pile 2, and red on pile 1. He is informed after every classification whether it was correct or not. The relevant dimension is changed by the experimenter after 10 correct classifications. In some experiments forewarning is given that such shifts will occur (Nelson, 1976; Brown and Marsden, 1988). In the original version, the

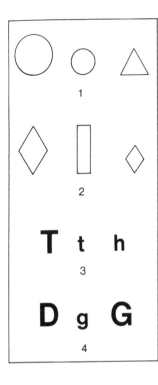

Figure 6-2 The Odd Man Out Test. Subjects have to indicate which of the three items on each card they think is different from the other two, using one of two possible rules. *Shapes sets, 1* and *2*: subjects choose either according to shape (triangle in *1*, rectangle in *2*) or according to size (large circle in *1*, small diamond in *2*). *Letter sets, 3* and *4*: subjects choose either according to letter (h in *3*, D in *4*) or according to size (T in *3*, g in *4*). Subjects are free to choose either rule on the first set, but must then apply it consistently throughout Trial 1. They must then apply the other rule on Trial 2, and alternate the two rules on later trials. (From Flowers and Robertson, 1985, with permission.)

shift following 10 consecutive correct choices was not announced (Milner, 1963; A. E. Taylor et al., 1987). The WCST was originally used to study difficulties with concept formation and concept shifting in neurological patients suffering frontal lobe damage. Later studies have shown that poor performance on the WCST alone cannot be interpreted as an index of frontal lobe damage (Anderson et al., 1991).

Parkinson patients achieve fewer sorting categories and make more errors than controls, but the deficits are much smaller than those associated with frontal lobe lesions (see Downes et al., 1989, and Goldenberg et al., 1990, for reviews). Parkinson patients are significantly impaired on this test, even those selected after rigorous screening for diffuse cognitive impairment (Caltagirone et al., 1989). Set shifting problems have also been demonstrated with other sorting tasks, such as the Odd Man Out Test (Flowers and Robertson, 1985) (see Figure 6-2).

Extradimensional Shifting

One of the problems with card sorting tests is that impaired performance may be based on multiple deficits. The large demand they place on WM capacity is most relevant to our discussion. For example, in a number of studies PD patients and controls already differ significantly in the number of cards it takes them to obtain the first correct category before any shifting is required (Taylor et al., 1986; Karyandis, 1989). Downes and coworkers (1989) suggested four possible causes of poor performance and stated that such tests "appear most analogous to the paradigms of intra- and extradimensional shift used in the human and animal learning literature" (p. 1330). In intradimensional shift, a sorting dimension, for example, color, remains valid but the cards have to be sorted according to a different feature of that dimension. For example, cards with red figures have to be sorted into one pile and cards with other colors into a second pile; after the switch, cards with blue figures must be sorted into the first pile and all other colors into the second. The WCST does not include this condition.

With extradimensional shift (EDS), the sorting dimension itself is switched. Downes and colleagues (1989) stated that "the WCST can be seen as comprising a form of EDS but one in which the contingencies are not controlled with the same rigor as in studies on dimensional shifts and, because only a restricted set of four values are used for each dimension, true transfer to novel exemplars cannot be evaluated" (p. 1330). Also, the WCST is a difficult task because the high number of combinations of colors, shapes and numbers place a large demand on working memory. Downes and colleagues (1989) subsequently developed a computerized test of visual discrimination learning following intra- and extra-dimensional shifts which does not have these disadvantages. In addition to dimensional switching, this test requires searching and matching-to-sample of complex visual stimuli. A separate computerized test was designed to study the effects of figural complexity on visual search and matching-to-sample as a control condition.

Downes and colleagues' concept-shifting task had nine stages. At each stage four boxes were displayed on a screen, one in each quadrant. Two different boxes at each stage contained a pattern, either solid or lined. The subjects' task was to indicate the correct box; audiovisual feedback was given about the choice. For each of the two dimensions there were six values, filled or lined patterns, two of which matched. A subject proceeded to the next stage when six consecutive matches had been made. The test was aborted when more than 50 choices were needed to complete a stage.

Stage 1: simple simultaneous discrimination. Subjects were presented with one dimension, half of the subjects with solid patterns, the other half with line drawings. A dimension had two values, pattern 1 or 2 or line drawing 1 or 2. The subject must consistently point to one of these values.

Stage 2: value switch. The dimension stays the same, but the relevant value is switched. The subject must consistently point to the other value.

Stage 3: compound discrimination—separate. As stage 2, simultaneous presentation (in the same boxes) of two stimuli (values) from the other dimension. The stimuli are irrelevant and the subject must respond according to the instruction given for stage 2.

Stage 4: compound discrimination. As stage 3, but the stimuli of the two dimensions are superimposed, a line drawing on a filled pattern. The subject must respond according to instructions given for stages 2 and 3.

Stage 5: compound discrimination—reversal. The relevant dimension stays the same, but the relevant value is switched again so that the subject must consistently point to the other value (as in stage 1).

Stage 6: intradimensional-shift. New stimuli (values) are used for both dimensions, but the relevant dimension stays the same. The subject must consistently point to one of two new values.

Stage 7: reversal after intradimensional shift. The dimension stays the same but the relevance of the values is switched.

Stage 8: extradimensional shift. The previously relevant dimension becomes irrelevant and new values are offered for each new dimension. The subject must consistently point to one of the values of the new relevant dimension.

Stage 9: reversal after extradimensional shift. The dimension stays the same but the relevance of the values is switched.

The dimensional shift series and the control test were administered to three groups: mildly affected, unmedicated patients; patients at a more advanced stage of the disease who were currently on antiparkinsonian medication; and a group of healthy controls. The three groups were matched for age and verbal IQ (WAIS) and neither patient group showed signs of global cognitive deterioration.

In the control condition, the matching-to-sample/visual search paradigm revealed only minor impairment in the patients. Although they moved more slowly and made slightly more errors overall, they were not disproportionally impaired in selection of the matching stimulus when the level of difficulty was increased.

It appeared that the "simple" reversals at stages 2, 5, 7, and 9 were not a problem for the patients, nor was the intradimensional shift. In contrast, the extradimensional shift at stage 8 was very problematic for them. The experiment had to be aborted at the extradimensional shift stage in 35 percent of the medicated patients, and in 65 percent of the unmedicated patients. In the control group this occurred in only 10 percent.

Downes and colleagues (1989) pointed to the interesting fact that the problem appears to be greater in the unmedicated mild group. They also referred to a pilot study that demonstrated a double dissociation between Alzheimer's and Parkinson's diseases. Early Alzheimer patients were poor in the matching-to-sample tasks but good in extradimensional shift, while the reverse was seen in Parkinson patients. These two preliminary results revealed a very specific effect of Parkinson's Disease which cannot be attributed to negative effects of medication or global cognitive deterioration.

Although Downes and colleagues thought that the poor extradimensional shift performance in Parkinson patients may be caused by a form of frontal lobe dysfunction, they cautioned against an interpretation based on perseverative tendencies, as neither intradimensional shift nor other reversals of values posed problems for the patients; and because visual search in the matching-to-sample tasks was normal (see also Freedman, 1990). Also "From the subjective reports of many of the subjects who failed the EDS, it is apparent that they were not perseverating with the previously relevant dimension but were entertaining a large number of diverse and sophisticated rules, based mainly on presumptions about sequences of failure and success."

The investigators discussed the possibility that Parkinson patients are abnormally sensitive to the phenomenon of "learned irrelevance": "Thus it is possible that failure to complete the EDS may result from an enhanced tendency to ignore a previously irrelevant stimulus dimension, rather than a failure to shift from the one previously relevant" (p. 1341).

Whatever the precise cause of the problem with extradimensional shift, it appears that for the Parkinson patient it is not so much the strength of the previously relevant concept, but the weakness of the new alternatives. This leads to instability of the response set, but not necessarily to increased perseveration (see also Flowers et al., 1985 and Freedman, 1990). It is possible that the supervisory attentional system is able to inhibit irrelevant response tendencies, but unable to plan alternative strategies and/or regulate their execution.

Cognitive Planning

One manner of assessing the ability to generate and execute goal-directed strategies in non-routine situations is with the aid of The Tower of London Test (Shallice, 1982). This is a look-ahead puzzle, specifically constructed to assess the role of supervisory attentional system in planning, without confounding by capacity limitations. Solving the more difficult problems correctly involves planning several steps ahead and pursuing subgoals that initially appear to lead away from the final solution. (This test is described in greater detail in Chapter 5.)

In the two studies by Morris and colleagues (1988) and Goldenberg and colleagues (1990), the test was not, regrettably, administered in the form described by Shallice. Thus, the data cannot be compared directly with that from left prefrontal patients. In the original version, the subject is told the number of moves needed to solve each problem. The important dependent variables are the number of problems solved at one attempt and the total number of problems solved. In the two studies on non-demented Parkinson patients, the number of moves was not specified in advance but was taken as a dependent variable. No difference between patients and healthy controls was found in either study using this variable.

Morris and colleagues (1988) also found that the patients needed significantly more decision time for correct solutions. They concluded that "the results are clear in showing a specific planning deficit in this group." Goldenberg and colleagues (1990) disagreed with this conclusion and argued that slowness could be the consequence of a particularly self-critical attitude. It might also be said that the use of time as a dependent variable introduces an external resource limitation (namely, time), limiting the value of the test as a method for studying a specific ability, independent of resource limitations. In left frontal patients, the planning deficit is seen in situations without time-pressure (Shallice, 1982; Owen et al., 1990). Taking these two arguments into account, no evidence exists as yet to show that Parkinson patients have impaired planning ability. The problem must lie in regulating the execution of planned strategies rather than in forming the strategies.

To summarize this section, it has been shown that Parkinson patients perform poorly on categorization tasks in which the dimension to categorize on is frequently shifted. This impairment is also seen in patients with damage to the prefrontal cortex. Poor performance cannot be explained by perseverance with the previous set, nor by impaired ability to plan an alternative strategy. In this respect, performance of PD patients clearly differs from the performance of patients with orbitofrontal damage or Alzheimer's disease (Freedman, 1990).

The relationships between impaired performance in extradimensional shift tasks and impaired memory for temporal information might provide an interesting subject for study (Sahakian et al., 1988). Sagar and colleagues (1988) showed that temporal information (ranging between 1 and 150 s) was retained relatively more poorly than content information in Parkinson patients (an unselected group of 15 medicated patients) than in healthy controls. Fifteen early Alzheimer patients were also tested and performed poorly both on content and temporal information. The performance pattern in Parkinson patients is reminiscent of source amnesia (forgetting the origin but not the content) and the impaired temporal order recall that follows restricted surgical lesions of the prefrontal cortex (see Taylor et al., 1990). In an extradimensional shifting task, such a problem could result in the memory that a category is irrelevant without the qualification *when* it is irrelevant. This time cue is very important in any situation where the relevance of dimensions is regularly switched and in which no clear external cues are given. An impairment of this type might also increase sensitivity to proactive interference (e.g., Goldenberg et al., 1990) resulting in relatively poor performance in the uncued condition of the modified Stroop Test (Brown and Marsden, 1988).

SUMMARY

Research on cognitive impairments in PD patients was largely inspired by animal models of basal ganglia dysfunction. Consequently, research has focused on impaired concept-shifting aptitude and impairments resembling the effects of frontal lobe lesions.

Focused visual attention seems to be normal in PD. Aspects of focused attention which have been shown to be unimpaired are: inhibition of a dominant response tendency as revealed in the Stroop task, covert orienting of visual attention, both with internal and external cues, and sustaining a perceptual set, as in delayed match to sample tasks.

Speed of information processing is also apparently normal in Parkinson patients, that is, there is little evidence for decreased speed of cognitive operations. This has been demonstrated in choice reaction time tests, memory scanning tests and the PASAT. The slowness of PD patients in timed tasks could be explained by impaired movement preparation processes, for example, they are not able to benefit from precues for specific motor activities required in choice RT tasks.

Divided attention: although the motor problems of Parkinson patients are often aggravated when different actions have to be performed simultaneously, there is remarkably little evidence for impairment of divided attention in dual-tasks with low motor requirements. For example, in a dual task situation in which a simple RT task must be combined with a completely different task, that is, reading aloud, simple RT increases less in patients than in healthy controls.

The only cognitive tasks in which problems have been consistently observed are so-called *concept shifting* tasks. In such tasks stimuli must be categorized according to stimulus dimensions which vary in such a way that previously irrelevant dimensions become relevant, and vice versa. Extradimensional shifts, in particular, present a problem for PD patients. The main difficulty does not appear to be perseveration from previously valid dimension, but may be overcoming the irrelevance of the dimension which has become valid. Attempts have been made to explain the diminished shifting ability as a weakness of the supervisory attentional system, especially as a capacity limitation of this system. The evidence for this hypothesis is not convincing, however. We would suggest a more specific hypothesis to explain the problems that patients have with category shifting tasks: impaired memory for temporal context information. The time cue may be essential in a situation where the relevance of dimensions is regularly switched.

7

Epilepsy

The term *epilepsy* covers a wide variety of clinical phenomena. It does not refer to a disease but to a bioelectrical "symptom." Hughlings Jackson defined epilepsy as "an occasional, excessive and disorderly discharge of nerve tissue." Among laymen it is one of the better known neurological conditions. In earlier times it was regarded as a sacred disease; the fit caused by the excessive discharge of nerve tissue was assumed to indicate divine intervention in the activities of the victim.

Epilepsy is a fairly common neurological condition. Prevalence rates tend to cluster between 3 and 6 per 1000 population. According to Hauser (1978), this variance in prevalence is due to problems in selection and definition. As he points out, the numbers probably reflect the proportion of epileptic patients under active treatment with medication. It may be assumed, however, that a certain proportion of subtle epileptic phenomena remains unrecognized. The phenomena popularly known as fits, seizures, convulsions, or attacks vary widely in their appearance and are therefore not easily defined. A feature common to all epileptic phenomena is disturbed consciousness. This may range from a lowering of consciousness for a few seconds to a complete loss of consciousness for many minutes or even hours. The International Clinical and Electroencephalographic Classification of Epileptic Seizures (Dreifuss et al., 1981; see Table 7-1) makes a fundamental distinction between generalized seizures and partial seizures. The former are said to originate in pathology of a centrencephalic integrating system (Penfield, 1952). Abnormal electrical discharges in this pacemaker system would cause loss of consciousness and a generalized seizure. However, it has been suggested that some forms of generalized epilepsy are caused not by pathology in the centrencephalic pacemaker but by generalized hyperexcitability of cortical neurons (Gloor et al., 1979).

Partial seizures have their origin in a circumscribed focus, usually in the temporal or frontal lobe. Consciousness is not initially disturbed; hence the patients are aware of sensations caused by the abnormal discharges in part of their brain. Very frequently, however, a partial seizure develops into a generalized one, in which case consciousness is lost and the episode is described as a secondary generalized seizure. The clinical manifestations of partial seizures are heterogeneous, as shown in Table 7-1, and will not be expanded on here. Diagnosis of a particular kind of epilepsy is based on the clinical manifestation of

Table 7-1   The Revised Seizure Classification as Proposed by the Commission on Classification and Terminology

I. Partial (focal, local) seizures
   A. Simple partial seizures (consciousness not impaired)
     1. With motor signs
     2. With somatosensory or special sensory symptoms
     3. With autonomic symptoms or signs
     4. With psychic symptoms
   B. Complex partial seizures (impairment of consciousness)
     1. Simple partial onset, followed by impairment of consciousness
     2. With impairment of consciousness at onset
   C. Partial seizures evolving to secondarily generalized seizures
     1. Simple partial, evolving to generalized
     2. Complex partial, evolving to generalized
     3. Simple partial, evolving to complex partial, evolving to generalized seizures
II. Generalized seizures
   A. Absence seizures
     1. Typical absences
     2. Atypical absences
   B. Myoclonic seizures
   C. Clonic seizures
   D. Tonic seizures
   E. Tonic-clonic seizures
   F. Atonic seizures (astatic)
III. Unclassified epileptic seizures

From Dreifuss et al., 1981, with permission.

the seizures and on EEG patterns. In practice, the diagnosis often remains difficult, which explains the presence of the category "unclassifiable seizures" in the International Classification.

This classification is based on symptomatology rather than etiology. In the etiology of epilepsies, a major distinction is made between idiopathic and symptomatic epilepsy. In idiopathic epilepsy, sometimes also called essential or cryptogenic, the etiology is unknown. According to Hauser (1978), between 65 and 75 percent of identified cases are idiopathic.

Shorvon (1984) points out that an epileptic seizure is an expression of disordered physiology, and almost any condition affecting the fine balance of neural functioning may precipitate a seizure. Thus, almost all gray-matter diseases, many white-matter diseases, most metabolic disorders and many systemic diseases may cause epileptic seizures of some sort. Still, as noted above, most epilepsies are diagnosed as idiopathic as the actual cause cannot be determined. If the etiology is known, the epilepsy is called symptomatic. A common etiology is trauma where head injury leaves scar tissue in the brain that forms an epileptic focus (Jennett, 1982).

COGNITIVE IMPAIRMENT IN EPILEPSY

Most people with epilepsy can live completely normal lives. It is possible to control seizures in most patients with skillful use of clinical and electroencephalographic measures, and serum level monitoring. It has been reported that approximately 80 to 85 percent of all cases can be controlled. Although the statement has been challenged (Rodin, 1968; Laidlaw and Richens, 1982), the fact remains that most epileptic patients are never recognized as such within their social environments. People with epilepsy can write classic novels (Dostoyevsky), become proverbial for virtuosity (Paganini), or be able teachers, taxi drivers, and so on.

This suggests that epilepsy does not necessarily affect cognitive functions. Nevertheless, clinical observers in the nineteenth century were convinced that an intellectual decline occurred in patients who had suffered from epilepsy for many years. Reynolds (1861) concluded that two-thirds of chronic epileptic patients were in some way affected in their intellectual abilities. On the basis of such reports, it was generally assumed that people with epilepsy were prone to dementia, and the concept of *epileptic dementia* was a part of earlier psychiatric teaching (Betts, 1982). More recent research has indicated that a decline in cognitive functioning occurs only in patients with severe epilepsy and uncontrollable seizures (Dikmen and Matthews, 1977). In a 1986 literature review Lesser and associates found very little evidence for cognitive deterioration in the majority of epilepsy patients. Trimble (1988) observed: "It would seem that patients most at risk are those who have continuing seizures, mainly of a generalized tonic-clonic type, during which they fall and suffer recurrent head injuries."

Still, among students of cognitive functioning in epileptics there is a widespread belief that more subtle impairments may be found, even in patients whose seizures can be controlled. Dodrill (1978) introduced a neuropsychological test battery for epilepsy, an extended and improved version of the Halstead-Reitan battery (Reitan, 1966). The tests were specifically aimed at "neuropsychological impairments often seen in epileptics regardless of their sources (brain damage, anticonvulsants, seizures themselves, etc.) or associated variables (seizure type, age at onset, EEG epileptiform discharges, etc.)." Dodrill mentions memory, sustained attention and verbal problem solving as areas of special importance in clinical work with epileptics. Thompson and Huppert (1980) state that short-term memory impairment, mental slowing, and poor concentration are particularly common complaints among epileptics. By contrast, Alpherts (1986, in Brons and Arts, 1987) estimated that less than 5 percent of the outpatient population at a specialized epilepsy clinic in The Netherlands reported complaints about cognitive functioning. Surprisingly, a well-known textbook on epilepsy (Laidlaw and Richens, 1982) does not describe what, exactly, epileptic patients are complaining about in the cognitive domain. Moreover, in the index of this book the words attention, cognition, concentration, and vigilance are absent.

The impression exists that subjective *complaints* by epileptic patients have not as yet been studied on a large epidemiological scale. There is, of course, a special problem in the study of subjective complaints in epileptics: many patients have been suffering from epilepsy since childhood and are therefore unable to note subtle impairments in themselves. By contrast, adults who sustain severe head injuries or cerebrovascular accidents may experience a sudden reduction of cognitive skills. They can compare their present level of functioning with their personal past, and can usually give an accurate description of any changes.

Although much research has been aimed at *objective assessment* of cognitive impairments in epilepsy in the past 20 years, this has not yielded a clear and complete picture. This is largely due to severe methodological problems, that is, the fact that nearly all epileptics are under treatment with anticonvulsants, making it hard to distinguish between the effect of the epileptic condition and the effect of the drug on cognitive functioning. Further problematic variables in this area are the etiology, the frequency of seizures, age of onset, and duration of epilepsy, and interference of frequent seizures with education and intellectual development (Dikmen et al., 1975; Dikmen and Matthews, 1977).

In this chapter we review attention impairments in epileptics. Two approaches have been taken to the study of such impairments. First, groups of patients have been tested to determine whether they performed worse than control groups on tests sensitive to "attention," such as the Stroop Color Word Test, the Trail-making Test and dichotic listening. These results are mainly relevant to focused attention and divided attention. Secondly, investigators have shown a great and lasting interest in the disruption of cognitive processes by epileptic phenomena. While a manifest seizure will, of course, interrupt all attentive behavior, there are more subtle, subclinical phenomena affecting information processing. The diagnosis of epilepsy is primarily based on EEG recordings made between seizures, where the patient makes a perfectly "normal" impression on the clinical observer. In a vast majority of cases, these interictal recordings show disturbances of brain function, in particular short episodes of spike-wave bursts (see Figure 7-1). These episodes are accompanied by a lowering of consciousness known as a "trough of consciousness." At the behavioral level these episodes result in transitory cognitive impairments (Aarts et al., 1984). This concept is clearly related to attention lapses and will be reviewed in the section on sustained attention below.

An important question in neuropsychological research with epileptic patients is: Do anticonvulsants affect aspects of attention? While this issue may appear to be outside the scope of this book as the influence of chemical substances on the brain is not considered in the rest of the volume, anticonvulsants are so closely linked to epilepsy that the chapter would be incomplete without mentioning them.

FOCUSED ATTENTION

When Dodrill (1978) presented his neuropsychological battery for the assessment of epileptic patients, he included two tests that were assumed to tap certain aspects of attention: the Seashore Tonal Memory Test (Seashore et al., 1960) and the Stroop Color-Word Test (Stroop, 1935). The Trailmaking Test parts A and B were already part of the Halstead-Reitan battery. Dodrill did not specify which aspects of attention were assumed to be tested with these methods, although it is clear that all three of them demand "concentration" and a conscious

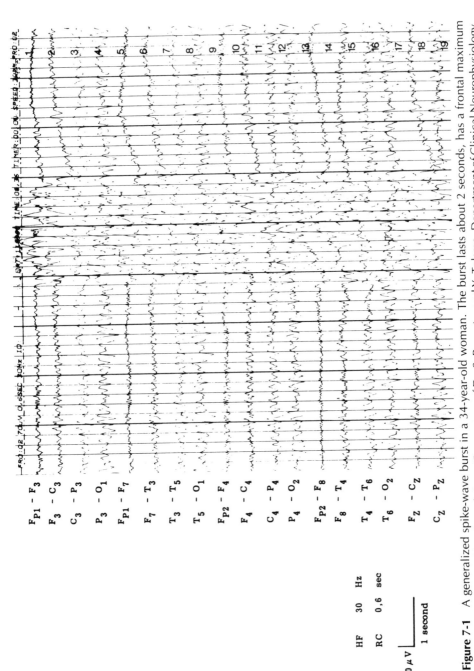

Figure 7-1 A generalized spike-wave burst in a 34-year-old woman. The burst lasts about 2 seconds, has a frontal maximum and is not accompanied by clinical signs. (By courtesy of Dr. S. Boonstra and Y. Talsma, Department of Clinical Neurophysiology, State University Groningen.)

effort. The Stroop Test can certainly be viewed as a test of focused attention, since one dimension of its stimuli serves as a distractor in the task.

In the form devised by Dodrill, the Color-Word Test consisted of a printed sheet with color names such as "blue" and "green," printed in incongruous colors such as red and orange. In the first part of the test, the subject simply read the words as printed, regardless of the colors in which they appeared. In the second part, however, the subject had to name the colors of the ink in which the words were printed and ignore the word meaning. This latter part requires extreme concentration, according to the author, in order to prevent "slipping" in to the major set (reading). Please note that this procedure is somewhat different from the usual one; Dodrill compared speed of reading to speed of color naming with distraction. The usual comparison is between color naming with and without distraction.

In the study, 50 epileptic patients were tested, with a mean age of 27.4 years and a mean duration of illness of 14.9 years. Etiology and type of seizure were mixed. EEGs were abnormal in 48 of the 50 subjects, and all patients were taking anticonvulsants. A control group of nonepileptic subjects well-matched for age, sex, and educational level was also tested.

The epileptics were significantly slower than the controls on both tasks. Reading the ambiguous words took an average of 88.6 seconds in the control group and 111.8 seconds in the patient group—a difference of 26 percent when taking the normal time score as a basis. Naming the colors of the same stimuli took 225.8 seconds in the control group and 307.7 seconds in the epileptic group—an increase of 36 percent. These findings indicate that focused attention was somewhat poorer in the group of epileptics of mixed etiology. Dodrill noted in the discussion of his study that no effort was made to separate the effects of anticonvulsants, brain damage, and/or seizures themselves, under the presumption that one would then be evaluating the net effects of the condition "epilepsy" on test performance.

DIVIDED ATTENTION

Divided attention cannot be assumed to be completely normal in epileptics during interictal periods. A certain slowness in RT tasks has been reported by several investigators, even where background EEG was normal at the time of performance (Prechtl et al., 1961; Bruhn and Parsons, 1977). This justifies the assumption that some epileptics will reveal divided attention deficits (DAD) in tasks that can be performed adequately by subjects in whom this mental slowness is absent. However, even if such an effect could be demonstrated, its cause remains unclear: the underlying factor might be the etiology of the epilepsy in the case of symptomatic epilepsies such as the posttraumatic epilepsy, or it might be a side effect of anticonvulsant drugs. An adequate test of DAD, the PASAT has been used in a study of epileptic patients (Reinvang et al., 1991). In this study, however, the test was used to determine the effects of serum concentrations of carbamazepine with the patients serving as their own controls. As a result, the findings cannot be compared with normal performance.

The dichotic listening paradigm can be considered a divided attention task as subjects are expected to attend to two input channels with simultaneous stimulation. Gorman and colleagues (1990) reported that dichotic listening was more sensitive to cerebral dysfunction in patients with multiple seizure symptoms than standard EEG. In a sample of 225 patients, 73 percent failed dichotic listening, while only 38 percent showed EEG abnormalities. The investigators thought that dichotic listening performance may have been disrupted by subclinical electrophysiological dysfunction. Roberts and colleagues (1990) studied 24 patients with multiple symptoms of untreated complex partial seizures. The patients performed poorly at a baseline assessment of dichotic word listening but their performance improved significantly following anticonvulsant therapy. These studies suggest that in the absence of macroscopic structural lesions, dynamic electrophysiological dysfunction may interfere with the processing and transmission of simultaneously presented auditory information.

From a theoretical point of view, it is interesting to consider spike-wave discharges as periods of increased "neural noise" in the brain. An increase of neural noise reduces the channel capacity of the information-processing system, resulting in a slowing of decision making. Roberts et al. thought that the anticonvulsant therapy improved dichotic listening by reducing electrophysiologic dysfunction, that is, reducing noise. This view is supported by earlier studies of Hutt and coworkers (1977), who found that the effect of spike-wave bursts was proportional to the information-processing demands of the task: "the greater the amount of information presented per stimulus, the greater the impairment."

If it is correct to say that dichotic listening in epileptic patients can be disrupted by a brief increase in neural noise, the question arises whether this should be called a divided attention deficit. One could say that it is a bit misleading to use the term DAD for impairments that are so clearly limited in duration, and that it should be applied instead when an individual's processing capacity falls short while his level of consciousness remains adequate for the task at hand. In other words, divided attention might be normal in an epileptic patient as long as his background EEG is normal. It may be assumed that an epileptic patient will be more vulnerable than a nonepileptic to DADs only when it can be demonstrated that the epileptic has prolonged reaction times even in the absence of abnormal electrophysiologic activity in his EEG during the test.

SUSTAINED ATTENTION

Studies on Task Level

In sustained attention studies, task performance is analyzed over periods that may range from a few minutes to several hours. The tasks involve three phenomena: time-on-task effects, intraindividual variability, and lapses of attention.

Pioneer work using the Continuous Performance Test (CPT) was done by Mirsky and coworkers (1960) (Rosvold et al., 1956). In their paper introducing this test, the authors stated that the design of the CPT was based on electroencephalographic evidence which suggested that brain-damaged individuals are less capable of performing tasks that require sustained attention or alertness. The waking EEGs of brain-damaged patients generally show either random bursts of hypersynchronous (high amplitude) activity intruding upon the normal activity of the brain or a general hypersynchronicity. Hypersynchronous activity is also evident in recordings from sleeping subjects. If hypersynchrony is associated with reduced vigilance, as its presence during sleep suggests, then the hypersynchronicity of brain-damaged patients might also indicate reduced attention. The authors assumed that the intermittent bursts of hypersynchronous activity would result in lapses of attention. Such lapses are usually not picked up by short-lasting attention tests such as Digit Span and Digit Symbol Substitution in the WAIS. Hence, a longer lasting test was required to assess vigilance, alertness or sustained attention.

The CPT was designed to provide two attention tasks, labeled X and AX. In the X task subjects faced a display on which a random series of letters appeared. They were instructed to respond to the appearance of the letter X by pressing a key. The A version lasted 10 minutes and contained 160 possible correct responses. In the AX version, X was considered a target letter only if it were preceded by an A—which in fact meant that the letter A began to function as a warning signal that was occasionally followed by the imperative X. The AX version likewise lasted 10 minutes and contained 120 possible correct responses.

Rosvold and colleagues tested 25 adults of mixed etiology with this procedure. The group consisted of "either epileptics being treated at a seizure clinic, or brain surgery patients being seen at a neurosurgery clinic." Results were presented as percentages of correct responses. In the X condition, a control group obtained a hit rate of 88 percent, while the mixed patient group had a hit rate of 79 percent, the difference being non-significant. In the AX condition, hit rates were somewhat lower in both groups: 79 percent in the control group, and 61 percent in the brain-damaged group ($p < .01$). The authors concluded that brain-damaged individuals perform poorly relative to non-brain-damaged controls on a task requiring continuous attention. The results also indicate, in their view, that on a task designed "to require even more sustained attention" brain-damaged individuals perform even more poorly. Rosvold et al. admit that the data do not allow for a distinction between lapses of attention and a lowering of the general level of signal detection as a cause of missing signals. Nor do their findings lead to the conclusion that impaired CPT performance is indeed related to hypersynchronicity, a relationship that could only be proven by means of on-line EEG recordings during the test.

Subsequent studies by the same group (Mirsky et al., 1960; Lansdell and Mirsky, 1964) specifically targeted attentional impairments in epileptics, with special emphasis on performance differences between patients with generalized seizures and patients with focal seizures. In the 1960 study, 19 patients with centrencephalic epilepsy performed worse on the CPT than patients with epileptic foci in the frontal or temporal lobes. Hit rate percentages on the AX condition of the CPT were as follows: controls 78.8 percent, frontal epileptics 82.5 percent, temporal epileptics 87.0 percent, and centrencephalics 57.7 percent. The results have been interpreted as showing that maintenance of attention as tested with the CPT is partly dependent on the integrity of central subcortical structures.

Bruhn (1970) studied sustained attention in patients with subcortical epilepsy by means of a continuous reaction test. His subjects were epileptics who exhibited generalized paroxysms of high amplitude, slow waves and spikes in their clinical EEGs. These patients, along with 15 hospital staff controls, were tested with an apparatus presenting 12 stimulus lights in a horizontal row. Stimuli appeared in random order and had to be switched off by pushing the lights as quickly as possible. The task was paced, with lights flashing at 1-second intervals whether or not the subject responded to the preceding stimulus. At this fixed rate 200 stimuli were presented over an interval of about 3.5 minutes. The optimal performance level (OPL) was determined for each individual as the shortest RT recorded at least 20 times. In the control group mean OPL was 510 ms, and in the epileptic group it was 570 ms. Next, the number of delayed reactions (DR) was calculated for each subject as the number of RTs exceeding the OPL by at least 100 ms. DRs were far more frequent in the patient group: in the control group 7.6 percent of responses were delayed, while in the patient group 37.1 percent of the responses were delayed. Even more striking was the frequency of nonreactions: of the 3000 responses recorded from the control group, on only 6 occasions did the subject not respond at all to a stimulus. In the epileptic group this occurred 216 times (or 7 percent of all reactions). In a further analysis of delayed reactions, Bruhn demonstrated that DRs tended to appear more frequently in clusters in the patient group. Assuming that DRs indicate fluctuations in vigilance, he pointed out that only one out of fifteen controls showed fluctuations exceeding 3 seconds, while almost all epileptics (14 out of 15) had fluctuations lasting more than 3 seconds. In his view these fluctuations reflected dysfunction of the reticular activating system related to "subcortical" epilepsy.

In a second investigation a wider range of epileptic patients was studied, again with a continuous reaction task (Bruhn and Parsons, 1977). The patient group consisted of 63 epileptics whose diagnosis was based solely on the presence of manifest epileptic seizures. No restrictions as to origin, etiology, type and frequency of seizures, or presence of EEG abnormalities were applied to this group. In fact, 25 of these patients had normal EEGs despite their clinically manifest epilepsy. The control group was comprised of patients diagnosed as having peripheral neurological disorders. The RT apparatus displayed three red diode lamps lighted in random order with a variable interstimulus interval. Subjects were instructed to terminate the stimuli as quickly as possible by depressing a thumb-key. In about 6.5 minutes, 100 consecutive RTs were measured.

Mean RT was longer in the epileptic group: 296 ms, against 257 ms in the control group. However, the authors were especially interested in the intraindividual variability of their patients' performances. Intraindividual variability was determined by calculating the distance between the 10th and the 90th percentile within the distribution of an individual's 100 reactions. This index of variability was significantly increased in the patient group: 130 ms compared with 90 ms in the control group ($p < .001$). It cannot be said that this increase is simply proportional to the increase in median RT in the patient group: intraindividual variability was 36 percent of the median RT value in the control group, and 46 percent in the epileptics. Bruhn and Parsons then analyzed the effect of several epilepsy variables on intraindividual variability. Etiology, age of onset and duration of illness had no impact. Surprisingly, the presence or absence of EEG abnormalities was also unrelated to variability in the RT task. In the group of subjects with abnormal EEGs, the type of electroencephalo-graphic abnormalities also had no effect. Only the type of seizure appeared to be relevant: the group of subjects with grand mal seizures had a median RT variability of 139.5 ms, which was significantly greater than the 119.5 ms in-traindividual variability in patients who did not have this type of seizure. In addition, frequency of seizures seemed to have some effect: RT variability in epileptic subjects with fewer than 4 seizures a year did not differ from controls'. A finding more difficult to explain is that the group with 4–12 seizures per year showed highly elevated RT variability, even when compared to the group having seizures more frequently than 12 times a year. Bruhn and Parsons cited Rodin's (1968) statement that a normal EEG in an epileptic does not automatically guarantee normal intellect and/or personality, but they added that neither does it guarantee stable RT performance. They pointed out that their findings were in line with the conclusion by Mirsky and colleagues (1960) that centrencephalics, i.e. epileptics with grand mal seizures without aura and with generalized par-oxysms in their EEGs, are the subgroup of patients with maximal attentional problems. The grand mal seizure is characterized by loss of consciousness, in-dicating that the basic arousal systems of the brain are temporarily affected. The differential performance found in the Mirsky studies and in their own in-vestigation led Bruhn and Parsons to conclude that interictal performance of these groups is characterized by the same kind of disturbance, although of less intensity, that is seen during actual seizures. Based on the performance of their total group, the authors emphasized that epilepsy results in both a general slowing (longer RT) and greater intraindividual variability.

Combined EEG/Behavioral Studies

The studies reviewed above show clearly that epileptics, particularly patients with centrencephalic epilepsy, have longer mean RTs and miss more signals in continuous tasks demanding sustained attention. In addition, their RT perfor-mance shows a greater intraindividual variability than is found in normals. How-ever, the methodology of these studies leaves open the possibility that epileptics perform normally at some points during testing and abnormally at others. To resolve this question it was necessary to combine bio-electrical data reflecting fluctuations in the assumed subcortical regulatory mechanism with behavioral data.

One of the first investigations combining on-line EEG recording with be-havior was carried out by Prechtl and coworkers (1961). These authors studied 12 epileptic patients, recording EEGs while the patients were performing a continuous RT task. The patients were a mixed group, 8 having grand mals (generalized seizures) and the remaining 4 having absences, psychomotor at-tacks, or aggressive bursts. The subjects were presented with a horizontal line of five lamps lighted in random order, which had to be switched off using switches below the lights. A light appeared immediately following the switching off of the preceding one, allowing the subjects to determine their own rates of response. The instruction was to proceed as rapidly as possible without making errors. The main variable in this experiment was the "push-button interval," the interval between two successive responses. In this case the push-button interval was equal to RT.

The performance of patients having epileptic discharges during the test was compared with that of a nonepileptic control group. For the epileptic subjects push-button intervals were analyzed separately for periods of normal background EEG and for periods with epileptic discharges. Push-button intervals with normal EEG background were somewhat longer in the patient group than in the control group; in fact, 6 of 10 patients had a mean push-button interval outside the normal range. Variability, however, was not significantly increased as long as the EEG had a normal background.

The investigators expected an increase in both push-button interval length and variability during spike-wave bursts, but their data analysis showed that there was no simple temporal correlation between epileptic activity in the EEG and the rate of performance on the test. For example, one patient made no errors and performed at his usual rate even during 10 seconds of generalized spike-wave activity. However, changes in performance were frequently associated with a very flat, undifferentiated wave pattern, often unrelated to but sometimes followed by unmistakable epileptic discharges. This *suppression* phenomenon clearly affected performance more than spike wave activity. When push-button intervals were analyzed for periods with and without spike wave discharge, only a slight increase was found for discharge-connected push-button intervals. On the contrary, comparison of push-button-interval values during normal periods and periods of EEG suppression revealed that in 6 out of 10 patients response speed decreased. Moreover, variability in push-button intervals increased significantly in all 10 patients during EG suppression. Prechtl et al. assume that the suppression phenomenon constitutes a manifestation of subcortical epileptic discharges. According to the authors a practical aspect of these findings would seem to be that epileptic patients whose EEGs no longer show epileptic discharges after anticonvulsant therapy but do show episodes of suppression may still be subject to considerable fluctuations in performance, for example, impaired reaction time at work or while driving a car.

An important finding in the Prechtl study was that push-button intervals recorded in patients during intervals with normal EEG were slightly longer than PIs in controls. The authors suggest that this effect might be caused by the prolonged use of anticonvulsants. On the other hand, as noted above, variability in patients' performance was normal as long as EEG remained normal.

Next, three EEG studies appeared which had three elements in common: they focused on the effect of *spike wave* discharges on behavior, they applied auditory RT and the patients served as their own controls. RT during spike waves was compared to RT with normal background EEG in the same individuals. Spike wave discharges can be subclinical phenomena, i.e. they are usually not accompanied by overt seizures. Grisell and colleagues (1964) investigated the relationship between this subclinical epileptic phenomenon and performance on a continuous auditory RT task. Six patients were studied. They had to press a key when a tone was presented, and to release the key when the tone stopped. In addition to RT, errors could also be related to EEG. Errors included failure to press the key when the tone came on, failure to release the key after cessation of the tone, premature presses, and premature releases of the key. RT was calculated for each subject in four conditions: during normal EEG, preburst, burst, and postburst. Preburst and postburst intervals were defined within 15-second limits, immediately preceding a burst and immediately following the end of a spike-wave discharge. A large increase in RT was noted during bursts. In addition, RT was also slightly increased in the pre- and postburst conditions, leading to the conclusion that the times just preceding and just following the appearance of seizure discharges may also be associated with some disruptive behavioral effects. RTs in this sample of patients were as follows: normal background 350 ms, preburst 430 ms, burst 630 ms, postburst 460 ms. Response errors occurred most frequently during bursts, although an illustration in the paper shows clearly that the majority of responses were correct during bursts, but with longer RTs. The dramatic increase of RT during spike wave discharges inspired the use of the term "trough of consciousness."

Porter and coworkers (1973) raised the question whether spike wave bursts and disturbance of consciousness are directly linked, or whether alterations in consciousness proceed in a more independent and less abrupt fashion than bursts. To answer this question they studied RT performance in an ingenious way during the beginning and the end of bursts, that is, during the downward and upward swing of the trough of consciousness. Presentation of stimuli was EEG-triggered in such a way that the appearance of a burst resulted in the presentation of a tone to the subject. Fourteen patients with petit mal seizures and generalized spike-wave discharges were tested.

The use of paroxysmal-controlled stimuli provided precise and reliable evaluation of responsiveness at particular times during the seizures. By varying the delay between onset of discharge and presentation of tone, Porter and colleagues could demonstrate that the maximal disturbing effect of spike wave bursts occurs between 0.5 and 1.5 seconds after discharge onset. The duration of discharges had no bearing on this effect: whether spike wave bursts are short or long lasting, the trough of consciousness occurs at the indicated interval.

These findings were confirmed by an investigation (Browne et al., 1974) in which 26 patients with absences were studied, again with an auditory RT task. Browne and colleagues found normal RTs up to 1 second before the onset of bursts, but during discharges abnormal RTS increased in number, according to this pattern:

Seconds	Percent normal reaction times
−1.0	100
0.0	43
0.5	20
4.0	52

The authors also report that responsiveness recovered quickly after discharges. When making a distinction between short bursts (1 to 3 seconds) and long bursts (more than 3 seconds) it was found that the maximal disturbing effect always occurred in the interval from 0.5 to 1.5 seconds, in accordance with the Porter study.

An interesting theoretical expansion of the on-line EEG approach was developed by Hutt (1972) and Hutt and colleagues (1977). Although their study used children as subjects, there is no a priori reason to believe that results would have been different with adults. Twenty-six children suffering from grand mal epilepsy were tested with a continuous choice RT task containing three levels of difficulty or task load: there were 2, 4, or 8 stimulus and response alternatives. Numbers referring to push-buttons appeared on a screen, indicating 1, 2, or 3 bits of information to be processed in the three conditions before subjects could respond. The children responded correctly in 95 percent of all trials. RTs were significantly longer during spike wave activity than during background EEG activity. Most important, however, was the finding that performance decrement caused by bursts was related to task difficulty. There was a clear and significant interaction between bits of information to be processed and negative effect of bursts, showing that in the 8-choice reaction RT in particular was strongly influenced by spike wave activity. Hutt et al. describe their findings as follows: "The data show that the effect of spike wave is not all-or-none, but is proportional to the information processing demands of the task: the greater the amount of information presented per stimulus, the greater the impairment . . . The primary dysfunction seems to be suffered by the internal decision stage in the information handling machinery." The latter statement refers to stages of information processing as they have been classically distinguished: stimulus perception, stimulus encoding, response selection, response execution. The assumed deficit in the Hutt investigation concerns the response selection stage.

The Continuous Performance Test (Rosvold et al., 1956) has also been used in combination with EEG recordings in epileptic subjects. Mirsky and Van Buren (1965) studied 18 subjects with centrencephalic epilepsy. The overall percentage of correct reactions was 84.8 percent, but this decreased to 24.1 percent during bursts. These authors questioned which function was actually disturbed by the burst—reception of information, integrative process, or motor output—paralleling Hutt's stages approach. Mirsky and Van Buren's results (1965) suggest that all of these functions may be affected by bursts.

Hutt and colleagues (1977) addressed this problem directly by testing 18 patients with an auditory signal detection task while spike-wave activity was provoked by means of stroboscopic light. During spike waves there was a decrease in the number of signals correctly responded to. Analysis of responses in terms of signal detection theory revealed that this was not due to a decrease in the detectability (d') of stimuli, but to an increase in the acceptability of a signal (β). This implies that the burst-related impairment was not located in an early, sensory stage of processing, but in the decision-making stage.

Despite the evidence from investigations reviewed so far, the precise *relationships between behavior, consciousness and bursts* remain unclear. As Prechtl and colleagues noted, subjects may continue to respond during spike-wave ac-

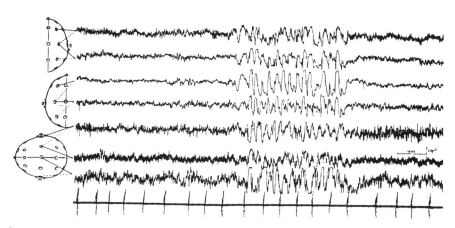

Figure 7-2 An illustration of the fact that spike-wave bursts cannot be equated with lapses of attention: in this 43-year-old male patient, reactions to stimuli continue (bottom line) despite the presence of a burst lasting 4 seconds. (From Prechtl et al., 1961, with permission.)

tivity in their EEG (see Figure 7-2). Mirsky and Van Buren (1965) addressed the problem in the discussion section of their paper on centrencephalic epilepsy:

> Three lines of evidence argue for the spike and wave pattern and attention impairment being considered as separable symptoms:
>
> 1. These patients showed impairment on the attention test in the absence of observable bursts.
> 2. The change in behavior tends to precede the electrographic symptom.
> 3. A lack of behavioral change was observed in some patients even in the presence of well-organized symmetric bursts.

Porter and coworkers (1973) addressed the same problem by asking whether alterations in consciousness are as abrupt in onset and cessation as the burst itself, or whether consciousness proceeds in a more independent fashion. The authors' own findings that performance decline is maximal from 0.5 to 1.5 seconds after burst onset, regardless of total length of bursts, indicate that spike wave discharges should not be equated with the behavioral impairment. In other words, spike-wave bursts are an electrophysiological phenomenon observable in the EEG, while lapses in attention are defined at the task level. These phenomena are clearly related but not identical.

It is remarkable that none of the studies reviewed above reported negative *time-on-task effects*. Possibly such effects were overlooked by the investigators as they were mainly interested in phasic effects and performance level per sé. However, we may assume that they have studied their data extensively: Bruhn (1970), for example, looked at performance curves over time, as may be seen in an illustration in his paper.

Some evidence from a related field is available. Aarts and coworkers (1984) studied cognitive impairment during focal and generalized epileptiform EEG activity. They tested 46 patients with two short-term memory tasks, one verbal and one nonverbal, somewhat resembling the Corsi-blocks procedure. Their test sessions could last an hour or more, depending on the subject's performance level. This implies that sustained attention was required, and a continuous processing of information. Still, the paper does not report any decline in performance over time, and the senior author (Aarts, personal communication, 1990) confirmed that no time-on-task effects had been noted during the experiments. At present the same task is still in use in a shorter version consisting of two 20-minute periods. Recent research has also failed to show an unusual decline in performance in epileptic subjects over these time intervals (Kasteleyn-Nolst Trenité, personal communication, 1990).

Hence the impression exists that, although centrencephalic epileptics perform less well than controls on sustained attention tasks, they maintain their initial level of performance as well as healthy subjects. Their main problems therefore consist of an increased intraindividual variability and lapses of attention.

Effect of Attentive Behavior on EEG

Clinical observation has suggested that activity, physical or mental, can suppress epileptic seizures. Prechtl and coworkers (1961) also noted this effect in their study with a continuous RT task. Their subjects were assessed with standard EEGs before the experiment, and comparison of standard EEG with EEG recordings in the experimental situation revealed a difference in frequency of epileptic discharges: "These were generally lower during the periods of concentrated attention and associated arousal than during routine procedures, when the patient is relaxed and shows alpha-waves."

This effect has been investigated systematically by Hutt (1972), who varied task difficulty in a study of 5 children with spike wave discharges. The subjects listened to a random series of digits presented at a rate of 1 per second. In the simplest condition, the subjects had only to listen, a situation that was characterized as "boring" by the investigator. In the other conditions subjects had to react by pushing a button to either one, two or three indicated digits. Many bursts were seen when the children were merely listening, but when a response was required to one or two digits there was a progressive decrease in spike wave bursts. However, there was an increase when responses were required for three digits. Hutt concluded that when the task exceeds a critical level of difficulty the amount of spike wave in the EEG rises again. These results were in line with findings when epileptic patients were surveyed about the frequency and occurrence of their seizures. Patients often reported that a state of concentration, whether on a physical or mental task, seemed to prevent seizures. Seizures appeared to be most frequent in two situations: states of tiredness and drowsiness; and states of intense emotion, anger, frustration, anxiety, and fear. In short, seizures seem to occur most frequently at either low or high arousal levels.

This effect seems to imply that the risk of a patient having a seizure is relatively low as long as he or she is engaged in some daily life activity (work, driving) which requires attention in the sense of conscious effort.

SUPERVISORY ATTENTIONAL CONTROL

No studies of the integrity of attentional strategies in the interictal behavior of epileptics have been published yet. Supervisory attentional control (SAC) poses a unique theoretical problem in the case of centrencephalic epilepsy: how does the epileptic cope with recurring disruptions of his cognitive activities? The evidence reviewed for sustained attention showed clearly that epileptics may react slower or not at all during spike-wave bursts and that they miss more signals in a continuous performance task during bursts than with normal background EEG. Are epileptic subjects aware of these changes, and can they reconstruct what has transpired during these short episodes? How do the bursts influence understanding an ongoing conversation; and what is their effect on car driving or any other form of road use? It should be kept in mind that epileptics are not rendered completely blind and deaf by spike-wave discharges: in many cases they continue to respond, albeit at a less efficient level. Basic to this issue is whether supervisory strategies enable the epileptic to minimize the change in task performance.

As far as conversational speech is concerned, lapses of attention resulting from spike-wave discharges need not have a dramatic effect; conversational speech is highly redundant. Even if 10 percent of the syllables or even words in a sentence are missing, we can generally pick up its global meaning. From a psychological standpoint there is the question of whether the articulatory loop (Baddeley, 1986) might partially bridge the gap caused in information processing by the trough of consciousness.

This articulatory loop, or "slave system," is an integrated part of working memory which allows phonological information to be stored for up to two seconds. Although we tend to view the articulatory loop as a memory mechanism, it partly determines the processing capacity in working memory and as such it is related to attention. It would seem worthwhile to investigate what epileptics can actually reconstruct from a stream of speech sound immediately after the occurrence of a burst. It would also be useful to study motor behavior during spike-wave discharges. It is a well-known clinical phenomenon that so-called automatic behaviors can occur during epileptic seizures, particularly during partial seizures when consciousness is merely clouded. It is possible that task performance is influenced only insofar as controlled processing is required; the more automatized components of a task being performed at the usual level. For example, in driving it might well be that tracking, that is, keeping the car in its correct position in a lane, is not seriously influenced by bursts, while interpretation of traffic signs and other less conspicuous elements might be delayed.

EFFECTS OF ANTIEPILEPTIC DRUGS ON ATTENTION

There is strong evidence that some anticonvulsant drugs (ACDs) can have negative effects on behavior, particularly cognition. Due to severe methodological problems in this area of research, it is difficult to offer general conclusions about such effects. In order to study the "pure" effects of ACDs, two approaches have been taken: testing cognition in human volunteers taking ACDs, and observing and testing animals under the influence of the same agents. Both approaches have their limitations. In laboratory rats one can study only relatively simple tasks and processes, making generalizations to the domains of, say, human education and traffic participation questionable. This problem can be circumvented by studying healthy volunteers, but here another methodological problem arises. Epileptic patients usually take their drugs over periods of many years, while experiments with normal volunteers study the effects of ACDs over periods of weeks, or months at the most. There is reason to believe, however, that the drugs' negative effects on cognition gradually wear off as patients develop tolerance.

In animal studies the effects of ACDs on motor activity and operant conditioning have been investigated. Kulig (1980) studied the effects of sodium valproate and phenobarbital administered to rats for two weeks. Initially these drugs had a negative influence on motor coordination and motor activity in the animals. However, within two weeks the rats developed a tolerance for the effect on motor coordination, while the effects on spontaneous activity did not diminish. In a review of available literature on ACD effects in animals and man, Kulig concluded that "drugs used in the treatment of epilepsy are a heterogenous class of psychoactive compounds and as such deserve serious consideration as a source of behavioral change in the clinic and systematic investigation."

In human studies with volunteers methodological designs can be applied that are not acceptable with patients, such as the double-blind crossover design with placebo and ACD. Hutt and coworkers (1968) studied the effect of phenobarbitone in this way over a period of three weeks. A variety of cognitive tasks were used. Performance on relatively simple tasks deteriorated only with very high blood levels of the drug, but in more difficult tasks a relationship between performance and blood level was found: the higher the level, the worse the performance. Hutt and colleagues also analyzed time-on-task effects and concluded that "tasks requiring sustained attention over a longer period of time were especially vulnerable to drug effects. The half-hour vigilance task, the key-pressing and the verbal learning task were of this nature. It appears that during phenobarbitone administration the subject is unable to maintain vigilance over long periods, but is capable of short bursts of attentiveness." Once more, it should be pointed out that this effect might be temporary, as 3 weeks is possibly not long enough to build up a tolerance for the drug effect on cognition. Thompson and colleagues (1981) studied the effects of phenytoin on measures of concentration, memory for verbal and nonverbal material, motor and perceptual speed and speed of decision-making. The Stroop was used here as a concentration task. It was found that subjects made significantly more errors on the Stroop in the phenytoin condition than with placebo. Speed of finger tapping was significantly reduced. On the decision-making test subjects took significantly longer in the phenytoin condition to answer questions both about the color of an object and category membership. Thompson and colleagues concluded that acute administration of the drug can impair some important aspects of cognition. Their observation that these deficits occurred at a mean serum level *below* the usual therapeutic range is very relevant. In a second study, Thompson and Trimble (1981) demonstrated that sodium valproate likewise had a negative effect on speed of decision making in healthy volunteers. The conclusion from experiments such as these seems to be that ACDs can have negative effects on cognition, including aspects of attention, in nonepileptic human brains. There is some evidence that these effects may occur at relatively low drug serum levels. A negative relationship has been observed between serum level and test performance with more complex activities.

Kulig (1980) remarked that findings in *clinical* ACDs research are difficult to interpret in the presence of many complicating factors. Epileptic patients' performance on cognitive tasks is not determined by drug serum levels alone, but also by brain lesions or other disturbances causing the epilepsy, by the frequency of seizures, and by subclinical epileptic discharges during performance. Moreover, serum levels of the target drug will vary greatly, even in a group of patients with the same type of seizure, as the medication dosage is always individually determined. Manipulation of the independent variable, that is, drug and dose, is usually limited or impossible by clinical considerations. In studying patients it is therefore often difficult to see whether the independent variable is the drug or the clinical condition (epileptic discharges) it purports to control (Hutt et al., 1968). In the search for medication with maximal therapeutic and minimal negative effects, a special feature of ACD research has been to compare various drugs with regard to their relative effects on cognition. As a result phenytoin has been replaced in many cases by carbamazepine, which seems to have fewer effects on memory, aspects of attention and motor functions. Another important finding has been that polytherapy should be avoided if possible; reduction of the number of ACDs taken by a given patient usually resulted in better performance on cognitive tests. Recent studies have shown that most epileptic patients can be controlled with single-drug therapy.

Notable research in this area was carried out by Trimble and Thompson (1983). Healthy volunteers and epileptic patients were studied for two weeks in a double-blind crossover design to determine the effects of four ACDs on cognitive function and behavior. The healthy volunteers experienced significant deficits in performance with phenytoin, carbamazepine, sodium valproate, and clobazam. The most widespread changes were seen with phenytoin. The results of several patient studies showed that

1. Cognitive function improves in patients receiving polytherapy when ACDs are reduced.
2. Patients with high serum levels of ACDs demonstrated more cognitive impairment than those with low levels.
3. When carbamazepine is substituted for another ACD cognitive function is improved.
4. In patients receiving monotherapy, high serum levels are linked to greater cognitive impairment than lower levels and the profile of changes differs between the drugs.

Several clinical studies have been done on the effects of ACD serum levels on cognition, in particular to determine whether fluctuations in serum levels over a patient's day result in variable performance on cognitive tests (pharmacokinetic effects). Aldenkamp and colleagues (1987) tested patients with a single-blind crossover design, comparing the effect of a standard carbamazepine dose with a slow-release form of the drug. The hypothesis was that with the standard medication cognitive defects might result from peak levels: short periods with high serum concentration. As the slow-release version prevented such peaks it was expected that patients would perform better on a variety of cognitive tests. Two of these, the Stroop Color Word Test and a Computerized Visual Search Task, were meant to assess aspects of attention. The findings showed a systematic tendency toward better performance in the slow-release condition for the battery as a whole. In the Stroop Test the slow-release condition resulted in fewer errors and the Visual Search Task was performed faster. The authors concluded that the smoothing effect of slow-release carbamazepine on serum levels had a favorable effect on cognitive functioning.

Reinvang and associates (1991) also studied the pharmacokinetic effects of carbamazepine, but in a standard medication regimen. Patients took two daily doses and they were tested twice, at times close to the expected maximum and minimum serum concentrations. Trailmaking A and B and PASAT were used to test attention. Although the patient group showed significant fluctuations in serum carbamazepine concentration, these had few significant effects on cognitive functioning. PASAT performance did not fluctuate with serum levels, nor did performance on Trailmaking A. There was a significant change on Trailmaking B, but the direction of this finding was contrary to expectation: the task was performed more slowly at the time of low serum concentration. The authors point out that their alternate forms of Trailmaking, used for retesting, were possibly not equivalent in difficulty. Based on their findings as a whole, they conclude that "the few and scattered differences do not show a systematic and consistent trend."

The results of the two studies described above are somewhat conflicting. If serum levels have no effect, as the Reinvang study suggests, how can the smoothing of fluctuations have a positive effect on cognitive functioning as reported by Aldenkamp and colleagues (1987)? Of course the attention tests were different in the two studies, and relevant differences may have existed between the patient samples—for example, the first seizure occurred at a mean age of 21 years in the Reinvang study and at 11.6 years in Aldenkamp's sample.

Reynolds (1983) points out that the side effects of ACDs can be troublesome in some areas of daily life, or in certain occupations: "Evidence has accumulated in the last few years that most of the major antiepileptic drugs, especially in combination, do interfere in subtle ways with cognitive function, including attention, concentration, memory, motor and mental speed, or mental processing. These sometimes slight effects are easily overlooked but can be a heavy price to pay on a long term basis for seizure control. This is especially true for children in the learning situations, and for the adult in occupations requiring prolonged concentration and high degrees of mental processing." Still, it should be realized that the effects of ACDs are limited in general. Many patients either do not experience the effects in their daily activities, or if they do, they accept them as being "all in the bargain." The minor effects on cognition seem a reasonable price to pay for the relief of psychological distress by suppression of their seizures.

COGNITIVE DECLINE REVISITED

In Section 7.2 the obsolete concept of epileptic dementia was mentioned. This ominous term has been abandoned, and Trimble (1988) even suggested that any cognitive decline must be an indirect effect of continuing seizures during which patients fall and suffer recurrent head injuries. Still, the question remains whether a more subtle decline in cognitive functioning must be expected during the lifetime of an epileptic patient. In fact the problem should be properly stated in two questions:

1. Do epileptic variables such as frequency and type of seizure effect cognitive functions over time?
2. Does anticonvulsive medication taken over many years result in cognitive deterioration?

The first question was the subject of a thesis from the University of Helsinki (Kalska, 1991): 69 adult patients were assessed with an extensive battery twice, at a mean interval of 9.4 years. Three tests from the battery may be considered as having an important attentional aspect: Digit Symbol and Digit Span from the WAIS, and the Stroop Color Word Test. The general outcome of the study was favorable, as most test scores showed no decline at all. For example, the full scale WAIS IQ of this group was 92.2 on the first occasion, and 95.8 on the second occasion. Memory quotient on the Wechsler Memory Scale went from 91.9 for the first test to 96.8 for the second test. Performance on the three tests relevant to attention was:

	Initial	Follow-up	Paired t-test
Digit symbol	8.6	8.3	1.16 NS
Digit span	10.0	9.6	$-2.55, p$ .01
Stroop			
Seconds	133.1	137.5	1.17 NS
Errors	3.2	2.5	1.23 NS

As the study did not include a control group (patients served as their own controls), it is difficult to judge the absolute level of performance in this epileptic sample. The time scores on the Stroop seem relatively high: 84 items in the colors green, black, red, yellow, and brown had to be named. At follow-up, only Digit Span showed a significant decrease, but the table shows clearly that the effect was not impressive despite its statistical significance.

The effect of epileptic variables on cognitive change was studied in detail. Etiology, age of onset, type of seizure, and number of anticonvulsant drugs used had no effect on cognitive change. However, disturbed background EEG was relevant for Stroop performance. Twenty-five patients had normal background

EEG both at initial assessment and follow-up; their mean Stroop score rose from 131.4 to 138.3 seconds. Fifteen patients had a pathological EEG background on both occasions, and their mean Stroop score rose from 136.5 to 164.1 seconds. On the other hand, normalization of background EEG was related to improvement on the Stroop test: 19 patients had an abnormal background EEG at the initial study, but a normal background at the follow-up. Their mean Stroop score decreased from 125.5 to 108.9 seconds.

Frequency of seizures had a slight effect on Stroop performance at follow-up. Patients were grouped according to number of seizures during the follow-up interval as follows: none, under ten, over ten, innumerable. An analysis of variance did not show an interaction between this variable and change in group performance, but those with innumerable seizures were slowest on the Stroop at follow-up. However, the relationship between frequency of seizures and Stroop score was not linear: the group with a frequency of seizures over ten was faster on the Stroop task than the group with fewer seizures.

The global conclusion from this study seems to be that, in general, attentional impairments in epileptics do not increase dramatically over time. A high frequency of seizures and a background EEG that is repeatedly disturbed might have a negative effect on attention as measured by the Stroop task.

Possible adverse *long-term effects of medication* on cognitive function have recently been addressed by Dodrill and Wilenski (1992). These authors carried out a detailed neuropsychological evaluation of 198 adult epileptics at the beginning and end of a five-year study. All were on medication and most had few seizures during this time. The subjects were divided into three subgroups: those on phenytoin (PHT) monotherapy, those taking PHT and other drugs, and those taking drugs other than PHT. The test battery included the Stroop Color Word Test and Trailmaking B. No negative effects of time were observed. In fact there were significant changes in three variables; Trailmaking B, WAIS Performance IQ and WAIS Full Scale IQ, and all represented improvements over the five-year period. The authors state their conclusion cautiously as follows: "We were unable to find evidence for insidious cognitive losses with PHT and other drugs over time, with normal therapeutic serum levels and in the absence of seizure disorders."

The results of these longitudinal studies appear to be reassuring. The first showed that most test performances in the areas of intelligence, memory, attention and motor function remained unchanged over time, and the second found no long-term effects of medication on cognitive functioning. Not only is the concept of epileptic dementia obsolete, even its modern counterpart, "insidious cognitive losses," seems to be of no practical importance.

SUMMARY

Epileptic phenomena can disturb consciousness and antiepileptic drugs can affect cognition. Studies of attentional impairments in epileptics have been hindered by the combination of these effects; task level deficits could be attributed to either the subclinical epileptic manifestations or the anticonvulsants.

Epileptic patients' subjective complaints have not been systematically studied. It seems that psychologists were more concerned with cognitive impairments than the patients themselves when psychology began to enter the field of epilepsy research. Early studies showed that epileptics in general have longer reaction times than control subjects and greater intra-individual variability in performance. Furthermore, there is evidence that focusing, as tested with the Stroop paradigm, may be poorer and that divided attention, as assessed with dichotic listening, is often deficient.

The bulk of neuropsychological research has been concerned with lapses of attention, often characterized as transient cognitive impairment. Behavioral measures combined with on-line EEG registrations allowed investigators to compare cognition during normal EEG with cognition during spike-wave bursts that result in a "trough of consciousness." This method showed that reaction time and variability are normal or near-normal as long as background EEG is normal. However, task performance suffers when spike-wave bursts occur; reaction time increases and signal detection becomes poorer. These changes are not completely time-locked to the electrophysiological phenomenon, indicating that the concepts of bursts, troughs of consciousness and lapses of attention are not synonymous. Time-on-task effects have not been reported in the literature on sustained attention in epileptics: even when patients occasionally react more slowly or miss more signals than controls, they seem able to maintain their original performance levels quite well during a task session. Thus, it must be concluded that lapses of attention are indeed the main attentional impairment in epilepsy. The effect of these lapses on daily life activities such as work or traffic participation has not yet been studied extensively. A theoretical question of considerable interest would be whether the disruption of attentive behavior by lapses requires a special kind of supervisory control.

In the last century it was believed that epileptics were bound to deteriorate mentally, ending in a state of epileptic dementia. Although this nosological entity is obsolete, some concern has lingered about the possibility of more subtle deficits. These might develop as the effect of either repeated seizures or lifelong medication with anticonvulsants. Evidence accumulated in recent years has shown that no cognitive deterioration occurs in the vast majority of patients. This is due in part to the fact that anticonvulsant drugs with demonstrable negative effects on cognition have been removed from the therapeutic arsenal as a result of neuropsychological research.

8

The Assessment of Attention

The assessment of attention has long been neglected in psychology; consequently very few tests that meet basic psychometric standards have been developed. Even when the concept of attention was taken up again by cognitive psychology, particularly within the framework of information processing models, it seldom penetrated clinical psychology and neuropsychology. In 1978, when Walsh published his valuable "Neuropsychology: A Clinical Approach," the word was completely absent from the index. In other well-known handbooks, attention is often casually mentioned without being treated as a separate topic. Lezak's text (1983) is an exception; it contains a section devoted to several forms of attention. Fortunately, since the 1980s attention has clearly made a comeback in neuropsychology (Van Zomeren, 1989). Nevertheless, the lag has not been overcome. Numerous tests are available for intelligence and memory that include satisfactory information about their psychometric qualities, such as reliability and validity. This is not the case for attention. Stuss and Benson (1986) stated: "Few tests are available, and these have not been carefully validated for different patient populations. The most frequently used tests are not derived from theories of attention, and improvement in the techniques for evaluating attention, particularly for clinical use, has been limited."

In Chapter 2, we applied the term attention to a broad class of phenomena that cannot be contained in a single definition, unless it is very general. It follows that attention cannot be assessed with a single test. We drew broad distinction between two types of definitions of attention in Chapter 2 and this distinction is important for categorizing tests of attention as well. In classical experimental psychology, attention is viewed as a selective mechanism enhancing or attenuating some part of available information for shorter or longer periods of time. Alternatively, attention is seen as the dynamic state that arises from preceding information processes and that determines selective behavior.

This distinction is also made implicitly in clinical practice. According to the classical view, tests of attention are only those tests that isolate the effects of specific selection processes on performance. Such tests must always have at least two conditions: one with a high attention requirement, the other a control condition that is as similar as possible with regard to all other psychological requirements except attention. The classic example is the Stroop Test, in which the quality of attention is indicated by the difference in time scores between the color and the color-word subtests. Without a control condition it cannot be concluded that poor performance on a task is related to an attentional requirement.

If attention is viewed as a dynamic cognitive state, a single-condition test would be a sufficient measure, for example, PASAT applied with only one interstimulus interval. In this case, poor attention would reflect nothing more than poor performance on a test of attention. Any limiting factors, that is, poor hearing, slow reaction time or poor motivation, would require separate assessment. Thus, no explanation can be found for poor performance on an attention test using this definition. It merely provides data that must be interpreted on the basis of other tests. For instance, severe CHI patients' poor PASAT performance would have to be explained by slow information processing.

Common to both views is the conclusion that performance on an attention task can never be interpreted in isolation. Data from other tasks or task conditions must always be taken into account.

A related problem is that each test will inevitably tap several aspects of attention. Thus, if we describe a test that seems appropriate for studying the capacity to divide attention, it should be borne in mind that the subject in this particular situation must be alert, perceiving selectively, and able to sustain attention for at least several minutes to finish the test. Also, the subject's supervisory attentional control must be active during testing. And let us hope that he will show no lapses of attention as a result of lack of sleep the preceding night. A nice account of the difficulties encountered in separating attention from other functions, and in separating aspects of attention, is given in Lezak's (1983) description of cancellation tests:

> These paper-and-pencil tests require visual selectivity at fast speed on a repetitive motor response task. They assess many functions, not least of which is the capacity for sustained attention. Visual scanning and activation and inhibition of rapid responses are also necessary to the successful performance of cancellation tasks. Lowered scores on these tasks can reflect the general response slowing and inattentiveness of diffuse damage or acute brain conditions, or more specific defects of response shifting and motor smoothness or of unilateral neglect.

The close relationship between attention and memory was discussed in Chapter 2. We made the point that distinguishing between these two functions is of little use when information processing is being studied on a second-to-second time scale (Baddeley, 1993). The fact that attention and memory are intertwined becomes apparent when an attempt is made to assess them. Some investigators may describe a given test as a test of short-term memory, while others may describe it as a test of attention. Digit Span, for example, is usually considered a test of immediate or working memory, but it appeared as a test of attention in a study by Wade and colleagues (1988). Stuss and Benson (1986) state categorically that: "The classic test of attention is the digit span." Stuss and associates (1987) also included a Brown-Peterson test of auditory short-term memory in a comparison of "three tests of attention." This should not be considered wrong or inconsistent, but it does illustrate that there are no pure tests of attention or short-term memory.

Psychological assessment has been computerized at an amazing rate in the last few years, and formal testing programs are now commercially available. This development has occurred in both clinical psychology and neuropsychology. The FEPSY program has become popular in Europe (Moerland et al., 1986; Alpherts and Aldenkamp, 1990). Computerized test batteries like FEPSY usually contain tests that have a loading on aspects of attention, such as visual search and choice-RT tasks. A special program for assessing attention that includes tests of selective attention, alertness, and vigilance is used widely in the German-speaking European countries (Zimmerman and Fimm, 1989). Comparable batteries, such as the Neurobehavioral Evaluation System (Baker et al., 1985) for the assessment of toxic effects of solvents on the central nervous system, have been developed in other fields. The reliability of these computerized batteries is often satisfactory, but in most cases normative data and validity studies are limited.

Many practitioners rely on their clinical eye and make impressionistic statements about attention in their patients if laboratory equipment is lacking. In principle, this is an acceptable pragmatic approach. In the same way that mild aphasia can be detected by simply listening to a patient, hemineglect can be detected by careful observation of a patient's behavior in a testing situation. As sophisticated laboratory techniques are not available in all settings and institutions, we will attempt to list all available techniques, whether or not they come under the formal heading of "tests," in our review of assessment methods.

ATTENTION IN DAILY LIFE: OBSERVATION AND INTERVIEW

Clinical assessment begins with observation. When meeting a patient with a cerebral lesion, the clinician will readily note peculiarities in behavior that seem to reflect attentional impairments. In addition, the relatives and caretakers often spontaneously report problems of concentration and mental fatigue in the patient. Hospital staff and professionals in rehabilitation can likewise contribute to a complete behavioral description of the patient. Whyte (1992) demonstrated "excellent inter-rater reliability" when videorecordings of head-injured patients in work tasks were judged by their on-task behavior, "fidgeting" and reaction to naturalistic distractions.

Attempts have been made to systematize these observations of attentional behavior by means of *rating scales*. Attentional items are usually found in scales aimed at a specific neurologic disease or syndrome. The Mattis Dementia Rating Scale (Mattis, 1976) and CAMDEX (Roth et al., 1986) were devised as diagnostic tools to be used with elderly patients, but they have been successfully applied in research as well (Kertesz et al., 1990). Levin and colleagues (1987b) devised the Neurobehavioral Rating Scale (NRS) for assessing the behavioral sequelae of head injury. Twenty-seven aspects of behavior can be measured on a 7-point scale, ranging from "not present" to "extremely severe." Table 8-1 gives the items from the NRS that appear to load on attention.

Levin and coworkers (1987b) reported satisfactory inter-observer reliability and some preliminary support for construct validity of the NRS. Corrigan and

Table 8-1   Items from the Neurobehavioral Rating Scale Related to Attentional Problems

---

1. Inattention/Reduced Alertness
   Fails to sustain attention, easily distracted, fails to notice aspects of environment, has difficulty directing attention, decreased alertness
7. Conceptual Disorganization
   Thought processes confused, disconnected, disorganized, disrupted, tangential social communication, perseverative
17. Fatigability
   Rapidly fatigues on challenging cognitive tasks or complex activities, lethargic

---

From Levin et al., 1987b, with permission.

Table 8-2   Ponsford and Kinsella's Attentional Rating Scale

---

1. Seemed lethargic, lacking energy	1.60
2. Tired easily	1.94
3. Was slow in movement	2.04
4. Was slow to respond verbally	2.16
5. Performed slowly on mental tasks	2.78
6. Needed prompting to get on with things	1.64
7. Stared into space for long periods	1.16
8. Had difficulty concentrating	2.02
9. Was easily distracted	2.14
10. Was unable to pay attention to more than one thing at once	2.44
11. Made mistakes because he/she was not paying attention properly	2.18
12. Missed important details in what he/she was doing	2.12
13. Was restless	1.18
14. Was unable to stick to an activity very long	1.42

From Ponsford and Kinsella, 1991, with permission.

Frequency of occurrence of impairments in head-injured rehabilitation patients as observed by speech pathologists. Note that slowness and inability to do two things simultaneously score highest.

coworkers (1990) carried out a validation study in an acute inpatient rehabilitation setting and found acceptable levels of interobserver reliability and validity. These authors analyzed the usefulness of NRS items according to three criteria: interobserver agreement, frequency of occurrence, and differential contribution to total NRS score. The three attentional items fared well in this analysis, with only Fatigability failing on the criterion "differential contribution."

The first attempt to construct and validate a rating scale specifically aimed at attentional impairments was made by Ponsford and Kinsella (1991). They devised a list of 14 items, mainly to be used with severely head-injured subjects in a rehabilitation hospital. Impairments were scored on a 5-point scale, according to their frequency of occurrence in a particular week. The scale ranged from "not at all" to "always." The interjudge reliability of this instrument was high. Table 8-2 gives the items, and the average score by speech therapists who judged the behavior of 50 patients.

Useful information about attentional impairments can also be acquired through a systematic *interview* or questionnaire. The Trauma Complaints List (TCL) (Van Zomeren and Van den Burg, 1985) was devised in Groningen to be filled

Table 8-3   Items from Van Zomeren and Van den Burg's Trauma Complaints List with Regard to Attentional Difficulties

---

11. Do you tire more easily when you have visitors, or in a crowded room?
12. Do you have more trouble concentrating or fixing your mind on things than you had before the accident?
13. Do you have more trouble now concentrating in a conversation with several people?
14. Do you have more trouble doing two things simultaneously, since the accident?
15. Do you have more problems now when you are disturbed during an activity, that is, if your work is interrupted?
26. Do you think, generally speaking, that you are slower now?
27. Do you think that you respond more slowly in a conversation?
28. Do you have more difficulty now with planning or organizing things?
29. Do you have more problems forming an overview in complicated matters since the accident?
36. Has your tolerance for bustle decreased?

From Van Zomeren and Van den Burg, 1985, with permission.

out by the clinician while interviewing head-injured patients, their relatives or a caretaker. The presence of complaints is scored on a 3-point scale: not present, mild to moderate, severe. The items in Table 8-3 focus on attentional impairments.

The Trauma Complaints List seems to have a satisfactory content validity and some predictive validity, but its reliability has not been studied (Van Zomeren and Van den Burg, 1985).

The investigator should take care to avoid semantic confusion, and when questioning laymen about the complex phenomena included in the global term, "attention," he should be very specific. One day, before giving a patient the Trauma Complaints List, we asked him whether he had a memory problem. His answer was: "Oh no, my memory is perfect—the only problem is that I forget everything." He was probably referring to his memory for past events as being perfect. This confusion about the common word "memory" shows that psychologist and patient may think of quite different things when questions are asked about unfamiliar concepts such as attention, distractibility, alertness, and so on.

TESTS OF MENTAL CONTROL

The so-called "tests of mental control" (Stuss and Benson, 1986) form a family of tests of attention that are clinical tools for bedside use. They stem mainly from behavioral neurology, where attention usually appears under two headings: confusional states and hemineglect (Geschwind, 1982; Mesulam, 1985). In general, neurologists assess patients with more severe pathologies than those encountered by neuropsychologists. A neurological assessment of attention is meant to be a quick procedure that can be carried out at the bedside without testing materials. It is largely meant to verify whether the patient is able to concentrate on a simple task demanding some mental effort. These tests have a certain face validity as they demand concentration and effort and place demands on the patient's working memory.

The simplest of these tests requires counting backwards from 10. The material is highly familiar to any patient, but the unusual direction demands some effort and concentration. The Serial Sevens task (Smith, 1967; Luria, 1966), in which the patient has to subtract 7 from a number near 100 (101–94–87–80, etc.) is used more frequently, followed by Digit Span Forward and Backward (Lezak, 1983). As noted above, Stuss and Benson (1986) consider Digit Span the classic test of attention. Factor analyses of WAIS and WAIS/R have established that Digit Span, together with Digit Symbol and Picture Arrangement, does indeed weight a factor called "attention/concentration" (Cohen, 1957; Lezak, 1983). Digit Span has a great advantage over clinical tests in that it is a subtest of the Wechsler Adult Intelligence Scale (Wechsler, 1955, 1981), which means that finely graded norms are available for various age groups. Digit Span could also be considered a "real" test of attention as it contains a highly demanding condition (digits backward) and a control condition with low demands (digits forward). The discrepancy between the two is a particularly interesting diagnostic sign with regard to attention (Rudel and Denckla, 1974; Goodglass and Kaplan, 1979; Lezak, 1983). Some patients who pass the Digit Span Forward may fail on Digit Span Backward. This effect has been noted after head injury (Mandleberg and Brooks, 1975; Brooks, 1984; Barth et al., 1989). Barth and colleagues found that performance on forward Digit Span was rarely impaired after mild head injury, while reversed Digit Span was sensitive in the early days after injury.

A new "mental control" test was designed by Weber (1988). This Attentional Capacity Test consists of eight subtasks of increasing difficulty, including steps such as:

1. Repeating a single number
4. Counting the number of 8's in a sequence of mixed numbers
7. Counting number of 8's, 5's, 4's and 7's in a sequence of mixed numbers
8. Counting the number of sequences of 5–3–8 in a sequence of mixed numbers

Weber described the ACT as a test of information processing capacity. It has been validated in that it discriminated between normal subjects and patients with brain damage of diverse etiology. In addition, it correlated .73 with a rating of patients' "attentional capacity" by hospital staff, on a five-point scale. Concurrent validity was demonstrated by positive correlations with PASAT. Weber pointed out the ACT has a special clinical advantage in that the mode of responding places minimal demands on the motor system. Responses on the test range from 1 to 10. The answers can be given orally or by pointing to the correct number in display, or even by repetitive eye blinking when speech and hand movements are impossible. The author provided some normative data in his article.

ALERTNESS

A *phasic* change in alertness, provoked by a warning signal, can be assessed on two levels: electrophysiologically and behaviorally. A phasic increase in alertness can be seen electrophysiologically in the CNV, and can be separated into motor preparation and stimulus anticipation using Brunia and Damen's (1988) paradigm. Normative data for these assessment techniques are not yet available, and may never be because of practical problems like differences in setup and equipment.

The effect of a phasic increase in alertness on behavior can be assessed by comparing reaction times with and without a warning signal within one subject. A warning signal increases reaction speed in simple RT tasks by reducing time uncertainty (Theios, 1975; Ponsford and Kinsella, 1992). This effect is thought to be based on response preparation between a warning signal and the stimulus. Hence the difference between warned and unwarned RT more or less parallels the motor preparation as registered in the CNV. However, normative data for this method are lacking. See Figure 8-1.

Recording *tonic changes* in alertness would also be difficult in a clinical setting as it requires long registrations with high-technology equipment. In most cases, observation of the patient's daily behavior can provide some information on his state of alertness. The first item in Levin's Neurobehavioral Rating Scale addresses Inattention/Reduced Alertness (Levin et al., 1987b). As noted, this aspect of behavior must be assessed with the aid of the following statements: "fails to sustain attention, easily distracted; fails to notice aspects of environment, difficulty directing attention, decreased alertness."

A testing session lasting several hours offers a special opportunity to observe tonic changes in alertness. During the session the patient's behavior may change

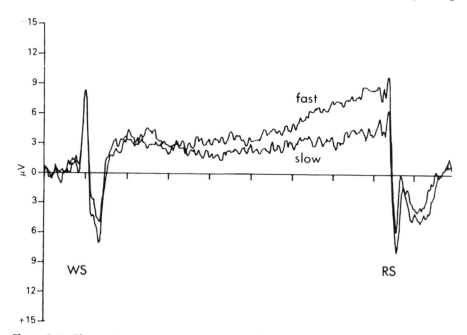

Figure 8-1   The contingent negative variation (CNV) in normal subjects. The upper curve represents CNVs preceding fast reactions to the imperative stimulus, the lower curve CNVs preceding slow reactions. A larger amplitude of CNV predicts a faster reaction. (From Brunia and Vingerhoets, 1981, with permission.)

in ways not recorded by separate tests. He may become less talkative and less alert, particularly in the short intervals between tests when left on his own. Such changes can indicate a global decline in attention or receptivity to information from outside. These observations have a practical relevance when the psychologist is asked to comment on the patient's chances of resuming his former work, where he will have to maintain an adequate level of alertness for at least several hours.

It is difficult to distinguish between effects of "fatigue," decreasing motivation and attentional deficits. Unfortunately, fatigue is hard to define and hard to record, and usually remains a purely subjective phenomenon. When an experimenter tries to categorize "fatigue," he generally focuses on decline in task performance (decreasing response speed, increasing errors). The approach assumes a somewhat circular character, as these same indices are thought to reflect deficits in sustained attention. It seems that we must accept the fact that fatigue, motivation and attention are intertwined in such a way that it is often impossible to separate them.

HEMINEGLECT

According to Heilman and colleagues (1985) a neglect syndrome is present when a patient fails to report, respond or orient to novel or meaningful stimuli presented to the side opposite a brain lesion and when this failure cannot be attributed to either sensory or motor defects. Lesions in the right hemisphere induce more frequent and severe neglect.

The major behavioral manifestations of hemineglect are hemi-inattention and hemispatial neglect. *Hemi-inattenion* is the failure to attend to stimuli presented contralaterally while *hemispatial neglect* is the neglect of one-half of space, even in the absence of specific stimuli. The latter phenomenon is clearly seen, for example, in drawings of common objects made by patients with hemineglect. The signs of hemineglect are most conspicuous in the visual sphere, although it can also manifest itself in hemi-somatagnosia or inattention to one half of the patient's own body. Visual hemi-inattention can exist without visual field defects. This dissociation is most apparent in the case of visual extinction: a patient may be able to perceive a stimulus when it is presented in isolation to one-half of his visual field, but no longer note the same stimulus when at the same time an identical stimulus is presented to the other half of his visual field. Like hemineglect, the extinction phenomenon is more often found in the left half field than in the right. The difference between the effects of left and right hemisphere lesions is less obvious in extinction than in other signs of hemi-inattention (Kinsbourne, 1987).

Observation of the patient's behavior may reveal hemineglect. He may bump into furniture to his left, or against the left door jamb. During testing, he may fail to note material on one half of the table, or start reading in the middle of a line of text. In an intelligence test like the Raven Progressive Matrices where multiple-choice responses are presented, the patient may fail to find the answer if it is shown on the left half of the page.

Formal testing of hemineglect may begin while the patient is still bedridden. Bedside methods for assessing various manifestations of hemineglect were described by Heilman and colleagues (1985) and Mesulam (1985). Psychological tests involving drawing and visual search are often applied once the patient is ambulatory. In his *drawing* the patient will show a tendency to neglect the left half. See Figure 8-2. Neglect may also become apparent when the patient has to copy complex Figures like the Rey-Osterrieth (Osterrieth, 1944).

The next tests involve *visual search* tasks. The patient is presented with an array of stimuli in which he has to detect target stimuli and tick them with a pencil. Albert's Test consists of a collection of one-inch lines randomly distributed over a 21 by 30 cm sheet of paper (Albert, 1973; Vanier et al., 1990). A more sensitive test was devised by Gauthier and colleagues (1989). In this Bells Test, 315 stimuli, familiar figures, such as house, horse, and key are randomly distributed over a 20 × 26 centimeter sheet of paper. Of these stimuli, 35 are targets (bells) and have to be circled by the subject, the rest are distractors. While they appear to be random, the bells among the distractors are organized into seven columns. Vanier and colleagues (1990) compared the discrimination power of Albert's test with the Bells Test and found the latter far better. In a group of 47 right-hemisphere stroke patients, the Albert's test revealed 7 cases of neglect (15 percent) while the Bells Test revealed 22 (47 percent). Both tests showed a gradient of omissions. The percentages of missed targets were higher in the extreme left column and diminished from left to right. The Bells Test permitted a finer scale of omissions than the Albert's Test.

In the two tasks described above, the field of search is unstructured. Tests in which targets and distractors are arranged horizontally are more widely used. A well-known example is the Letter Cancellation Task (Diller and Weinberg,

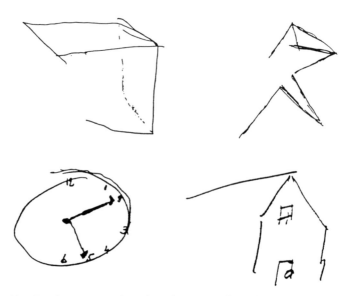

Figure 8-2 Hemineglect as manifested in drawings of a cube, star, clock and house. (From Glas, 1992, with permission.)

1977; Lezak, 1983) which consists of rows of letters with a randomly interspersed designated target letter. Search strategy is derived from the well-trained reading process, as subjects search from left to right, line by line, from top to bottom. Performance is scored for errors and time to complete. Diller and Weinberg included some normative data. Their stroke patients with right hemisphere lesions were not much slower than control subjects but made many more errors, always of omission and usually on the left side of the page. Patients with left hemisphere lesions made few errors but worked much more slowly than controls. Digit Cancellation Tasks have also been described as useful for assessing hemineglect. Wade and associates (1988) applied this method in a study of cognitive recovery after stroke and included normative data for elderly subjects. Performance was scored as a percentage, dividing the number of correctly cancelled digits on one side by the number correctly cancelled on the other side. All normal subjects scored between 90 and 110 percent. Wade et al. found this relative percentage scoring a simple way to score visual neglect. A retest of 12 elderly subjects, 2 to 4 weeks after their first assessment, indicated that the test had an acceptable reliability.

Reading can also be used to test visual neglect. When presented with a text, patients may skip the first word of the next line, indicating that the well-trained habit of picking up the beginning of the next line "at a glance" is disturbed by damage to their right hemisphere. Caplan (1987) refined this method with his Indented Paragraph Reading Test (IP). This is a passage consisting of 30 lines glorifying the beauty of trees. The left margin is intentionally constructed to be highly variable. The first word of each line is indented from 0 to 25 spaces, with the amount of indentation unpredictable from one line to the next. Thus, the layout of the text precludes the possibility that a neglecting subject could form a compensatory "spatial set," as each refixation from the end of one line to the beginning of the next requires a separate act of controlled scanning. Caplan reported that in some cases patients with neglect showed impairment on this task only, and he considered the test a valuable screening measure. However, Towle and Lincoln (1991) criticized the IP tests after finding no significant effect of paragraph layout in a group of right-hemisphere stroke patients. The authors indicated that more information on the validity of the IP cutoff scores was necessary as there was poor agreement beween IP and the Behavioral Inattention Test (Wilson et al., 1987).

The latter test comprises a series of fifteen tests of hemineglect. A basic and original feature of this battery is that it is composed partly of traditional hemineglect tests such as letter cancellation and line bisection, but also includes behavioral subtests such as telephone dialing and map navigation. Hence, it has a practical validity, as it makes use of standardized tests derived directly from daily life situations. Moreover, it has good interrater and test-retest reliability. It was published with satisfactory normative information (Halligan et al., 1991).

FOCUSED ATTENTION

Focused attention involves selectivity in perceiving and responding. An enormous number of tasks could be used to approach this aspect of cognitive func-

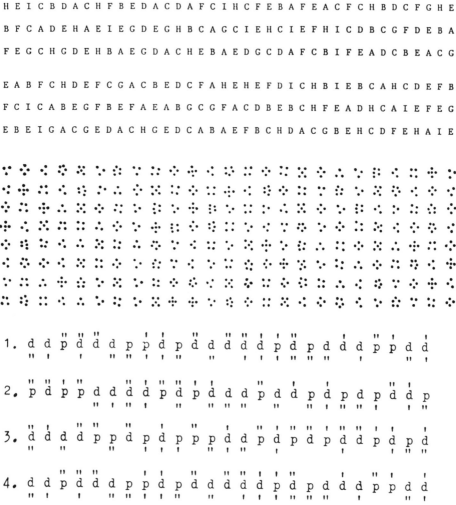

Figure 8-3 A selection of cancellation tests. **Top:** Letter Cancellation Test in which C's and E's must be cancelled (Diller et al., 1974). **Middle:** Bourdon Dot Cancellation Test in which groups of 4 dots have to be cancelled (Bourdon, 1895). **Bottom:** Brickenkamp d2 Test. Letters d have to be cancelled when they have two primes, either above or below, or one above and one below (Brickenkamp, 1981).

tioning, however, in practice, focused attention is usually assessed in the auditory and visual areas.

Auditory focused attention may be tested with dichotic listening tasks. Two different texts can be directed simultaneously to the left and right ears through earphones; one text is the target text, the other a distractor to be ignored. Examples of this method are described in several preceding chapters. Task difficulty can easily be varied by varying the similarity between the target and nontarget texts, either physically (e.g., male vs female voice), phonologically or semantically. Normative data are not available, but it is presumed that auditory focused attention in normal subjects is perfect, resulting in ceiling effects when they are required to listen selectively.

Visual focused attention is usually operationalized as visual search. Target stimuli have to be found in a field of distractor stimuli. Stimuli are usually arranged in horizontal rows. These tasks are self-paced, although the subjects are always instructed to complete the task as quickly as possible. The Letter Cancellation Task and the Digit Cancellation Task (also used to assess hemi-neglect) are well-known examples. Two further variations are also used in Europe, the Bourdon-Wiersma (Bourdon, 1895; Grewel, 1953; Deelman, 1972; Newcombe, 1982) and the Brickenkamp Test. The Bourdon-Wiersma uses groups of dots, either 3, 4, or 5, as stimuli. The dot groups are arranged in 50 horizontal lines. Subjects have to check each line as quickly as possible, and cross out groups of 4 dots. The Brickenkamp (1966, 1981) presents rows of p's and d's with some of the letters labeled with primes. The target stimulus is the letter d with 2 primes (see Figure 8-3). Norms are available on speed and efficiency of target detection for all of these tests.

In the tests described thus far, the subject's visual search pattern is almost entirely guided by the structure of the stimulus field. Just as in normal reading, his gaze follows the horizontal rows of stimuli in search of targets. This is not the case in the A-form of the Trailmaking Test (Reitan, 1958), in which circles numbered from 1 to 25 are randomly distributed on a page. Starting from circle 1, the circles have to be connected by a line as quickly as possible. Lezak presented detailed norm tables for the interpretation of results in her handbook

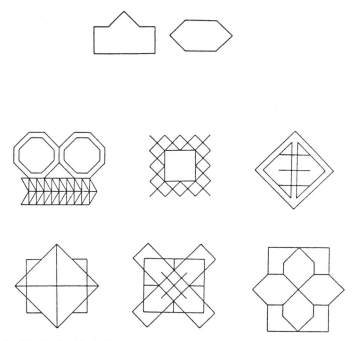

Figure 8-4 The Embedded Figures Test as designed by Gottschaldt (1928). The figures on top must be found in the patterns below, and indicated with a pencil.

(1983; see also LaRue, 1992). These tables reflect a clear effect of age on Trailmaking-A, older subjects being much slower. This effect was confirmed by Stuss and colleagues (1987), who supplied additional normative information. The European counterpart of the Trailmaking Test is the German Zahlen Verbindungs Test (Oswald and Roth, 1978) for which good normative data are available.

The Embedded Figures Test (Figure 8-4) is a more difficult test of visual focused attention. This test was developed from Gottschaldt's Hidden Figures Test (1928). It requires the subject to identify a simple figure embedded in a complex pattern. This is clearly an example of selective perception, as the combination of a few relevant lines has to be seen against the background of a multitude of irrelevant ones. Thurstone (1944) stated that successful performance in normals was related to the ability to form perceptual closure in the presence of distraction. The test has been shown to be sensitive to brain lesions in a variety of locations, caused by various etiologies (Teuber et al., 1960; Talland, 1965; Lezak, 1983). We found this test to be very sensitive to the effects of normal aging. Therefore, caution should be taken in interpreting very low scores as abnormal in very old subjects.

DIVIDED ATTENTION

As described in Chapter 2, the ability to divide attention is determined by three factors: processing resources, types of tasks to be combined, and attention allocation strategy. In many of the tests described in this chapter the relative contribution of each of these factors cannot easily be extracted. As a result, this section, although emphasizing processing capacity, overlaps somewhat with the section on supervisory attentional control. We will begin with the relatively pure tests, that is, reaction time tests in many variations.

In a "single channel" system with serial processing, capacity is measured as *processing speed*. With this in mind, psychology has always tended to measure latency and duration of mental activities. The rate of information processing can be assessed with a variety of tasks, although care must be taken that demands on the motor system are kept at a minimum. A suitable method is to record choice reaction times (Blackburn and Benton, 1955; Norrman and Svahn, 1961; Miller, 1970; Bruhn and Parsons, 1971; Van Zomeren and Deelman, 1978; Müller et al., 1991). From 30 to 40 trials, after some 10 practice trials, are sufficient for calculating the median as a stable index of the central tendency in an individual's responses. Visual stimuli are most widely used as they are easier to present and manipulate. Reaction Times using cross-modal shifts can also be used to assess *flexibility* (Benton, 1962). Analysis of a randomly presented combined series of visual and auditory stimuli can be used to determine whether a shift between modalities has a disproportionate effect on the patient. Reaction time to stimuli preceded by an identical stimulus are compared with RT to stimuli preceded by a signal from the alternative modality.

The introduction of computerized assessment in recent years has facilitated the recording and calculating of reaction times. While in the past choice-RT stimuli included only basic stimuli as lights and tones, it is now possible to display symbolic stimuli, that is, letters and digits, on a computer screen. The Sternberg paradigm (Sternberg, 1969) and various forms of visual search tasks based on the work of Shiffrin and Schneider (1977) are particularly elegant methods for measuring central reaction components.

When the clinical setting is not suited for recording RT, alternative methods for global assessment of information processing are possible. Timed tasks, such as reading word lists or naming colors (used as a precondition in the Stroop test) (Stroop, 1935), can give the investigator some idea about his patient's mental speed.

The Digit Symbols subtest from the Wechsler Adult Intelligence Scale or its counterpart, the Symbol Digit Modalities Test (Smith, 1982), are also useful for this purpose. The latter requires translation of symbols into digits, and has the advantage that no unfamiliar line figures have to be drawn by the subject (Morgan and Wheelock, 1992). The SDMT provides norms on various age groups (Lezak, 1983).

Form B of the Trailmaking Test (Reitan, 1958) is another measure of processing speed. In this test the subject has to connect numbered circles by lines drawn between them with a pencil, starting at circle 1. In Form B the visual search requirements are not much different from Form A, but there is a critical difference in cognitive requirements. In Form B two types of circles are presented: thirteen contain the numbers 1 to 13, and 12 contain the letters A to L. The subject has to connect the circles (requiring the same motor activity as in Form A), alternating between letters and numbers. Thus, the sequence becomes 1-A-2-B-3-C, etc., demanding flexibility of the subject in the continuous alternating. In this second part of the Trailmaking Test the patient's working memory is loaded with the double task of keeping track of both the alphabet and counting. Extensive normative data for several age groups were presented by Davies (1968; also in Lezak, 1983), Stuss et al. (1987) and LaRue (1992). As stated above, performance on the B Form should be judged in the light of performance on the simpler A version.

It must be emphasized that when measuring information processing speed care should be taken to account for any motor problems: dysarthria may impede reading speed, and a mild hemiparesis may prolong visual RT or performance on paper-and-pencil tests, even when processing speed is normal. The use of control conditions similar to the critical test conditions with regard to sensory and motor requirements, can be very helpful.

Many of these timed paper and pencil tests have elements of *divided attention tasks*, since their rapid execution is facilitated by opportunities for parallel processing. For example, in the Trailmaking Test it is efficient to locate the following target while drawing the line between the two previous ones. In the Digit-Symbols test the relationship between digits and symbols can be learned in parallel with the translation process. The visual search trajectories are less predictable in these tasks than in traditional reaction time tasks and more visual search is required. Possibly because of the cumulative effects of slow information processing on all of these components, these tests tend to be more sensitive to the effects of diffuse brain dysfunctions than standard RT tests.

Few clinical tests are formally classified as divided attention tests. Divided attention can be operationally defined by combining two or more tasks in one test, or by combining two sources of information, both relevant to the same task. A divided attention test with a rather long history, comparatively speaking, is dichotic listening, now however with very *short* texts, and instructions to repeat *both* texts immediately after presentation. Impaired divided attention is indicated by a disproportionate loss of information from the ear reported last. The use of this test in dementia and normal aging is described in Chapter 5.

Another well known test of divided attention is the Paced Auditory Serial Addition Task or PASAT, devised by Gronwall and Sampson (1974). This test requires division of attention between subtasks. The authors described their test as follows:

> A random series of digits from 1 to 9 is presented to the subject, who is instructed to add pairs of numbers such that each number is added to the one immediately preceding it. The second digit is added to the first, the third to the second, and so on. To be correct, a response must be made before presentation of the next stimulus. PASAT thus yields an estimate of the subject's ability to register sensory input, respond verbally, and retain and use a complex set of instructions. He must also hold each item after processing, retrieve the held item for addition to the next digit, and perform at an externally determined pace.

Thus, the subject has to perform several subtasks within one test, under considerable time pressure. At a low presentation rate, for example, one digit every 4 seconds, the task is fairly easy for normal subjects. When the rate is increased to one digit every 2 seconds, subjects begin to make errors as their processing capacity is exceeded. Some normative data for PASAT can be derived from work by Gronwall and her coworkers, mainly on the effects of head injury (Gronwall, 1977, 1987, 1991; Gronwall and Wrightson, 1974) and by Stuss and coworkers (1987; 1988). Rate of presentation is, of course, critical in this test. Gronwall's publications suggested that an interstimulus interval of 2 seconds discriminated best between normal controls and subjects who had sustained mild head injuries. PASAT has also proven useful for monitoring recovery after such injuries by retesting patients over the course of several weeks or months. However, findings from retests should be corrected for a practice effect demonstrated by Stuss and coworkers (1987).

Gronwall and Wrightson (1981) originally claimed that PASAT performance was not significantly correlated with either general intelligence or arithmetical ability. This view was challenged by Egan (1988) who found a correlation of .63 between PASAT scores and IQ on Raven's Standard Progressive Matrices, in a nonclinical group of 28 young adults. In our own department (Bruins and Van Nieuwenhuizen, 1990) we found a Pearson correlation of .40 ($p = .012$) between Raven-IQ and PASAT scores in a group of 32 normal subjects. In addition, a correlation of .42 was found between PASAT and adding speed (adding three numbers under 100, for 1 minute). Women performed significantly better than men in this group. Stuss and coworkers (1987) reported a positive correlation between years of education and PASAT performance. These findings suggest that norm tables for PASAT should control for level of education, intelligence, and possibly gender.

De Vries and colleagues (1992) studied the feasibility of the PASAT for testing elderly subjects (48 to 74 years). They found that the inter-stimulus intervals of 3 and 4 seconds are feasible, provided sufficient opportunity for practice is given. The PASAT had some concurrent validity, as both series correlated well with two other attention tests, that is, .53 with Digit Symbol from the WAIS and .67 with Brickenkamp's d2 test. The correlations with decision time in an RT task were weak (.29 and .33). De Vries and colleagues also studied the relationship between PASAT and Digit Span, and found that correlations were somewhat higher for Digit Span Backwards. PASAT-3 correlated .20 (nonsignificant) with Digit Span Forward, and .29 with Digit Span Backward. PASAT-4 correlated .35 with Digit Span Forward and .41 with Digit Span Backward. When subjects were retested 2 months later, a significant practice effect was noted. Test-retest reliability was not high, as the test-retest correlation was only .61 for PASAT-3 and .54 for PASAT-4. The authors concluded that the test is not appropriate for individual diagnostic purposes—but one could argue that this statement is too general and that it applies to elderly subjects only.

SUSTAINED ATTENTION

For the clinician, all three aspects of sustained attention as described in Chapter 2 may be relevant: time-on-task effects, lapses of attention and intraindividual variability.

Time-on-Task Effects

As every task has an attentional aspect, in principle, every test could be extended to last 15 minutes and claim to assess "sustained attention." In practice, two categories of tasks have widely been used to study attention over time periods up to 1 hour, that is, vigilance and monitoring. The study of vigilance began with the classical investigation of N.H. Mackworth (1950) who placed his subjects "alone in a cubicle for two hours, watching a clock hand jerking round in regular jumps, one jump a second, one hundred jumps per revolution. The signal was a jump of twice the usual distance. The interval between successive signals varied from .75 to 10 minutes (!), twelve signals being presented each half hour." (J.F. Mackworth, 1970). It is clear that this classical vigilance task presented an extremely boring situation to the subjects. Vigilance tests of such long duration are, however, hardly feasible in a clinical setting. Fortunately, for time-on-task effects, half an hour appears to be enough time to provoke a decrease in signal detection (Sanders, 1983; Brouwer and Van Wolffelaar, 1985). However, setting up a vigilance task is a laborious enterprise, and therefore commercially available tests of monitoring play a more important role in present clinical neuropsychology.

In this chapter, *monitoring* refers to a situation in which suprathreshold stimuli are presented at a high rate, and at a high signal to nonsignal ratio. The most widely used test of monitoring is probably the Continuous Performance Test (CPT) devised by Rosvold and Mirsky (Rosvold et al. 1956). In this test the subject faces a visual display on which a random series of letters appear at intervals of approximatley 0.92 seconds. The subject is instructed to press a button when the letter X appears. In a second condition, the subject is instructed to respond only if the X is preceded by an A. Thus the A serves as a warning signal that is sometimes followed by the target stimulus, and sometimes not. The Continuous Performance Test has been used with patient groups of various neurologic etiologies, including epileptics and head-injured patients (Greber and Perret, 1985). There is an auditory version of the CPT called the A-test (Strub and Black, 1985; Grafman et al., 1990). In this test subjects listen to a long random series of letters and are required to respond each time they hear the letter A.

Zimmermann and Fimm's (1989) computerized program for the assessment of attention deficits also contains a Vigilance task. These authors made a distinction between "sustained attention" with high frequency of targets, and "vigilance" with low frequency of targets. We would prefer to call the high-frequency target task a test of monitoring, applying the more general term, sustained attention, to a variety of task situations and phenomena, including vigilance, monitoring, intraindividual variability, and lapses of attention.

Working with vigilance or monitoring tests presents a particular problem in that poor performance on these tests does not necessarily reflect impaired vigilance or monitoring. Of course, brain-damaged subjects will often do poorly on these tests, responding slowly or missing more signals than healthy subjects. However, if they maintain a level of performance over time in a way comparable to healthy subjects, there is no indication of "decreased vigilance." The most parsimonious explanation for poor test performance is slow information processing. Initial performance in the early part of a sustained attention task may be viewed as a control condition for later parts. An impairment is indicated only if performance is substantially poorer for the later parts than the early ones.

The rate of stimulus presentation is fixed by the experimenter, both in vigilance and monitoring tests. This is not the case for prolonged *cancellation* tasks, which are another approach for studying sustained attention (Lezak, 1983). From a clinical point of view, cancellation tasks have the advantage that they are self-paced; the subject can determine his own rate of working and speed/accuracy trade-off. This facilitates generalization of test findings to real life situations like monotonous low-level office work.

Some cancellation tasks were mentioned in the sections on hemineglect and focused attention. The Bourdon-Wiersma, the Letter Cancellation Task (Diller et al. 1974) and the Digit Vigilance Test (Lewis and Kupke, 1977) can all be applied as tests of sustained attention. In our own laboratory we doubled the duration of the Bourdon by simply combining two test forms to get a task of at least 15 minutes' duration. Some normative data are available for the above-mentioned tests.

Lapses of Attention

Lapses in sustained attention tasks with a high response frequency may occur as missed responses or series of responses. In continuous RT tasks, lapses are defined as reaction times that exceed the mean by at least two standard deviations. Lapses can, in principle, be recorded in self-paced cancellation tasks. When the task consists of blocks or rows of stimuli, a lapse in attention may be reflected by an increase of time per block. In the Bourdon-Wiersma, time is recorded in seconds per line of 25 dot configurations; normal times range from 10 to 14 seconds per line. The definition of a lapse is more or less arbitrary, although in this case the criterion might be a deviation of 2 seconds or more from average time per line. This approach is clearly less sensitive than a high-frequency continuous RT task. If a lapse during a cancellation task lasts only a few seconds, it may be lost in the variance of time-per-line or block.

Intraindividual Variability

The variability of a subject's responses can be analyzed in a sustained attention task. The simplest behavioral measure for such an analysis is the rate of response. In continuous RT tasks, intraindividual variability (IIV) can be calculated over blocks of a certain duration. The question remains which index of variability will work best. In our experience, standard deviation is not the index of choice, as RT distributions are highly skewed to the slower side by the occurrence of extremely slow reactions or where the target push button is missed on the first attempt. For that reason, we prefer the median as the index of central tendency, and the interquartile deviation or Q as the index of variability. Q is calculated as half the distance between the 25th and 75th percentile in the distribution of a subject's RTs. Bruhn and Parsons (1977) suggested that the difference between the 10th and 90th percentile is a more sensitive index, as the use of Q implies a serious reduction of information taken from the distribution.

Time is not the only dimension with which variability can be analyzed. Variation in the quality of response or efficiency in signal detection might also be considered in a sustained attention task. For the sake of completeness, it must be noted that IIV could be used for the assessment of time-on-task effects. Instead of looking at a decline in performance, changes in variability in prolonged task conditions could be considered.

Regarding the relationship between IIV and attentional lapses, it can be stated that lapses are merely one possible aspect of IIV. In principle, however, the concepts are independent. Even when a subject shows no lapses of attention at all, his or her performance will show some variability from response to response.

SUPERVISORY ATTENTIONAL CONTROL

It is not current standard practice in clinical neuropsychology to assess this aspect of attention. However, supervisory attentional control activity can be discerned in the performance of subjects on many of the tests mentioned above, particularly those that put high demands on working memory, for example, Digits-Backward, Serial Sevens, PASAT and Trailmaking-B.

Some tests that are assumed to assess "frontal functions," or the executive functions, apparently touch on supervisory control, particularly if they require shifting between sets and attending to changes in stimulation. For example, subjects must react flexibly to changes in feedback from the experimenter in the Wisconsin Card Sorting Test (Heaton, 1981). These tests are not patient-friendly, to say the least, and poor performance can have many different causes (see Chapter 6). Techniques that test supervisory control directly are not yet available in a clinically useful form. Hence the clinical neuropsychologist must rely primarily on personal observations to estimate a subject's ability to cope with tasks that exceed his processing capacity or that force him to set priorities when he can no longer maintain an optimal task performance level. It is hoped that cognitive psychology will contribute to and participate in clinical investigations leading to the development of useful tests for assessing supervisory control, such as tests for adaptive strategies in tasks with a stepwise increase in loading on the subject, and systematic feedback on his level of performance.

Some attempts to assess supervisory attentional control (SAC) have been published. Shallice (1982) described the use of his Tower of London Test in a problem-solving study with patients suffering unilateral localized brain lesions. It appeared that left anterior patients performed significantly worse than patients with lesions at other sites. This difference could not be explained by differences between the patients' spatial and verbal abilities. In a subsequent study, however, the test failed to discriminate between frontal patients with normal WAIS IQs and normal subjects (Shallice, 1988). This doesn't necessarily invalidate the usefulness of the test as an indicator of impaired SAC, as these patients may have been unimpaired, but it certainly raises some doubts. Shallice also attempted to assess the integrity of SAC with tests that required nonobvious approaches to novel problems and of checking the plausibility of one's response (see Shallice, 1988). It might well be asked whether such tests are concerned with "attention," or whether the borderline between attention and intelligence is crossed. The introduction of the SAC concept has indeed widened the concept of attention considerably.

SUGGESTIONS FOR A CLINICAL APPROACH

What general guidelines can be given for assessing attention in the neurologic patient? The fundamental difficulty in answering this question lies in the *variety of symptoms* that stems from the variety of etiologies encountered by clinicians. An epileptic patient presents a picture of attentional impairment that is very different from that of a patient with Alzheimers disease or CVA. Thus, general statements are hardly justifiable. Another problem concerns the *time of examination* when acute brain damage has been caused by CVA, head injury, cerebral anoxia etc. At a very early stage, alertness may be the aspect of attention most affected as most patients are comatose. During the recovery period alertness may slowly increase to the point that the patient is aware of his surroundings, but tends to return to a somnolent state (drifting attention; see Stuss and Benson, 1986). He may later appear to be stimulus-bound, reacting only to objects in his surroundings. In fact, this could be considered a form of distractibility when, for example, the patient grasps the investigator's pen instead of answering his questions. In a subacute stage, the patient may be behaving adequately, but be hindered by divided attention deficits due to mental slowness. In the case of progressive disease, the time of the examination might dictate which impairments to assess. In Chapter 5, the description of the development of Alzheimer's disease suggested that various attentional impairments may appear at different stages.

Still, it can safely be said that the assessment of attention should begin with *observation* of the patient's behavior from the very first moment of contact. Alertness can be estimated. A normal reaction on the part of the patient to the appearance of the investigator should be increased alertness. The patient's interest in the test situation, manifested by exploratory eye movements and questions, is a further area for observation. Hemineglect may be noted, or at least suspected, on the basis of observation. The investigator can form an impression of what used to be called "attention span," that is, the patient's ability to maintain an adequate level of alertness over the course of an interview or test session within a few minutes. Finally, the patient's distractibility—his reactions to irrelevant sounds from outside the room or to irrelevant features of the testing material—may also be observed. An *interview* that includes questions about possible attentional problems should be conducted with the patient and the relatives and/or caretakers. Some guidelines for a structured interview can be found in the section "Attention in Daily Life" in this chapter.

Mental slowness is one of the various aspects of attention that can be assessed with standardized tests. This seems to be relevant for all subjects with cerebral lesions and diseases. Mental slowness is a nonspecific, very frequent result of brain damage (Hicks and Birren, 1970; Benton, 1986). In a readily observable form, it is known by psychiatrists and neurologists as bradyphrenia. Even if a patient's behavior does not appear to be particularly slow, any delay in response can be revealed with timed tests which contain adequate age-adjusted norms. As stated above, mental slowness may cause divided attention deficits in many daily activities. Recording choice RT, in combination with more traditional neuropsychological tests like the Trailmaking and the Symbol-Digits Tests may provide valuable additional information. For recording RT, the splitting up of total reaction time in decision time and movement time is recommended (see apparatus in Figure 4-1 in Chapter 4). The use of the PASAT is also recommended, preferably with varied interstimulus intervals. As noted above, a 2-second interval has proven useful in head injury research, but for older populations intervals of up to 4 seconds seem more feasible.

Spatial attention and supervisory attentional control can be tested when focal lesions involving areas of the brain relevant for attention are suspected. Hemineglect can be determined by one of the visual search or reading tasks described earlier or by the Rivermead Behavioral Inattention Test. Impairments in planning and regulation can be studied with the Tower of London and tests that put a high demand on working memory, particularly the central executive aspect.

Finally, *time-on-task effects* may be seen in patients with varying etiologies. To increase its practical validity, a laboratory task should last at least 15 minutes, and preferably up to 1 hour—although here we encounter the problem of boredom when the task has no face validity for the patient. It might also be worthwhile to assess lapses of attention in epileptic and narcoleptic patients (Valley and Broughton, 1983).

Generally speaking, a clinical neuropsychologist might use the following traditional tests: Trailmaking A and B, Digit Span and Digit Symbol from the WAIS-R, and the Stroop Color Word Test. Three of these four tests permit the manipulation of an essential variable while input and response mode remain more or less unchanged. In Trailmaking, performance on B can be compared with performance on the relatively simple A. The backward condition in Digit Span can be compared to the forward condition. Finally, in the Stroop Test, performance on the ambiguous color words can be compared to simple color naming.

An attention battery should also include a visual search task with adequate normative data. If time and money permit, an extended Continuous Performance Test would be helpful, preferably a version of the test consisting of a series of 3-minute blocks. The CPT can easily be programmed on a personal computer. An apparatus for recording RT is a great help to clinical neuropsychologists as it combines several measures of attention in one test: processing speed in simple and choice RT; flexibility, when cross-modal shifts are built into the program; time-on-task effect; intraindividual variability and lapses of attention, if the test is extended to at least 15 minutes. In addition, an RT task combining two response modes and two stimulus modalities can be used to assess divided attention. PASAT has also proven to be a useful tool in clinical neuropsychology in this regard. Finally, the Rivermead Behavioral Inattention Test would be a worthwhile investment in clinical settings where many stroke patients must be assessed.

9

Behavioral and Social Consequences of Attentional Deficits

Attentional impairments are frequent sequelae of brain damage resulting from disease or injury and it is important to understand how they influence the daily lives of patients. It is also necessary to consider whether tests of attention have predictive validity outside the laboratory, that is, ecological validity. Data on predictive validity are surprisingly scarce and, in many areas, nonexistent. Moreover, findings are often reported in a global manner. For example, in one of our earlier studies of head-injured patients correlations were found between visual reaction time and social outcome (Van Zomeren and Deelman, 1978). Simple and choice RT assessed 5 months after injury, correlated .41 and .48 with the social situation 1 year after injury. Although these correlations indicate that RT tests have some predictive value, the usefulness of the data was limited by the fact that "social outcome" was assessed by a compound score that included such factors as leisure activities, work situation, alcohol abuse, and marital problems. More specific indices of functioning in specific social areas are clearly necessary for proving the ecological validity of attentional measures. The evidence available at present will be reviewed under the headings of Memory and Attention, Work, Driving, and Social Skills.

MEMORY AND ATTENTION

Attention leaves traces, and those we call memories. Although cognitive psychologists may frown at this simplification, it serves to underline the intimate relationship between attention and memory. There is overwhelming evidence that the quality of memory traces is largely determined by the amount and type of processing given to the information to be remembered (Craik and Lockhart, 1972; Baddeley, 1990). Items that escape attention cannot be remembered. However, as soon as we pay attention, even with no intention to learn, some information will be retained in what has been called "incidental memory." The strength of the trace appears to be directly proportional to the duration and intensity of the attention given to the material (Russell, 1981).

The relationship between attention and memory has been used successfully in devising memory training techniques, particularly strategy training, in which

brain-damaged patients and elderly persons with memory problems are instructed to spend more time actively handling information relevant to their daily
lives (Koning-Haanstra et al., 1990; Berg et al., 1991). This strategy requires
giving more attention, in the sense of controlled processing, to material to be
remembered. The connection between attention and memory is sometimes recognized by patients themselves. A severely head-injured young man, G.D.,
spontaneously related how he had learned to cope with forgetfulness. He had
discovered that his attitude at the time information was presented to him determined his ability to remember it later. He described his strategy as "taking
in things at a quiet pace, and hoping they will stick." This seems to suggest that
he had learned to avoid information overload in order to learn and remember
better.

As mentioned in Chapter 2, the close connection between attention and
memory is prominent in the concept of *working memory* (Baddeley and Hitch,
1974). Recently, Baddeley (1993) has raised the question whether the term
"working memory" is a misnomer that could better be replaced by "working
attention." The reason for raising this question was his assumption that the most
crucial component of working memory, i.e., the central executive, is concerned
with attention and coordination rather than storage. Finally, however, Baddeley
proposed to continue to use the term "working memory" for the system as a
whole, as temporary storage is an absolutely essential feature of it.

In a paper on the effects of severe closed head injury, we speculated on the
relationship between processing speed and the quality of memory traces: "The
slowing of information processing after closed head injury implies that patients
cannot store information in memory with the efficiency they had before the
injury" (Van Zomeren et al., 1984). It has been demonstrated that the number
of words remembered in a multitrial free recall task is strongly dependent on
the subjective organization of the material during the acquisition stage (Baddeley, 1976; Deelman et al., 1980). However, subjective organization takes time.
It is reasonable to assume that much of this subjective organization is a "controlled" working memory process, presumably constrained by the speed of working memory operations and by the efficiency of its central executive component.
On the basis of a connection between speed and memory, we surmised that
some of the memory problems CHI patients experience might be the result of
slow controlled processing which would limit elaboration of information during
encoding. The point is illustrated by a report in which the efficiency of the
encoding and retrieval processes was seen to be limited by a poor central executive component in frontal patients (Luria, 1971).

Our reasoning about the role of speed of information processing in the
etiology of memory problems was based on the notion that a general faculty,
controlled processing, is specifically impaired in CHI patients and that this impairment is responsible for their problems in time-limited attention and memory
tasks. In a subsequent study, however, we found little specific evidence of slowness in controlled processing (Brouwer, 1985; Van Zomeren and Brouwer, 1987;
see Chapter 4). The data suggested a more global slowness indicating that the
activation of any long-term memory representation might take more time in
CHI patients. This was explained in terms of a decreased association strength

between conceptual nodes in an associative network. This theory would also explain the problems CHI patients have in memory tasks like verbal multitrial free recall tests and category naming. In the free-recall test there is less spread of activation through the network, and consequently less rich elaboration of the material. In the category-naming test, less salient items, in particular, tend to be missed (Deelman and Saan, 1990). If this theory is compared to the previous one, it appears that slow information processing is used in a more general way now, and is not restricted to controlled processing operations. Then, slow information processing is seen as the result of a very basic impairment, reduced strength of association between conceptual nodes in an associative network. Common to both theories is the suggestion that a relationship exists between speed of information processing and memory.

Gauggel and colleagues (1991) studied the relationship between speed of processing and memory in brain-damaged subjects. They assessed information processing and memory in a large group of 231 patients referred to the neuropsychological department of a university hospital. Most of these patients had suffered head injuries or cerebrovascular accidents. Information processing was assessed with three tasks: a German version of the Trailmaking Test (Zahlenverbindungs Test), simple visual RT, and a continuous choice RT task (Wiener Determinationsgerät). Memory was assessed with an extensive battery that included Digit Span forward, Corsi Block Tapping Test, immediate recall of a 10-word list, Benton Visual Retention Test recognition form, face recognition, logical memory (story recall), paired associate learning, face-name paired associate learning, and objects paired associate learning. Correlations between processing speed and memory scores were generally low, ranging from .01 to .55. Choice RT and age of the patients accounted on average for only 11 percent of the variance in memory scores in a multiple linear regression analysis. These weak relationships might be explained by assuming that only some of the memory tests were time-critical, or that they required little controlled processing, for example, face recognition. However, correlations were also low for those memory tests that appear most demanding of cognitive processing and organization. Immediate recall of a short paragraph of text correlated only .05 with simple RT, .26 with choice RT, and −.34 with the German Trailmaking (the latter two coefficients were significant). The multiple choice recognition version of the Benton Visual Retention Test correlated best with measures of processing speed. Performance on this task correlated nonsignificantly with simple RT, but the correlations with choice RT and the German Trailmaking were .44 and −.55, respectively. These data may be seen as lending weak support to the link between processing speed and memory: in the Benton VRT, subjects viewed a pattern of geometric figures for 10 seconds, probably verbalizing and rehearsing their nature. Speed of processing may have been a critical factor, partly determining the quality of reproduction. Still, Gauggel's conclusion that: "Reaction time was not a good predictor of the memory performance in these patients, or alternatively, our memory tests were not sensitive to a general reduction in speed of performance" cannot be rejected.

The correlational research described above raises a question: If a theory states that slow information processing, or slow access of memory, is the basic impairment in a certain category of patients, does this imply that the correlations between RT tests and scores on more complex cognitive tasks are higher in such patients than in healthy subjects? We think this is not the case. If the impairment is diffuse, it appears more likely that it will retard information processing on any cognitive process proportionate to the preinjury speed of that process, leaving the factorial structure of cognitive abilities intact and the correlations between test scores fundamentally unchanged. A better test of the role of speed of information processing in memory problems would be one in which both types of measurement are made within the same cognitive area. Such a study can be done using healthy normals as well as brain-injured patients.

Peeters (1986) and Godfrey and colleagues (1989) reported slow reactions in brain-damaged subjects presented with verbal stimuli in lexical decision or word recognition tasks. Slowness has also been shown in retrieving overlearned knowledge, such as answers to simple additions of digits below 10 (Brouwer, 1985), verifying "silly" sentences, and in category retrieval (e.g., Deelman and Saan, 1990). It is likely that such domain-specific slowness is more strongly related to poor verbal memory scores than to slowness in visual reaction time tasks. Again, we would not expect the correlations in patient groups suffering diffuse brain damage to differ from those in normal healthy controls.

WORK

Almost every work setting contains irrelevant, distracting stimuli and requires *focused attention*. This is most obvious with auditory stimuli. In vision, the act of focusing on task-relevant stimuli automatically precludes interference from the bulk of irrelevant stimulation. We are not distracted by stimuli outside our visual field. In contrast, sounds from behind us are not automatically excluded. Sounds such as human voices and mechanical noises can be heard in most job situations. When these sounds are constant and monotonous, the worker habituates to them quickly and completely. Even brain-damaged people never complain of the disturbing effect of a ticking clock or a humming air conditioner on their work activities. More important is the question whether focusing is affected by irregular non-task-relevant stimuli, e.g., colleagues discussing the local baseball team and its latest victory. Not only is this kind of stimulus irregular in pitch and volume, its verbal content may also have a distracting effect, especially since language processing is largely automatic and easily intrusive in the domain of controlled processing.

As far as we know, no studies relating focusing in attention tasks to distractibility in work situations have been published. The evidence for this is largely anecdotical, that is, patients often report that they cannot concentrate in noisy environments. As pointed out in Chapter 4, this is puzzling to the investigator. Head-injured patients are usually able to react selectively in the presence of distracting stimuli in laboratory tasks. It seems peculiar that they complain of noise disturbance, while at the same time demonstrating good selectivity. One possible explanation for this could be the effects of task duration. Gronwall (1987) quotes a head-injured student who complained about his inability to concentrate during lectures: "Fine for the first part, then I just kind of drifted off." It could be that investigators have been studying focusing for too-short periods of time and that susceptibility to distraction increases over time. Distractibility may be related to fatigue; even people without brain damage find it harder to concentrate when they are tired.

Another possibility might be that distraction becomes irritating only *after* concentration is lost. Maintaining an updated schema of the ongoing mental situation makes it easier to interpret incoming information. The schema generates expectations of what will follow and this works as an attentional filter. Through a cumulative loss of information due to mental slowness and memory problems as time-on-task increases, the schema may become less accurate, making it a less effective information filter. As a result, irrelevant information is more likely to dominate thinking. What appears to be a problem with focused attention could instead be a secondary symptom, i.e. the results of combined impairments in information processing and memory.

Most occupations include *divided attention tasks*. This is obvious for a bus driver in a downtown rush hour, but it is also true for the secretary in a busy office with telephones ringing, typing to be done and people asking questions. One of our patients, a head-injured ticket clerk for the national railway company, complained that he was frequently short of money at the end of his shift as he was no longer able to handle money efficiently while selling tickets and giving information to travelers.

There is some indirect evidence from subjective reports of head-injured patients on the influence of divided attention deficits in work situations. Van Zomeren and Van den Burg (1985) found a correlation of .62 between "return to work" and the complaint "inability to do two things simultaneously." This complaint is assumed to reflect divided attention deficit, and the correlation indicates that patients reporting such problems have a poorer chance of resuming their former work than patients who do not. In the same study, visual 4-choice RT correlated .49 with "return to work." This implies that about a quarter of the variance in the variable "return to work" was explained by the mental slowness as measured with choice RT. Rattok and colleagues (1992) have reported that visual processing skills in a neuropsychological rehabilitation program predicted vocational outcome, i.e., employment status at 9 months post-treatment.

Some ecological validity has also been claimed for the PASAT. Gronwall and Wrightson (1974) reported that speed and efficiency of information processing in this task were related to readiness to return to work in cases of mild CHI. This relationship was not found in more severe head injury. Hart and coworkers (1985) studied 28 severely head-injured patients, with a mean duration of PTA of 4 weeks, in a therapeutic job trial. The subjects were rated by their job supervisors while working in a full-time vocational placement within a hospital setting by means of a detailed check list. The most frequently observed problem involved memory. Supervisors often remarked: "When new material or information is presented, trainee is unable to recall and use the information." Another frequent problem involved time-sharing and dividing attention: "Trainee is unable to work on several tasks at the same time, alternating from one to another, and maintain good performance on each task." Speed on single tasks was also deficient in many trainees. Although this pattern is recognizable to anyone familiar with the mental sequelae of severe head injury, it was not related to PASAT performance. When trainees were grouped as being acceptable/un-acceptable for the work setting, the unacceptable group did not score lower on PASAT. In contrast, the classification was significantly related to memory per-formance on the Continuous Recognition Memory Task (Hannay et al., 1979). This could mean that acceptability was mainly determined by the absence of memory problems. Even when subjects were grouped according to their time-sharing abilities, it was found that trainees who had difficulties in doing two tasks simultaneously were *not* performing significantly poorer on the PASAT. Hart and colleagues (1985) concluded that vocational failure was most often due to problems with on-the-job memory, and that these problems could be predicted by clinical measures of memory.

Brooks and colleagues (1987) studied the relationship between return to work and cognitive status in a group of 98 severely head-injured patients. As late as 5 years after injury, 70 percent of patients were unemployed, and a convincing connection with cognitive impairments was demonstrated. Brooks and colleagues also reported that memory problems were predictive of failure to return to work. Of the patients who did well on Logical Memory from the Wechsler Memory Scale, 49 percent were unemployed at the time of follow-up. Of those who did poorly on Logical Memory, 89 percent failed to return to work. However, findings on attention measured with the PASAT did not agree with the study by Hart and colleagues (1985). The divided attention task had a considerable predictive power in the British study. The variable, "longest string recalled," in a version of the test presenting one digit every 2 seconds, clearly distinguished between workers and nonworkers in the patient sample. When scores on PASAT were reduced to three categories (low, medium and high) at the 33rd and 66th percentiles, it was found that 32 percent of the patients scoring "high" had failed to return to work. In the subgroup scoring "medium," 64 percent were unem-ployed, and in the subgroup scoring "low," 74 percent had not returned to work. Brooks and coworkers concluded that the PASAT appeared to be particularly sensitive for revealing the critical effects of attention deficits in hindering return to work.

Although the findings of the Brooks group appear more convincing on the basis of their much larger sample, the question remains how to explain the discrepancy between these two studies using the PASAT. Severity of injury was comparable in the two sample groups: median PTA duration was 4 weeks in the study by Hart and coworkers, while half of Brooks and colleagues' sample had been in PTA for more than 28 days. Vocational status was an obvious difference between the studies. Hart's patients were evaluated by their job supervisors after at least 1 week in a therapeutic job trial while Brooks' patients were assessed after many years during which they had had the opportunity to demonstrate their fitness to work in nontherapeutic job trials. Finally, there may have been differences in the formats of PASAT used. Brooks and colleagues used the 1 digit per 2 seconds presentation rate, taking the longest string recalled as the central index. It is not known which presentation rate was applied in the study by Hart and coworkers, but several studies have indicated that rate of presentation is a critical factor in PASAT performance after head injury (Thomas, 1977; Gronwall, 1987).

Level of task performance must be maintained over many hours in nearly all work situations. Nevertheless, no studies on the relationship between impairments of *sustained attention* and work have been published. This is remarkable, given the subjective complaints of patients such as the one quoted by Gronwall (1987) about a head-injured student "drifting off" during lectures. Furthermore, lapses of attention typical of patients with centrencephalic epilepsy must have consequences for their jobs, but we have found no studies addressing this problem.

The subjective reports of brain damaged patients also suggest that impairments in higher aspects of attention affect daily functioning, particularly task situations and work. However, the related concepts of Supervisory Attentional Control and Executive Functions are relatively new, and are only beginning to be applied to work situations. A promising new approach is the combination of a sophisticated measurement of attentional and supervisory function with a study of performance in a simulated work situation (Crepeau, 1992). Figure 9-1 illustrates another problem of supervisory attentional control in an occupational situation: a young woman realized, when she had partially recovered from a severe head injury, that she was lacking "overview" in her working situation. She then devised a schedule that she called a "prothesis," and that enabled her to regain control.

DRIVING

Driving competence is traditionally divided into driving skill and medical/psychological fitness to drive. *Driving skill* refers to the smoothness and safety of driving in actual traffic, using one's knowledge, basic abilities and resources efficiently, and it is assumed to depend heavily on learning and experience. *Fitness to drive* is defined as having the necessary mental and physical abilities and resources required for driving a motor vehicle safely and without unduly hindering the progress of other traffic. It is assumed that brain damage affects fitness to drive rather than driving skill per sé.

Theoretically, fitness to drive is not considered dependent on learning and experience. However, safe driving probably demands less basic ability and fewer resources of the experienced driver than of the beginner. In severely brain-damaged patients we have observed moderately high correlations between driving experience (distance driven) and driving quality and safety as assessed by driving experts on the basis of a one-hour ride in the subject's own car. The assessment was based largely on overall judgment and the items headed "traffic insight and perception" (Van Zomeren et al., 1988; Van Wolffelaar et al., 1988). These correlations were stronger than the correlations between expert judgment and neurological and neuropsychological impairment indices. Caution should be taken when relating test performance to everyday driving performance as impairments that are quite limiting for beginners may not be so for experienced

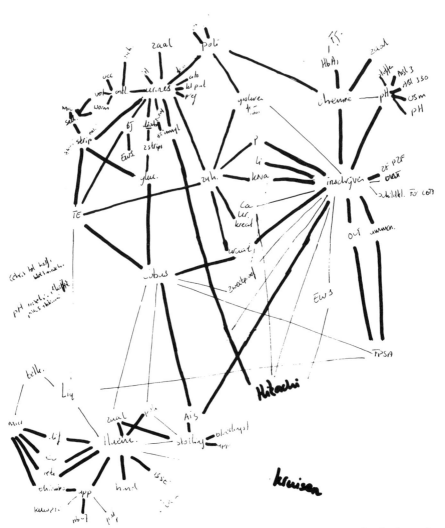

Figure 9-1 The reconstruction of structure. A 29-year-old laboratory worker had sustained a severe head injury. After resuming her work (part-time) she realized that she was lacking an overview, in her mind, of the multitude of subtasks and details in her work. She then constructed this ergogram, by putting together everything she could remember, clustering it around a few nuclei (urines, hematology, registration). Originally she drew thin lines only. As soon as she felt that a certain connection had once more become "natural" in her experience, she replaced the thin line by a thick one. The names Cobas and Hitachi refer to apparatuses for automatized biochemical analyses. The woman invented this approach without any professional coaching; she called her ergogram a "prothesis." Her prothesis turned out to be effective. It is presented here in the state where she abandoned it, as she felt confident again in her job.

drivers. It should be noted that our findings were derived from patients with very severe CHI. According to Hartje and coworkers (1991a), the effect of driving experience might not be as strong in patients who had suffered CVAs.

Specific effects of brain damage on driving skill can be demonstrated in experienced drivers despite the influence of driving experience. This is most apparent in more elementary elements of driving skill, which are not immediately related to traffic safety. Driving skill may be studied in two ways. In the first, driving behavior is observed in a *natural setting*; the subject drives in a variety of traffic situations representative of everyday traffic. Scoring is basically qualitative (e.g., Gregory, 1989; Hartje et al., 1991b). The second approach uses one or more critical driving subtasks, singled out for detailed quantitative study in a *quasi-experimental* manner, for example, the measurement of lateral position control during straight-road highway driving (Van Wolffelaar et al., 1988). As the following brief literature review shows, correlations between tests of information processing and driving skill are much higher in the second approach.

Attention and Global Indicators of Driving Skill

Laymen tend to see fast reaction times as predictors of driving skill. From this standpoint, *slow information processing* should be one of the global indicators of reduced driving quality. That this general assumption is untenable is demonstrated by the fact that very young drivers, who have the best RTs, also have the highest accident rates (McFarland et al., 1954; Hopewell and Van Zomeren, 1990). Obviously, a tendency for sensation seeking (generally associated with youth) is more relevant than RT. On the other hand, the complex cognitive structure of driving skill allows ample compensatory behavior when basic information processing abilities have slowed (Brouwer et al., 1990, 1991). However, there is a limit to this compensation. There is, for example, a definite increase in accident risk for drivers over 75 (Transportation in an Aging Society, 1988). More specifically, in a study of driving performance in older drivers, we found evidence to support the notion that test scores for information processing speed become relevant when the scores are quite bad (Brouwer et al., 1988).

In a study involving 60 healthy drivers between 60 and 80 years of age, the two main variables were speed of information processing and cognitive flexibility. Speed of information processing was operationally defined in terms of a composite variable based on a number of uncomplicated speed tasks, for example, Trailmaking-A and visual choice reaction. We measured flexibility independent of speed of information processing using adaptive tasks: 5 very slow subjects with very low flexibility, 5 very slow subjects with high flexibility, 5 very fast subjects with low flexibility, and 5 very fast subjects with high flexibility were selected from the sample of 60 older drivers. These subjects were rated by a driving expert who rode with them for 1 hour in their own cars and rated them according to his standard method. The result was a clear relationship between performance on timed tasks and the expert's overall judgment of driving quality (Table 9-1). In the total sample of 60 drivers, however, there was no significant correlation between the speed variable and the expert judgment.

Table 9-1   Relationship Between Overall Driver Quality and Psychological Test Results in a Selected Group of Elderly Drivers

Judgments	Groups			
	I + S +	I + S −	I − S +	I − S −
Insufficient	—	—	2	4
Doubtful	—	3	1	1
Sufficient	2	2	2	—
Amply sufficient	2	—	—	—

From Brouwer et al., 1988, with permission.

A test battery independently measured speed of information processing (I) and supervisory attentional control (S). For I a composite score was obtained as the average z-score of constituent subtasks, both paper-and-pencil and computerized tests. The S score was a mental flexibility score corrected for slow information processing. It was derived from the efficiency of adapting to changing task demands in a dynamic driving simulator. On the basis of these composite scores, four subgroups consisting of 5 subjects each were selected from a total group of 60 drivers (60–80 years old), viz. very good on I and S (I + S +), very good on I and very poor on S (I + S −), very poor on I and very good on S (I − S +), and very poor on both aspects (I − S −). The selected drivers were judged by an independent expert in a driving test in their own cars in actual traffic. In these extreme groups the relationship between test scores and expert judgment was quite strong.

Another candidate for the role of global indicator of driving skill might be flexibility, demonstrated by an *ability to switch attention*. In the study of elderly drivers described above, simple speed tests appeared to be more important than tests of cognitive flexibility. However, a number of studies of the relationship between accidents and test performance suggest that flexibility in switching attention to task-relevant sources of information is of greater importance. Kahneman and colleagues (1973) used a dichotic listening test with words and digits presented simultaneously in a study of young bus drivers. In one condition these subjects were required to switch attention from one ear to the other upon receiving a cue. A correlation of .37 was found between errors in the switching condition and accident rate. Parasuraman and Nestor (1991) suggested that the essential element in switching ability is the *disengagement* component of attention, described extensively by Posner and his colleagues (Posner and Petersen, 1990, see Chapter 3).

The existence of a significant relationship between accident rate and switching efficiency in laboratory tests was confirmed by several later studies. All reported correlations between .30 and .40 (see Parasuraman and Nestor, 1991, for a review). The problem with a number of these studies is that the effects of aging were not controlled for. The highest correlations were found in studies that included older drivers (up to 65). It is possible that the correlation between attention and accident rate could be spurious (McKenna et al., 1986), the result of an underlying relationship of both with age. Nevertheless, Parasuraman and Nestor concluded that the evidence for a relationship between attention and accidents is greater for switching selective attention and less for divided and sustained attention.

Parasuraman and Nestor (1991) stated that impaired switching is also conspicuous in Alzheimer's disease. A number of recent publications have shown that AD patients are a specific risk group with regard to driving (Friedland et al., 1988; Lucas-Blaustein et al., 1988; Kaszniak et al., 1990, 1991). In an early study of patients with "senile dementia," Waller (1967) concluded that the accident rate of individuals suffering from dementia was approximately two times that of normal older drivers. Although it is likely that AD patients' high accident involvement is related to impairments of attention (see Chapter 5), we think that the claim that it is related to impairments of switching attention is too specific. Current studies on the relationship between global indicators of driving skill and test performance in older drivers indicate a critical role of divided attention and supervisory attentional control.

Ball and Owsley (1991) measured peripheral detection in a divided attention situation using perceptual tasks with very short presentation of peripheral stimuli. In a sample of older drivers, they found a significant negative correlation between a measure of peripheral detection [the so-called Useful Field of View (UFOV)] and involvement in intersection accidents (intersection accidents, particularly at intersections with a major road, are typical for older and demented drivers). The UFOV score was based on performance both in single- and dual-task situations; the attentional and sensory/perceptual contributors to the effect cannot be separated out. By measuring various aspects of eye-health and elementary visual function (e.g., visual acuity and contrast sensitivity) along with UFOV, they were able to show that poor UFOV could occur both in persons with and without significant elementary visual dysfunction.

Their explanation of intersection accidents in older drivers implies that older drivers may suffer from a kind of "visual extinction" phenomenon, in which peripheral information is neglected in the presence of relevant central information. Following Parasuraman and Davies's line, the explanation for this could be an impaired ability to disengage attention from the central source of information. This compares with the effect described in right-parietal patients with symptoms of hemineglect (see Chapter 3), but in this case it is not related to lateralization of the stimulus. Eye disease may also be a factor, as well as change in information processing strategy and general resource limitations (Myerson et al., 1990).

Ball and Owsley (1991) found that the scores on a test of mental status, a screening instrument for dementia (Mattis, 1976), correlated significantly with involvement in intersection accidents (mental status and the UFOV contributed independently to the multiple prediction of accident involvement). As part of their mental status examination consisted of tests of mental control, this suggests that very poor supervisory attentional control may also play a role in the etiology of accidents. All investigators pointed out that driving by patients with dementing diseases may be a serious public health problem. It was found that many patients often continue to drive as long as seven years after the onset of illness. Friedland and coworkers (1988) confirmed the increased frequency of crashes and reported that most crashes involved driving errors at intersections, traffic signals or while changing lanes. All of these accidents suggested that the Alzheimer patients were "not paying attention." Lucas-Blaustein and colleagues (1988) reported that patients often lose their way while driving, implying that AD spatial disorientation may also result in hazardous situations.

The ability to *sustain attention* might be seen as a global indicator of driving skill, particularly during long boring rides. This would appear most relevant for epileptic patients; however, it has been shown that epileptic seizures are responsible for a negligible proportion of traffic accidents (Van der Lugt, 1975; Hansotia and Broste, 1991). Compared to the problem of drunk drivers, the problem of epileptic drivers is minor. Moreover, accidents resulting from epileptic seizures usually involve only the driver's car. Statistics have shown that the epileptic driver tends to have a seizure in low event rate situations. It is well known that mental activity can suppress seizures and subclinical epileptic manifestations. Kasteleyn-Nolst Trenité and colleagues (1991) recorded the EEGs of 19 epileptics while driving. A *decrease* of spontaneous EEG discharges was noted in 15 of the subjects during driving, compared to the frequency of discharges when subjects were sitting in a stationary car. Suppression of seizures by mental activity results in the epileptic seldom if ever experiencing a seizure while driving in dense traffic. Seizures are more likely to occur during long boring drives on empty roads (Van der Lugt, 1975; Fountain et al., 1983). Moreover, in some epileptic patients seizures are preceded by an aura that enables them to stop driving in time. Gastaut and Zifkin (1987) reported that immediate alterations of consciousness were significantly more likely to lead to accidents than seizures beginning with an aura.

Finally, the *hemi-inattention* that follows a stroke may impair driving skill. It is unlikely that a patient with gross neglect will be driving as this is usually a transient disorder which will have passed by the time the patient has resumed independent living. However, subtle effects may remain, becoming evident only when two or more sources of relevant information are presented simultaneously. In this situation information sources more to the left may tend to be missed. This so-called extinction phenomenon, mentioned above, particularly effects stimuli to the left of other conspicuous stimuli (see also Chapter 3). It is obvious that failure to note traffic coming from the left may cause accidents, but the frequency of accidents due to visual extinction in right hemisphere CVA patients is completely unknown. Observations concerning this effect are indeed included in the rehabilitation literature on driving, but these are based on impressions only (Van Zomeren et al., 1987).

Attention and Specific Indicators of Driving Skill

The preceding section addressed the relationship between broad concepts of attention, such as slowness of information processing, and overall driving skill. More specific relationships between aspects of attention and subtasks in driving will be discussed below.

A number of studies in the area of *head injury* have attempted to relate specific driving skills to test performance (Sivak et al., 1981; Stokx and Gaillard, 1986; van Zomeren et al., 1988; Korteling, 1988). Psychological tests of information processing and movement speed were found to have a reasonable predictive value for certain aspects of driving.

Van Wolffelaar and coworkers (1988, 1990) demonstrated that choice RT in the laboratory predicts speed of decision making in a traffic merging task mod-

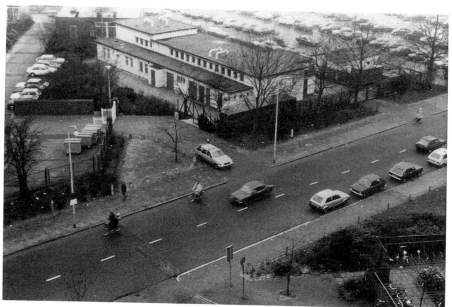

Figure 9-2   Field of view of the video camera used to record the positions and velocities of other traffic in the merging task described in the text. To ensure synchronization between the video signal and stimuli and responses by subjects in the car, lights on the roof of the car blinked whenever a subject received a signal to decide on merging, and when he made a decision.

erately well. Head-injured subjects seated in a stationary car at an intersection with a major road, had to decide whether it was possible to merge with traffic when a small signal lamp in the car flashed. See Figure 9-2. The patients needed significantly more time to decide than a control group; this slowness in a real-traffic situation correlated .60 with the decision time component of a visual four-choice RT in the lab. The authors also found that simple tests of visual motor speed like the Minnesota Rate of Manipulation Test and Trailmaking-A correlated moderately highly with lateral position control, a measure of steering precision recorded during actual highway driving. This result was also found by Van Zomeren and colleagues (1988).

Stokx and Gaillard (1986) reported appreciable correlations between a visual RT task and aspects of real driving. Their head-injured patients had to drive a slalom on a closed course, and they had to accelerate from 0 km/h to a speed of 60 km/h, with repeated shifting of gears. The time required for both tasks was predicted well by RT measures in the laboratory.

Gouvier and colleagues (1989) studied able-bodied, head-injured, and spinal cord-injured groups. Subjects were given a variety of laboratory tests, and drove on a closed course that included slalom courses marked by rows of cones. The authors reported that nearly all the measures in their test battery were significant predictors of driving ability. The best of these was the oral version of the Symbol Digit Modalities Test, "a task that appears to measure information processing capability." Korteling (1988) demonstrated that choice RT in a laboratory task predicted the RT of head-injured drivers to brake lights and changes in speed in a car-following test. A special feature of his laboratory task was the fact that it implied estimation of time duration: the imperative stimulus, a yellow light, was preceded by a green light. If the green light was on for 3 seconds or longer, subjects had to respond to the yellow light by pressing a button on the right. If the green light was on for less than 3 seconds subjects had to press a button on the left. Thus, the task required estimation of time duration, relevant in traffic as duration is linked to the perception of speed.

In the area of epilepsy and driving it has been shown that minor epileptic phenomena, such as *subclinical spike-wave bursts* with lapses of attention, can affect specific driving skills, although their effects are not dramatic in terms of driver safety. During a ride on a straight and empty road in the countryside, a lapse of attention will probably have no effect on the driver. In such a situation little action is required of him. (The reader can easily discover this for himself by closing his eyes for 2 seconds while driving on a straight rural road.) As Hutt and coworkers (1977) demonstrated, it is mainly the information processing stage of decision making that fails during a spike wave burst in epileptics; driving a straight course does not significantly load this stage. Kasteleyn-Nolst Trenité and colleagues (1987) showed that lane tracking ability decreases slightly in some patients during short-lasting discharges. In a study of six patients driving an instrumented car with an on-line EEG-registration, three of the patients' lateral deviation increased relative to discharges. It may be that this short lasting impairment has no practical importance. Van Zomeren and coworkers (1988), using a similarly instrumented car, found an increase in lateral deviation in patients who had sustained severe head injuries several years before, but concluded that this increase had no effect on safe driving in 8 of their 9 subjects.

Compensation for Decreased Fitness to Drive

In summary, tests of speed of information processing and attention have a certain predictive validity for assessing fitness to drive as they correlate moderately highly with *specific* driving skills in real traffic. However, the step from this finding to the medicolegal judgment of fitness to drive should be made with caution. Real driving offers many opportunities to compensate for slow information processing and other attentional deficits. As mentioned above, the amount and quality of driving experience may be important factors in this context. As the level of skill advances, the degree to which performance taxes basic abilities and resources is reduced.

Several studies have established the fact that poor test performance is not necessarily related to poor driving as assessed by global ratings of actual quality of driving (Simms, 1986; Van Zomeren et al., 1987, 1988; Hopewell and Van Zomeren, 1990; Hartje et al. 1991b). Engum and coworkers (1988a) assessed fitness to drive in brain-damaged patients with the Cognitive Behavioral Driver's Inventory (CBDI). The CBDI contains attention tests such as Digit Symbol Substitution from the WAIS-R, Trailmaking and visual RT. The investigators included normative data and decision-making rules (Engum et al., 1988b) and added several validity studies to their original report (Engum et al., 1990; Lambert and Engum, 1992). The three attention tests named above revealed significant differences (tested over group averages) between controls, patients who had passed an on-the-road test and patients who had failed this driving test. Although agreement between CBDI performance and the on-the-road driving test was impressive in the earlier studies, a final cluster analysis of 232 patients from two rehabilitation centers revealed two problematic groups of patients. The first was a cluster of 36 young head-injured patients who had passed the CBDI and were judged by the psychologist as potentially safe to drive. Still, these "young trauma's" had only an average probability of passing the road test, which implies a discrepancy between CBDI scores and actual driving in many cases. Engum et al. pointed out that good neuropsychological recovery as seen in the tests does not guarantee good driving, and that caution should be exercised when evaluating young drivers who have sustained head injuries. The cluster analysis also revealed a second group of 23 "elderly passes." These were patients aged 63 years or older with a variety of diagnoses who had obtained borderline CBDI scores, and all of whom had passed the road test.

An obvious difference between elderly drivers and young head injury patients, apart from the nature of the brain dysfunction, is age. As age is strongly correlated with driving experience (distance driven), this factor might explain part of the difference in the pattern of prediction errors in the validation studies. The modifying effect of driving skill, premorbid experience, and experience gained after injury, should be systematically taken into account in future studies on driving and neurologic disease. A practical consequence of the relatively weak relationships between test performance and driving performance in neurologic patients and older drivers is the need for a practical on-road driving examination (Gregory, 1989; Hartje et al., 1991b; Fox et al., 1992). This statement is based on the further consideration that patients themselves seem unable to judge their own driver qualities (see also Rebok et al., 1990).

A very important compensation mechanism for impaired driving skills was suggested by a hierarchical task analysis of driving modeled by Michon (Michon, 1979; Van Zomeren et al., 1987). This model describes traffic behavior as a hierarchy of subtasks at strategic, tactical, and operational levels. At the *strategic* level, choices and decisions are made concerning route, time of day, and so on. These decisions are usually made without time pressure and often before engaging in actual driving. At the *tactical* level, preparatory actions are taken while driving, for example, deciding to slow down when a traffic sign indicates the vicinity of a school or hospital. A slight time pressure is usually present at this level. Finally, the *operational* level comprises the numerous perceptions and actions performed from second to second to hold the car on course, to avoid parked vehicles, and so on. At this level the task exerts constant time pressure, as the driver has only limited time for avoiding or dealing with dangerous situations.

Analysis of driving in terms of this model shows that time pressure exists particularly at the operational level (escaping from acute danger). However, decisions at higher levels can strongly influence the risk of running into time pressure on lower levels. The strategic decision not to drive into the city during rush hours may prevent potential traffic conflicts with time pressure. The tactical decision not to overtake on a winding rural road will also prevent serious traffic hazards. Such strategic and tactical compensations could be important mechanisms for a brain-damaged driver, particularly in coping with impairments which reduce the speed of information processing either in a global or specific way.

SOCIAL SKILLS

What was said above about the lack of useful data applies even more forcefully to the present topic. The relationships between impairments of attention and social behavior have hardly been studied. What follows is therefore mainly speculative and draws on our experience in interviewing patients and relatives.

The main problem for brain-damaged people in social situations seems to be that *they do not note relevant cues* (Kreutzer, 1993). A social situation is by definition complex; it involves at least two people, usually more. This implies that visual and auditory information from various sources must be processed, while at the same time the subject may be performing a formal task, for example, working with two colleagues while talking about their family problems. In such situations, adequate social behavior requires the ability to perceive subtle cues in facial expression, verbal intonation, emotional content of remarks, and so on. With regard to head-injured subjects, we have heard many reports of "childish" and "self-centered behavior" that seem related to an incomplete perception of social situations.

Examples are easy for any clinician to find. The mother of a severely head-injured boy complained that her son no longer noted when she was wearing a new dress, which was painful to her as she interpreted it as a sign of decreased interest. A couple of parents told us about the blunting of their daughter's behavior, describing how the girl entered the kitchen where her parents were sitting at the table in a depressed mood, discussing the troublesome financial situation of their farm. The girl began to tell, in a childish way, about her experiences at school that morning. The parents were quite sure that this was "unlike her," that before her accident she would have noted their mood.

In these examples, the behavior of the patients can be explained as the result of incomplete analysis: the patients saw their parents, but not their dress or mood. An alternative explanation for the second example might be that the brain-damaged patient had a specific deficit in the perception of emotion. This phenomenon has been well-documented, and related to right hemisphere damage (De Kosky et al., 1980; Etcoff, 1991). It has also been noted in cases of severe head injury (Braun et al., 1989a). However, it is our opinion that these social failures are frequently based on an attentional deficit, i.e failure to attend to secondary cues, and may be related to reduced information processing resources.

The *laborious verbal production* of many brain-damaged patients may also be a factor. Expressing thoughts and feelings seems to be difficult for many patients, even in the absence of manifest aphasia. In particular, after severe head injury patients may speak slowly, have to search for words, and frown in an effort to grasp the situation. We have seen many patients who stared down at the table or past the interviewer's head, probably in an attempt to concentrate fully on their words and not be distracted by the eyes of the interviewer. It is very likely that patients with this kind of language problem simply have no "spare capacity" to pay attention to the mood, facial expression or other non-verbal cues in the behavior of their conversation partners.

Godfrey and colleagues (1989) studied the language production of severely head-injured patients. They videotaped and analyzed the behavior of 18 male subjects, all out-patients of a rehabilitation hospital, in two social situations. The first of these was a "friendly chat" with a female research assistant who offered the patient tea or coffee. The assistant was instructed to maintain a relaxed conversation with the subject for at least 10 minutes. In the second situation, the subject took part in an extended role play of a difficult job interview situation with the interviewer asking nasty questions "to place the interviewee under moderate stress." The video recordings were rated by two independent raters, using categories of social competence (interesting, pleasant, likeable, skillful, apathetic). An additional 10 rating scales were used to assess specific verbal and nonverbal microbehaviors: speech rate, speech duration, spontaneity, emotion, question frequency, speech pitch, looking, gesture frequency, smiling frequency and laughing frequency. In the comparison with a control group, means on all scales of social skill favored the normal subjects. The head-injured group was rated as significantly less interesting, less likeable and less socially skilled. An additional finding was that both control subjects and patients were significantly more lively during the "pleasant chat" than in the job interview. As Godfrey and colleagues put it: "The mean ratings favoured the opposite sex interaction over the stressful interview."

More relevant to the present topic were verbal data. The head-injury group spoke significantly slower, were less spontaneous, spoke more monotonously, and for shorter periods than the control group. Only in the job interview setting did the head injury group look at the interactor significantly less than the control group. This latter finding fits our own clinical impressions when interviewing patients, although it does not confirm our speculation that patients prefer to avoid eye contact in order to concentrate better on their verbal statements.

Godfrey's group also studied speed of information processing in the same 18 patients. Subjects were required to locate a target digit on a display containing 2, 4, or 6 digits, arranged randomly. Oral responses were recorded by a voice-activated relay. Patients reacted significantly slower than controls in this visual search paradigm. Moreover, there was a significant interaction between groups and numbers of digits; the absolute difference in RT between groups increased with the number of digits (proportionally, the difference remained roughly the same; patients were about 40 percent slower than controls in all conditions). Correlations between speed of search and social skills ratings were nonsignificant. Likewise, no significant relationships were found between speed of search and ratings of nonverbal and verbal social behavior. This seems to conflict with our hypothesis that reduced information processing capacity plays an important role in the etiology of problems in social skills. However the case for domain specificity proposed in the section on memory may be raised in defense. It appears likely that diffuse brain injury slows information processing on any cognitive process proportionately to the preinjury speed of that process, leaving the factorial structure of cognitive abilities intact, and consequently, the correlations between test scores unchanged.

Another explanation for the discrepancy between test scores and the quality of social skills was suggested by Godfrey and colleagues, that is, whether the nature of the information processing task precluded finding a significant association. RT tasks typically require subjects to make quick, simple and discrete decisions, unlike social interactions where sustained and complex information handling is required. This sounds plausible as verbal production in a conversation requires far more complex programming of responses than an RT task. It is also conceivable that subtle verbal impairments after head injury do not affect the recognition and naming of digits, while they may slow conversational speech. Godfrey and colleagues' study points the way to a most interesting approach, linking cognition and social behavior in the study of head injury. Furthermore, their findings produced objective evidence of reduced social skills after severe head injury. In the past such evidence was mainly impressionistic and clinical. The authors point out the negative consequences of this reduction: "It seems likely that very severely head-injured adults are not reinforcing people to interact with them, and that this reflects behavioral deficits in social skill. This may account for their often reported social isolation" (Thomsen, 1974; Elsass and Kinsella, 1987). Godfrey and colleagues stressed the importance of social skills training in the rehabilitation of these neurologic patients.

One further speculation based on clinical experiences is warranted before closing this chapter. Some head-injured patients indicate that they are consciously screening themselves off from social contacts. During convalescence patients may state that they already have more problems than they can handle, using this as a rationale for lowered interest in or decreased sensitivity to the problems of others, particularly, nonsignificant others. Although such statements may be a rationalization, it is possible that a decrease in social contacts may be a psychological compensation mechanism in individuals who do not feel strong enough to attend to their wider social environment. A theoretical framework for understanding this type of compensation can possibly be found in the concept of a hierarchical task-analysis such as the one proposed by Michon for driving (discussed above in the section on driving competence).

SUMMARY

Attention and memory have an intimate relationship, which is stressed in the concept of working memory. It can be argued on theoretical grounds that slowed information processing results in the formation of poor-quality memory traces. From a connectionist viewpoint, slowness of information processing and memory impairments can both be explained by reduced association strength between conceptual nodes in an associative network. Despite these theoretical relationships, empirical data have not revealed a close working relationship. The performance of brain-damaged patients on memory tests cannot be predicted to any useful degree from their performance on timed tests, such as RT and Trailmaking. Still, it is conceivable that speed of processing and memory will show a stronger relationship in more specific areas, for example, RT to verbal stimuli and recall of the same material.

Little is known about the consequences of attentional deficits in work situations. Although it seems plausible that such deficits could cause serious problems, the evidence is mainly anecdotal. Few studies have addressed this question directly. Choice RT and PASAT appear to have a certain predictive validity for return to work after head injury.

Some effects of attentional deficits on driving have been determined. Although from the layman's point of view mental slowness should reduce driver quality, empirical studies have demonstrated that RT is not strongly related to driving skill; only extreme slowness affects overall driver quality. There is some evidence that flexibility—the ability to switch attention effectively—is related to driving skill in normals. The relationships between performance on attention tests and driving are much clearer with regard to specific aspects of driving. RT in the laboratory, for example, satisfactorily predicts speed of decision-making in traffic, speed of slalom driving, speed of gear shifting, and brake RT. The fact that attention tests cannot predict overall driver quality can be explained via two mechanisms. The first is driver experience; an experienced driver may be less vulnerable to the effects of brain damage or disease. The second is theoretical; in a hierarchical model of driving, higher-level decisions will reduce time pressure and workload on lower levels, allowing the brain-damaged driver to compensate for slowness that might lead to fatal consequences at the lowest (operational) level of task performance.

The effects of impairments of attention on social skills have hardly been explored. On the basis of clinical observations, we hypothesized that the main problem lies in the fact that brain-damaged people do not note socially relevant cues. Theoretically, this could be linked to a reduced processing capacity. In some patients, laborious verbal production seems to play a role; putting thoughts into words apparently uses so much of their resources that no capacity remains to note subtle cues in the behavior of a conversation partner.

10

Rehabilitation of Attentional Impairments

Psychology's contribution to the field of rehabilitation dates back at least to 1947, when Zangwill described three broad approaches to rehabilitation which were to be rediscovered by later generations of psychologists: retraining, compensation and substitution (Brooks, 1990). An explosive growth in cognitive rehabilitation occurred in the 1980s, and various training programs for attentional deficits were developed. This is easy to understand since such deficits affect every area of functional independence and they can seriously hinder physical rehabilitation and occupational retraining. The training programs were mainly developed in rehabilitation centers, with great enthusiasm and inventiveness. Very often they made use of computers, which have many practical advantages and are appealing to the trainees.

For several reasons it is difficult to judge the efficacy of attention training programs. Three problems are encountered in a review of the literature:

1. Programs are seldom based on theoretical frameworks of attention. Instead, investigators describe the functions to be trained in colloquial terms that have an apparent face validity. Hence the field of attention retraining suffers from that general curse of attention research, confused terminology.
2. Training methods are usually based on more than one principle. Simple repetition, systematic feedback based on learning theory, praise, verbal mediation, application of new strategy, and so on, are combined, and it remains unclear which component deserves the credit for any improvement in performance.
3. Training programs can focus on different aspects of attention; subjects may be trained to work faster, to spend longer periods at a task, or to work more accurately.

Cognitive rehabilitation of attentional impairments is based, often tacitly, on three models: stimulation therapy, behavioral conditioning, and strategy substitution (Gross et al., 1986). The literature on attention training will be reviewed in this chapter under these headings. First, however, the training of hemi-inattention will be discussed separately. The reason for this separate treatment is that hemi-inattention is a clear nosological entity, mainly manifested in one sensory modality. It contrasts strongly in this regard with the less well-defined, more general impairments that are discussed in the second part of this chapter.

REHABILITATION OF HEMI-INATTENTION

Hemi-inattention, or unilateral neglect, is the failure of brain-damaged individuals to report, respond or orient to stimuli on the side of the brain contralateral to a lesion (see Chapter 3). This condition is a common impairment, particularly in stroke patients. In 1962, Lawson described an attempt to train two patients by frequently reminding them to "look to the left." The problem of retraining was extensively studied in the 1970s by Weinberg and coworkers (1977, 1979). Their general approach was aimed at restoring the scanning habits of patients to the affected side of the field of vision. One method for achieving this was the use of end-anchoring, that is, giving the left margin in reading and in cancellation tasks extra emphasis by means of a thick red vertical line. A "scanning machine" with a moving target was also used for training. The patients showed some improvement in performance compared with untrained control groups. Using the same remedial program, Diller and Weinberg (1977) found that training visual scanning had a positive effect on reading ability. However, it was evident in this series of investigations that improvement was strongest in evaluation tasks that resembled the trained tasks. In other words, the training effects seemed rather specific and showed little generalization, a problem that Lawson (1962) had noted in his pioneer study.

Weinberg's approach was adapted by Webster and coworkers (Webster et al. 1984; Gouvier et al., 1984), who also used the scanning machine. Their evaluation of training effects, however, was original. Webster and colleagues studied the performance of patients in wheelchairs navigating an obstacle course by counting the number of collisions with markers along the track. The scanning training indeed resulted in improved wheelchair navigation. These results were confirmed by a second study (Gouvier et al., 1984) that likewise demonstrated improved performance in wheelchair navigating and on the scanning board. However, this effect did not generalize to a letter cancellation task, which again indicates that the effects of training can be very specific.

Gordon and colleagues (1985) applied Weinberg's approach to fairly large groups: 48 experimental subjects and 29 nontrained controls. After 35 hours of training, the experimental group performed significantly better than the control group on a cancellation task, line bisection, and a search task. Unfortunately, the training effect seems to have been temporary. Four months later there were no significant differences between the two groups on these tasks.

Robertson and coworkers (1990) used a computerized form of the Weinberg method. They trained 20 patients with left-sided visual neglect by means of a computer screen displaying targets and verbal instructions. A target was presented at the top of the screen and a series of matching targets and distractors below. The task was to locate and touch the targets as quickly as possible. Before each response, the subjects had to touch a red bar at the far left of the screen which then immediately turned green. Failure to do this caused the computer to flash the message "Touch left" across the screen, along with a flashing arrow, until the subject touched the red bar. The bar was gradually faded until the subject touched left without any visual cue. Thus, the method was partially aimed at habit formation by verbal mediation. A control group of 16 subjects were given a comparable amount of time for recreational computing. Blind follow-up at the end of the training and 6 months later revealed no statistically significant or clinically relevant differences between groups on a wide range of relevant tests.

These negative results contrasted with positive findings in an earlier series of case studies by the same authors (Robertson et al., 1988). Gray (1990) raises the question whether the discrepancy could be explained by insight learning in the relatively short and intensive training of the patients in the case studies.

Gray (1990) summarized the effect of neglect rehabilitation as follows: "The results with patients suffering from unilateral neglect were disappointing. Initial success with the single-case studies was replaced by total failure in the group studies. Yet there is abundant evidence that neglect is remediable. The most likely explanation seems to be that while the single-case studies showed the effects of one sort of learning (insight learning), the group studies failed because the experimental procedures did not produce any useful form of incremental, motor learning."

Robertson and colleagues (1990) concluded that training strategies for hemi-inattention may be more cue-specific than has previously been suggested. In his view, chronic neglect patients are capable of learning specific compensatory scanning responses to specific stimuli, but much less able to learn general scanning strategies. According to the author, an implication of this should be that training must be tied to specific cues that are likely to be present in the everyday

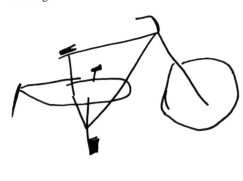

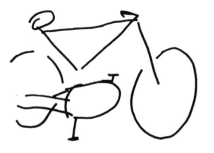

Figure 10-1 Drawings of a bicycle by a patient with hemineglect, before and after training. The author observed a slight effect of training in 5 patients, particularly in their drawings. In this case, the rear wheel is more pronounced after training. (From Glas, 1992, with permission.)

life of the trainee. In search of "a stimulus which is reliably present in all the different situations in which the sufferer must operate," Robertson and North (1992) eventually settled on the patient's *left arm*. They taught a patient with left-sided neglect to use his hemiplegic arm as a perceptual anchor by placing it immediately to the left of the area in which he was working. Training in this use of the limb, which appeared to have residual power sufficient for holding it in the necessary position, was applied in a variety of tasks such as reading, eating and working in occupational therapy. Clear improvements were seen in a number of "tests" such as dialing telephone numbers, reading and letter cancellation. A related method is contralesional limb activation (Robertson and North, 1992; Robertson et al., 1992). Visual neglect was reduced in three patients by means of left-arm activation. During training, a Neglect Alert Device was used—a small metal box with a buzzer and a red light. This device was placed close by the hemiplegic left hand, and the subject had to press a switch within a pre-determined time interval to prevent the Neglect Alert Device from buzzing. This method of contralateral limb activation clearly improved visual neglect, and the effect was generalized to the level of everyday functioning in the patients. Of course this method requires some residual motor function in the left hand, but Robertson and colleagues point out that the movements required were the kind of residual minimal responses which are not uncommon in hemiplegic patients. Moreover, even when there is no movement whatsoever in the left arm, the possibility of using it as a passive perceptual anchor remains.

Robertson and Cashman (1991) demonstrated the efficacy of an external feedback loop in sensory neglect. A woman with unilateral left sensory neglect who was walking with her left foot heel-up in a highly unstable plantarflex position was equipped with a pressure-sensitive switch under her heel. A buzzer on her belt supplied feedback about contact between heel and floor. Although various physiotherapeutic approaches had failed to improve this patient's walking, the feedback method resulted in an increased number of heel-strikes within 5 days, probably due to the patient's increased awareness of her left leg. Clinical observation showed that the effect remained after training was terminated.

In conclusion, it seems that hemineglect as such cannot be helped by training. No permanent general effects of training on hemi-inattention have been reported so far. What has been demonstrated is the effect of task-specific training by means of special cues or feedback, which may help the patient in certain daily life situations. The use of the patient's left arm as an always present cue seems particularly promising. See Figure 10-1.

GENERAL ATTENTIONAL DEFICITS

Stimulation Therapy

The major premise of the stimulation model is that attentional impairments can be alleviated by means of direct stimulation of brain structures assumed to be involved in attention or in a particular aspect of attention. Treatment is based on submitting patients to repetitive exercises and providing them with feedback about their performance. Although they were not the first to take this approach, Ben-Yishay and colleagues (1987) have been some of its chief exponents. Repeated stimulation of brain structures would supposedly facilitate neuronal growth or regeneration (Powell, 1981), and attention would respond like a "mental muscle" whose function, as in the case of real muscles, could be improved by repeated exercise (Harris and Sunderland, 1981).

The effect of training can be measured in three ways: at the task level, at the level of task-related psychometric tests, and at the level of daily functioning (Van Zomeren and Fasotti, 1992).

Task-Level Measures

All studies in which improvement on trained tasks was systematically measured have shown progress. Wood and Fussey (1987) trained very severely head-injured patients to scan moving symbols on a computer screen. They found a gradual and significant increase in the number of correct responses during the first 7 days. They also noted a halving of variability in individual performances. In the case study of a radiologist with a right temporal lobectomy, Rao and Bieliauskas (1983) noted a considerable training effect in a Symbol Cancellation Task. Ben-Yishay and coworkers (1987) applied the Orientation Remedial Module, a computerized series of five tasks forming an overlapping hierarchy in complexity of reception/response demands, to a group of severely head-injured patients. The training resulted in a progression from initially impaired performance to the average normal range.

What can be concluded from these investigations? That patients with severe brain damage *can* learn to carry out specific tasks in the visuomotor domain or in visual search. This in itself is an important finding for the social reintegration of patients as it would appear that they could be taught certain skills, such as those demanded by a new occupation. However, any optimism must be tempered by the fact that these training effects are task-specific. An essential question is: Does the effect of training generalize? This question must be answered by means of the next two evaluation methods.

Psychometric Measures

Stimulation studies often use psychometric tests to determine any generalization effects of training. Results have been somewhat conflicting. In the Wood and Fussey study (1987), psychomotor and vigilance measures did not reveal significant changes after training on the scanning task. Malec and coworkers (1984) employed video games to improve sustained attention in patients with traumatic brain injury. Three tests of sustained attention and a reaction time task were used as dependent variables. The only measure that approached significance was the reaction time task. Ponsford and Kinsella (1988) also trained a group of severely head-injured patients, who had to respond rapidly and selectively to information presented on a computer screen. Progress on psychometric measures of information processing speed did not exceed spontaneous recovery levels. See Figure 10-2.

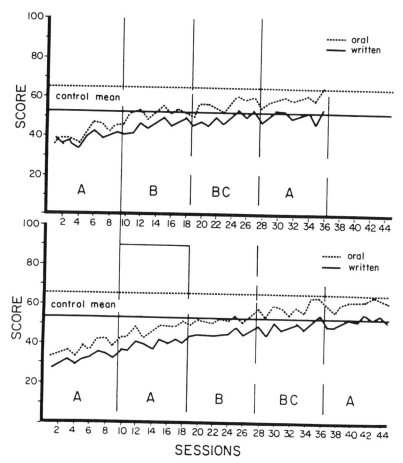

Figure 10-2 Improvement on the Symbol Digits Modalities Test (SDMT) in head-injured patients receiving stimulation training. Effect of training was assessed thrice weekly with an oral and a written form of this test. Performance of the patients improved steadily, regardless of training condition. *A*, baseline assessment, prolonged for the group in the lower half of the picture; *B*, stimulation training lasting 3 weeks; *BC*, stimulation training during 3 more weeks, with additional feedback and systematic reinforcement by therapist. Ponsford and Kinsella concluded that subjects showed no significant response to remedial intervention. The steady increase in SDMT score is explained by them as a combined effect of practice on this task and spontaneous recovery. (From Ponsford and Kinsella, 1988, with permission.)

On the other hand, a few studies *do* report training effects visible in psychometric evaluations. Ben-Yishay and colleagues (1987) trained a very severely head-injured subject with the Orientation Remedial Module and found significant improvements in visual reaction times, auditory digits and the WAIS verbal IQ. Two studies in which head-injured patients were trained with various visuomotor, visual search and reaction time tasks (Sivak et al., 1984a, 1984b) reported improved performance, after training, on a variety of psychological tests, including Trailmaking A and B and a Letter Cancellation Task (Diller et al., 1974).

Sohlberg and Mateer (1987) designed Attention Process Training, a hierarchical, multilevel computer-program for improving various aspects of attention. Four brain-damaged subjects underwent 5 to 10 weeks' training and all showed significant and stable gains in PASAT performance. Gray and colleagues (1992) reported that a group of traumatic and nontraumatic brain damaged patients improved more than a control group on PASAT, Backward Digit Span, and the WAIS subtests Block Design, Arithmetic and Picture Completion. Their study included patients with attentional problems according to explicit, although mixed, criteria: either subjective reports of difficulties in concentrating in real-life situations such as reading or following a conversation; either a score of one standard deviation below the mean or lower on the PASAT; or more than five errors on the Wisconsin Card Sorting Test. The authors considered the latter a test of certain higher aspects of attention, that is, integrity of the control processes involved in the maintenance and switching of attention or set. Training comprised RT tasks (simple and discrimination), rapid number comparison (Braun et al., 1985), Digit Symbol Transfer (Braun et al., 1985) an alternating Stroop task (Dyer, 1973) and divided attention tasks. The divided attention tasks were computer games which combined the sort of visuomotor demands of "space invaders" with mental arithmetic under time pressure.

When experimental and control groups were evaluated after the training period, the experimental subjects performed significantly better on PASAT and on Arithmetic from the WAIS. The authors state that the effects of training were by no means trivial: the experimental group improved by an average of 2.14 on Arithmetic versus 0.7 for the control group. For Forward and Backward Digit Span, Picture Completion, Block Design and Arithmetic, performance in the experimental group had become virtually normal. The authors argue convincingly that the difference between groups could not be explained on the basis of spontaneous recovery, motivational factors, and so on. They believe that verbal-mediated strategies for self-arousal and for combating interference effects in working memory are involved in their training tasks, and that this can produce improvement in nontrained tests of attention.

Niemann and colleagues (1990) reported the results of computer-assisted attention retraining in 26 head-injured patients. These patients enrolled in a training and testing program lasting 14 weeks, and all of the patients were at least 1 year postinjury (which implies that spontaneous recovery effects could not play an important role in any changes during the program). The subjects were outpatients, that is, they were no longer hospitalized or in rehabilitation centers.

The study was methodologically well done, with multiple baseline measures and a random assignment of patients to either attention training or memory training. The latter condition served as a control condition. Attention training consisted of auditory and visual choice reactions, including reactions to green stimuli between red distractors. In addition, a task for shifting attention was used in which the subjects had to react to various dimensions of stimuli. The effect of this training was assessed with two sets of tests. Each set was a combination of attention and memory tests. For example, in the first set the Brick-enkamp d2, the PASAT, a digit-digit matching task, and Trailmaking B measured attention. The Rey Auditory Verbal Learning Test (a list of 15 words) and a Block Span Learning Test measured memory.

Niemann and coworkers (1990) found a significant effect of attention training on the attention part of the evaluation set, and no effect on the two memory tests. However, the effect on the four attention measures was mainly determined by the effect on Trailmaking.

As mentioned above, there was a second set of evaluation measures; this one contained a Digit Cancellation Test as an attention measure. Niemann and coworkers did not describe this test, but they called it the "2 and 7 test," so it may be assumed that the twos and sevens in rows of digits had to be ticked. While this evaluation measure bore some resemblance to the Brickenkamp in the first evaluation set, it did not work. So here we have another riddle: one cancellation test suggests a training effect while the other does not. Moreover, as far as can be judged from a figure in the paper, the training effect on the Brickenkamp was modest in comparison to retest effects.

It would seem that stimulation training effects are found only if the tests used for evaluation resemble the training tasks. Sturm and coworkers (1983) employed a series of 16 psychometric tests to evaluate training with reaction time and memory-search tasks in head-injured patients. Improvement was most evident in the tests resembling the training tasks. This problem of *limited generalization* was even more conspicuous in a later study by the same authors (Sturm and Willmes, 1991) of patients with cerebrovascular lesions. The authors report: "Whereas for the tests resembling the training there were improvements for up to 100 percent of the patients, the proportion of 'improvers' decreased with decreasing similarity to the training." Recently, Sturm and coworkers (1993) have argued that stimulation training can be effective when it is aimed at specific aspects of attention, such as phasic alertness, selective attention, divided attention and vigilance. The authors designed computer-assisted training for each of these four domains, attempting "to construct tasks that represented the underlying attention paradigms as purely as possible." Training of 38 stroke patients made clear that significant improvements in "alertness" and "vigilance" were indeed found only after applying the respective training programs, and not with the other ones.

It is difficult to get an overview of the evidence and to draw a conclusion. Three of the ten studies described do not report progress on psychometric measures after stimulation therapy, while some of the other studies are either based on a single case, poorly controlled for spontaneous recovery, or show effects mainly in psychometric measures resembling the trained tasks. This latter point presents a problem for the evaluation of stimulation effects. If generalization of training effects to psychometric tests is absent or limited, can we expect stimulation training to have an effect in areas that are even further removed from the laboratory, that is, on daily life activities?

Effects on Daily Functioning

Three studies evaluated the effects of stimulation therapy on daily life functioning. Wood and Fussey (1987) recorded "attention to task" during patients' *therapy activities*. This measure produced significant differences between base-line and posttreatment assessment.

Ponsford and Kinsella (1988) used a rating scale for day-to-day attentional behavior. Like Wood and Fussey, these authors asked occupational therapists to rate the behavior of head-injured patients in a rehab setting by means of a Rating Scale of Attentional Behavior. This scale contained 15 items relating to different aspects of attentional behavior, such as slowness, distractibility, and attention to detail (see also Chapter 8). In addition, a 30-minute video recording of patients performing a *clerical task* was used to analyze and quantify their attentional behavior. Percentage of time spent directed to the task, defined by the patient's eyes being focused on it, was recorded. Improvements on the rating scale and on the video recordings were mainly due to spontaneous recovery. When spontaneous recovery and practice effect were controlled for, the patients showed little response to training in terms of these independent measures.

The training of perceptual skills given by Sivak and colleagues (1984b) resulted in improved *driving* performance. Eight head-injured patients underwent 8 to 10 hours' training of perceptual skills such as visual scanning and attentional capacity. This had a positive effect on their performance in a number of attention tasks, including the Symbol Digits Modalities Test (Smith, 1982), Trailmaking A and B, and the Letter Cancellation Task (Diller et al., 1974). The degree of improvement on cognitive tests was related to the degree of improvement in driving. Sivak and colleagues (1984b) report that 53 percent of the variance in the driving performance improvement was accounted for by the perceptual improvement. A problem in judging this investigation is the fact that the attentional components in the training program, the test battery and the driving, cannot clearly be distinguished. Driving quality was judged in five categories, one of them called "Observation." It may be assumed that this category, which included the use of mirrors and paying attention to signs, had a load on "attention."

The effects of stimulation therapy on attentional behavior in daily life remain unconvincing on the basis of this limited evidence. When Ponsford (1990) reviewed the evidence on the efficacy of computerized stimulation in the rehabilitation of attention disorders, she concluded:

> No studies published to date have conclusively demonstrated that training on computer mediated tasks, whether they be video games or tasks focusing on specific aspects of attention, has an impact on the everyday attentional problems of head-injured subjects. This has been so whether the intervention has been made during the early phase of recovery, less than 12 months post-injury or after recovery has plateaued.

Strategy Substitution

This therapy model is based on the assumption that patients can be helped by providing them with compensatory strategies, in the form of either external aids, for example, a checklist, or internal procedures such as self-instruction. *Verbal mediation* techniques are frequently used compensatory strategies (Meichenbaum, 1977). These are based on Luria's idea (1966) that the regulation of attention is largely dependent on subvocal, or inner, speech. Webster and Scott

(1983) trained a construction worker 2 years after a severe head injury, to use self-instructional statements to focus attention during reading or listening. Results suggested that not only attention, but also recall of information improved significantly.

Two more case studies have described positive effects of verbal mediation on cognition, although the link with attention is less clear in these reports. Barry and Riley (1987) introduced verbal mediation while teaching a young woman with a severe closed head injury hand movement patterns. Significant improvements were found which could be partially attributed to the assimilation of the verbal strategy. In Rao and Bieliauskas' study (1983) stimulation therapy was combined with verbal mediation techniques. The patient-radiologist was encouraged to use his verbal skills to solve nonverbal tasks, and to write verbal summaries immediately after seeing movies. After training, improvement was noted in several areas. Most relevant was the improvement in the patient's professional skills: his accuracy rate in reading radionuclide scans increased from 80 to 100 percent.

Although these three case studies seem to indicate that strategy substitution can be effective, further research on groups is needed to confirm the benefits of this training model. However, two advantages of strategy substitution are undeniable: the model is explicitly based on a theoretical idea, and the exercises are directly aimed at problem behavior and consequently avoid the generalization problems that are so prominent in stimulation therapy.

Behavioral Conditioning

Wood (1987) applied contingent reinforcement in the form of tokens to improve attention during therapy tasks. He used the term "span of attention" to indicate the amount of uninterrupted time a subject can spend on a given task. In our terminology, "span of attention" would be classified under the heading of sustained attention. Wood commented that very severely head-injured patients often seem unable to generate enough effort to sustain sufficient concentration to attend and cooperate during treatment sessions. In order to prolong the span of attention, a token was presented to a patient if, and only if, his head and eyes were directed at the therapist at the end of a 2-minute interval. In two out of three patients with very severe head injuries, including frontal lobe damage, the method resulted in significant changes in attention to task. Wood emphasized in his report that the treatment was in fact aimed at "attentiveness" which he characterized as the behavioral component of attention. This observable aspect should be distinguished from the cognitive, or information processing component. He also remarked that there was no evidence that improving attentive behavior led to a parallel increase in information processing capacity. Still, it is clear that the method described was successful in establishing the first step of a learning process, allowing greater cooperation between patient and therapist and an increase in time spent engaged in the therapy activity. Moreover, the training effect showed some generalization to other therapy activities.

Behavioral conditioning techniques presumably will be most appropriate for patients with very severe brain damage whose extensive cognitive impairments impede the application of strategy substitution. Still, related techniques might be applied in many daily life tasks to improve "attention to task." Wilson and Robertson (1992) described a training program based on a simple behavioral shaping technique used with a severely head-injured man who had complained of "losing concentration while reading." He was taught to identify his involuntary slips in attention which occurred while reading a novel, and to record their frequency with a golf counter. Slips were defined as those times when he found that he needed to reread a word or sentence, or when he became aware that his mind had wandered from the text to a different train of thought. After baseline assessment, training began in which reading the novel was practiced for the minimum period sustainable without an attention slip. This was followed by a planned break. The length of the reading period was gradually increased. This proved to be effective: the subject was able to increase the time for which he could read a novel without a slip from 1.5 to 5 minutes. However, once more a generalization problem was noted: although the subject reported that after the training he was "reading for pleasure now," he still could not sustain his attention when reading an accountancy text that he wanted to master in order to return to his clerical job.

THE FUTURE OF ATTENTION TRAINING

The efficacy of cognitive rehabilitation is as yet not widely accepted. In a discussion in the *Archives of Neurology*, Hachinski (1990) raised the question whether specific cognitive therapy is better than general rehabilitation. He summarized the opinions from the discussants as follows: "Berrol believes it is, Volpe and McDowell doubt it, and Levin thinks it is unproved but promising" (Berrol, 1990; Volpe and McDowell, 1990; Levin, 1990).

Limiting our opinion to impairments of attention, we tend to state that the efficacy of stimulation training for these deficits has not been proven convincingly. It has been demonstrated that one can teach brain-damaged patients the visuomotor skills required in many computer games but these skills do not always generalize to psychometric tests, and seldom to daily life. Again, experience in the area of cognitive rehabilitation clearly shows that attention is not a unitary mechanism. We simply cannot expect that a patient's "attention" will improve when he or she is trained on a few tasks that tap certain aspects of attention.

What remains then? What can be done for the brain-damaged patient with attentional problems? As the effects of stimulation therapy are limited, it seems there is no other choice but to move on to a higher cognitive level of training— *strategy training*. We see an analogy here with memory training. It has been shown that rote learning is ineffective in memory rehabilitation, that one can only try to teach patients either the use of external memory aids or the use of strategies to optimize their remaining memory capacity (Koning-Haanstra et al., 1990; Berg et al., 1991). Von Cramon and colleagues (1991) described a training program for problem-solving deficits. In a group of 61 patients of mixed etiologies, they demonstrated that patients can learn to apply methods such as "problem definition and formulation," "generating alternatives," and "solution verification." These positive experiences with memory and problem-solving seem to indicate that attention training might profit from a change in approach. This idea is not entirely new. Robertson and coworkers (1990) expressed the belief that verbal-mediated strategies for self-arousal and for combating interference effects in working memory were involved in their training program. Kreutzer (1993; Kreutzer et al., 1991) has pointed to the crucial role of compensatory strategies in return to work after brain injury.

When we talk about strategies of attention, we are in fact talking about supervisory attentional control. Theoretically, we might improve supervisory control by means of verbal instruction. The simplest form of strategy training is by giving general guidelines to the brain-damaged. One can think of at least four broad recommendations for these patients:

Avoid time pressure
Analyze priorities
Create structure
Prevent interruptions

However, such instructions are too broad and general, and in our opinion they should be adjusted for each patient and each of his or her specific tasks. The problem of work resumption illustrates this point well. Ideally, a complete task analysis should be made, and recommendations with regard to resumption of work should be based on the patient's known deficits. The process should involve the following steps:

1. *Task analysis*: It is essential that the mental load in the job be known. Is there time-pressure, are interruptions expected, how well structured is the task, does it consist of several subtasks? If so, can priorities be defined? Which kinds of information have to be processed, what sources of information have to be monitored? Does the job require overview and planning ability? Does it require verbal skills or social interactions?

2. *Analysis of impairments*: Is the patient suffering from mental slowness or lack of flexibility? Is he or she easily distracted? Does the patient have additional cognitive problems, such as memory deficits, that may complicate job performance? Are there additional neurophysical problems such as poor balance or motor coordination? Is tolerance of stress decreased? And, very important, does the patient know his or her shortcomings?

3. *Analysis of compensatory potential*: The insight factor mentioned above is crucial here as only if the patient recognizes his or her shortcomings will it be possible to compensate for them. The patient's motivation and his or her personality resources are likewise important. A minimal level of general intelligence is required for the understanding of strategies and instructions.

4. *Adaptation to task and/or environment*: Time pressure should be reduced and structure improved. A basic step might be to reduce the number of subtasks in the job. Interruptions should be minimized. Checklists of sequential subtasks can be very useful. Supervision should be standardized.

5. *Estimation of risk of nonoptimal task performance*: Errors in task performance may result in risk, although the magnitude will vary greatly with the contents of the job. Divided attention deficits may have a fatal effect in a pilot flying a passenger airplane. Less obvious is the risk in a teacher whose social attentiveness is reduced in such a way that she does not pick up on a mood of boredom in her pupils, or subtle signs of emotional problems in an individual child. In a more general sense, the costs of errors should be estimated.

A stepwise analysis of these items is not the responsibility of employers, who often show good intentions but lack specific knowledge of the shortcomings of brain-damaged individuals. In our experience, a kind employer may give his convalescent employee so-called "light work," for example sorting mail in the mailroom of a large business company. However, if this unfamiliar task which seems so easy to healthy people must be carried out under time pressure, the poor patient may well ask permission, with trembling hands, to return to his regular job—even if it demands a greater physical effort than sorting mail.

Cognitive rehabilitation of attention at the strategy level is linked to steps 3 and 4 in the approach described above. The patient's compensatory potential should be activated by training, combined with an adaptation to the working situation if necessary (Kreutzer, 1993). A study by Burke and colleagues (1991) should be mentioned as an example of this approach. Although their report concerned executive functions in occupational situations, the method they used might also be useful with attentional impairments. Burke and coauthors used checklists dictating the sequence of subtasks in a vocational training (woodshop, restaurant kitchen) for head-injured patients with task-sequencing difficulties. Initiation cues from supervisors were gradually replaced by self-initiated ones. Of course checklists can also be considered external memory aids as well as supporting executive functions. As we observed above (see Chapter 9), the distinction between memory, attention and executive functions is vague in practical situations where tasks inevitably contain components that could be classified in all three categories. Take the example of a brain-damaged engineer who must "check engine temperature" regularly. If he fails to do so, it can be said that he forgets to check, or that he is not attending to the engine thermometer. Whatever the theoretical wording, the problem can be solved by supplying the worker with a checklist that enables him to learn a routine sequence until the time when he is able to do his job without the aid of the checklist—as was the case in the Burke study.

SOCIAL ATTENTION

A major problem in the social lives of many brain-damaged people is their poor social perception. They seem to be suffering from *social inattentiveness*. As described in the section "Social Skills" in Chapter 9, relatives of severely head-injured patients may complain that these patients seem to be insensitive or uninterested. Such behavior is characterized in the literature as signs of "blunting of social behavior" or "impaired social awareness" (Prigatano, 1987).

In our opinion, this is an attentional impairment. The point is that the patients do not make use of social cues. In a similar vein, others have described how patients fail to recognize subtle jokes or funny remarks; they hear the words but not the irony in the voice of the speaker. This deficit probably is determined in part by reduced processing capacity; as has been expressed elsewhere, patients have less attention to pay than healthy people.

At issue is whether it is possible to increase head-injured patients' social attentiveness through coaching. Can they be trained to pay attention not only to another's location in a room, but also to that person's behavior, whether it is tense or relaxed? Is it possible to teach patients to pay attention not only to the wording of a message, but also to the tone in which it is delivered? It should be stressed that social attention could be a critical factor in work resumption. Success in vocational training or in actually returning to work can be hindered by poor social perception, that is, by the convalescent's failure to pick up signs of irritation and frustration in colleagues who are confronted with his slow work pace or errors (Kreutzer, 1993). Written instructions for trainees might well contain an item such as "checking colleagues' mood," analogous to that of the engineer and his thermometer. Theoretically, it should be possible to improve social attention in some patients, but there are built-in limitations in the approach. If we assume that the information-processing capacity of a patient is permanently reduced, he cannot be expected to react sensitively in a social situation where verbal information is presented to him at a high rate. In such a situation, social attentiveness is a "luxury" that the patient cannot afford. Another problem is that patients often understand instructions given to them and are able to repeat them verbatim, but unable to apply them. One of our patients, a severely head-injured young man with a striking verbal disinhibition, developed the habit of saying after every second phrase, "I am verbally disinhibited again," with no apparent effect on the rest of his discourse. This behavior can be observed in particular in patients with frontal lobe damage (Luria, 1963). On the problem of self-monitoring deficits (Stuss and Benson, 1986), McGlynn (1990) says: "These deficits may prohibit patients from effectively using self-talk or self-instructional procedures even if they were able to learn and understand the principles behind such a technique."

The problem of limited processing capacity could theoretically be circumvented by training to the point of automatization. Training should continue until patients can automatically perceive additional social cues as well as nonbrain-damaged subjects. However, this would probably require long-term intensive training. Nevertheless, there are a few encouraging reports in this area. Hopewell and associates (1990) described a program of behavioral learning therapies for traumatically brain-injured patients, including social skills training using video-taped role playing and "flashcard" cues presented by the trainer which prompt the patient to review an alternative response repertoire. This social competence training had a significant effect that seemed permanent over a 10-week follow-up period. Prigatano (1985) has also described effective social skills training that seems relevant for the problem of "social attentiveness."

BASIC QUESTIONS

It is hard to predict what the possibilities are for using the interventions sketched out above. The first problem in strategy training is based on a peculiar dilemma. We know that our patients have a limited information processing capacity, yet we supply them with a set of rules to keep in mind while working at a task or in a social situation. We are reminded of the patient with a memory impairment: we know he can't remember things, but we expect him to remember the strategies we give him for remembering. Malec (1984) pointed out that the complex techniques he used to train verbal skills in a head-injured woman can only be taught to brain-injured patients without severe cognitive deficits. In their study of problem-solving training, Von Cramon and colleagues (1991) noted that some patients did not profit at all from treatment. When interviewed afterward, these subjects stressed the point that they felt confused "with all these things to consider."

It is clear from these observations that research on the cognitive rehabilitation of attention should answer the question, *Who can be trained?* In reports about attentional training that supply results on individual patients (e.g., Rattok et al., 1992; Sturm et al., 1993), it can usually be seen that significant improvement is found in about half of the trainees only, or even in a minority only. It is tempting to select the more intelligent and better motivated patients with sufficient verbal skills and a favorable social background. A more fundamental variable might be the severity of the injury. As noted above, very severely injured patients with extensive cognitive impairments might be unable to profit from strategy training. In stroke patients, side of lesion might also be a critical factor, as there is some evidence that unilateral lesions may produce different patterns of attentional impairments (Sturm and Willmes, 1991).

Another basic question to be addressed is, *What should be trained?* A review of the literature shows clearly that, as generalization of training effects remains problematic, training tasks should resemble the target behavior as closely as possible. In fact, in many cases the best approach might be to train the target behavior directly, that is, to train occupational skills on the spot or to retrain in real traffic those who want to resume driving. If generalization is the problem, goal-specific training should be the solution.

The next question is, *How should attentional problems be trained?* As pointed out in the previous section, strategy training relying on verbal mediation seems the best approach at present. This does not imply that stimulation training should be abolished completely. Rather, one might consider continuing to use stimulation methods that seemed to have a certain effect, in combination with strategy training.

When should attention be trained? As far as we can tell, no guidelines can be formulated yet. In research on the efficacy of training, investigators have usually preferred, for obvious methodological reasons, to postpone training until spontaneous recovery had plateaued. However, animal studies of recovery of function after experimental lesions have suggested that training may enhance recovery, at least at the level of basic learning processes in rodents (Finger and

Stein, 1982). Although these experiments are far removed from the aims of cognitive rehabilitation in humans, the possibility that training in an early stage might be beneficial should not be ignored. On the other hand, it is also very clear that it is never too late to start cognitive rehabilitation: the evidence reviewed above shows that patients can learn new skills or profit from strategy training for memory and problem solving many years after sustaining brain damage.

Finally, one might ask, *What makes attention training effective?* Robertson (personal communication, 1992) suggested that specific cognitive training procedures might actually have a general impact on attentional functions by improving motivation and emotional states in patients. It is interesting to note that individual case studies of cognitive rehabilitation report success more often than group studies. Of course, this could be explained by selective publication: case studies with negative results do not appear in press. An alternative explanation of practical importance could be that cooperation between trainer and trainee is more intensive in individual case studies, resulting in stronger motivation and greater optimism in the patient. If this is correct, it seems to imply that a close working relationship between trainer and trainees should be a goal in any training program, be it with groups or individuals.

SUMMARY

The boom in cognitive rehabilitation that began in the 1980s led to several evaluation studies of the efficacy of attention-training programs. Most of these studies were concerned with the effect of stimulation training, and evaluation was based either on task-level measures, psychometric measures or indices of daily functioning. Clear effects of training have been found with task-level measures, indicating that the performance of brain-damaged individuals in a given task or skill will improve with practice. However, data on the two other evaluation methods have been conflicting. The core problem here is generalization of training effect: generalization decreases when the resemblance between training program and evaluation method decreases. This leads to the conclusion that "attention" in a broad sense cannot be trained. The case of hemi-inattention illustrates this point quite well: training can overcome hemineglect in specific tasks or by means of specific cues, but the general impairment remains. There is some evidence that behavioral conditioning can improve attention to task, but as this approach also concerns specific behaviors it does not conflict with the previous conclusion.

In our view, the questionable efficacy of stimulation training forces us in the direction of training strategies of attention. Strategy training has been applied with some success in the areas of memory and problem-solving. It is mainly based on verbal mediation, teaching the trainees self-talk for the execution of daily life tasks, often combined with external aids and adaptation to the task situation. The training of attentional strategies requires a careful analysis of the target behavior and of impairments and compensatory capacities in the individual patient. Given the problematic generalization of training effects, aims in this sector of cognitive rehabilitation should be modestly phrased. Attention remains a complex set of phenomena, and a general effect of training on all attentive behavior cannot be expected. One aspect of attention that seems to be of great practical importance for patients, in both vocational and social activities, is social attention. Training that enhances a brain-damaged individual's sensitivity to social cues would be most rewarding and helpful for his or her reintegration in society.

Glossary

ALERTNESS A variable state of the central nervous system which affects general receptivity to stimulation. This state may vary from a very low level in sleep, to a high level in wakefulness. Changes in alertness are either phasic or tonic.

AROUSAL A nonspecific response of the central nervous system to a change in stimulation. This response usually consists of a desynchronization of cortical alpha rhythm and a number of vegetative changes. Arousal is characterized behaviorally by head or body movements which orient the receptors to the parts of the environment in which stimulus changes are occurring.

ATTENTION Traditionally seen as a selective mechanism favoring the processing of one class of internal or external stimuli at the expense of other ones. Presently the word refers to a cognitive state characterized by a selective bias for processing certain internal or external stimuli. Important aspects of attention in this sense are selectivity, intensity, and its dynamic character.

AUTOMATIC PROCESSING A mode of information processing that occurs independent of strategic control and in parallel with other processing without interference from the latter (automatic processes are unlimited in capacity). Automatic processing is triggered by the appropriate stimulation and does not require effort to proceed. It is based on wired-in or inborn connections and on extensive learning experience.

CAPACITY A functional limitation of the number of information processes that can occur simultaneously. Time, space, and energy are the limiting factors. The concept of "resources" is often used as a synonym for capacity.

CENTRAL EXECUTIVE A hypothetical agent situated in working memory whose function is supervisory attentional control.

CONCENTRATION A lay term synonymous with attention; also used to describe a state of intensive focused attention.

CONNECTIONISM An approach to information processing in which it is assumed that information is processed and stored in a network of excitatory and inhibitory connections between nodes designating features or patterns. While earlier models of information processing were inspired by electronic communication systems and computers, connectionism was inspired by the study of the human brain. Distinctive features are parallel processing, flexibility of organization by learning effects, and variable states.

CONTENTION SCHEDULING   An automatic conflict resolution process within the process of routine selection between routine actions or thought operations. It selects one of a number of conflicting actions (schemas) according to priorities and environmental cues. By means of lateral inhibition and facilitation, contention scheduling prevents incompatible and chaotic behavior in situations where task performance is based on automatic processing.

CONTROLLED PROCESSING   An information processing mode for nonroutine situations. It is thought to be a slow, predominantly serial processing mode, requiring effort and having severe capacity limitations. The concept is related to supervisory attentional control but does not include the formation of a strategy.

DISTRACTION   Irrelevant stimulation in a task environment. Distraction may have a strong negative effect on task performance if overlearned response tendencies are associated with the distraction and if there is a close resemblance between responses required by the task and those suggested by the distraction.

DIVIDED ATTENTION   Refers to the situation where a subject has to attend to two or more kinds of stimuli or sources of stimulation, or to various components within one task. Performance in divided attention tasks is determined by capacity and strategy. Performance can also be described in terms of flexibility as the focus of attention is switching continuously in these situations.

DIVIDED ATTENTION DEFICIT   A decrease in task performance in a dual task as a consequence of capacity limitations alone.

EFFORT   The capacity invested in task performance. Also used to describe the process and the subjective experience of staying attentive in the presence of distraction and time pressure.

FLEXIBILITY   The ability to switch attention rapidly in reaction to changing task demands.

FOCUSED ATTENTION   Refers to a situation where reacting to only one source of stimulation is required, usually in the presence of distraction.

FOCUSED ATTENTION DEFICIT   A decrease in task performance in a focused attention task because of distraction.

HEMI-INATTENTION   A clinical condition in which the individual fails to report, respond, or orient to novel or meaningful stimuli presented to the side opposite a brain lesion. Also called hemineglect. The syndrome occurs more often after a right-hemisphere lesion than after a left-hemisphere lesion.

INFORMATION PROCESSING APPROACH   A functionalist approach to psychology, increasingly influential after 1950, that seeks to study the mind in terms of mental representations and processes that underlie observable behavior. Relative shortcomings of the approach are its lack of interest in individual differences, both between subjects and within subjects (e.g., effects of fatigue, mood) and its uncommitted character with regard to the neural hardware.

LAPSE OF ATTENTION   A short-lasting decrease in task performance due to a (phasic) change in alertness.

STRATEGY   A consciously accessible plan of action.

SUPERVISORY ATTENTIONAL CONTROL   The formation of a strategy (planning) and, accordingly, the regulation of information processing when the routine selection of actions by contention scheduling is inadequate. It operates not by directly controlling behavior, but by modulating the elicitability of particular actions in either an excitatory or inhibitory manner.

SUSTAINED ATTENTION   Any aspect of attention that is characterized by its duration, particularly time-on-task effects. Although sustained attention can be studied on a short time scale, investigators usually follow the tradition of vigilance research, using time scales of minutes to hours. Apart from time-on-task effects, lapses of attention and intra-individual variability in performance can be viewed as sustained attention phenomena.

TIME-ON-TASK EFFECTS   Changes in performance over time. Although these can be positive (improvement by practice), psychology has emphasized negative time-on-task effects such as the decrease of signal detection in vigilance studies.

VIGILANCE   The ability to remain alert in a low-event-rate situation. Early vigilance investigations made use of monotonous situations with little stimulation and target stimuli that differed only slightly from nontarget stimuli. The term "vigilance" has been broadened considerably and is now also used for performance in high-event-rate situations involving clear stimuli (monitoring).

WORKING MEMORY   Refers to a brain system that provides temporary storage and manipulation of the information necessary for complex cognitive tasks. It can be divided into the following three subcomponents: 1) the central executive, which is assumed to be an attentional controlling system, and two slave systems, namely 2) the visuospatial sketchpad, which manipulates visual images, and 3) the phonological loop, which stores and rehearses speech-based information.

References

Aarts JHP, Binnie CD, Smit AM, Wilkins AJ (1984) Selective cognitive impairment during focal and generalized epileptiform EEG activity. *Brain, 107,* 293–308.

Adams JH, Graham DI, Murray LS, Scott G (1982) Diffuse axonal injury due to non-missile head injury in humans: An analysis of 45 cases. *Annals of Neurology, 12,* 557–563.

Albert ML (1973) A simple test of visual neglect. *Neurology, 23,* 658–664.

Albert ML, Silverberg R, Reches A, Berman M (1976) Cerebral dominance for consciousness. *Archives of Neurology, 33,* 453–454.

Aldenkamp AP, Alpherts WCJ, Moerland MC, Ottevanger N, Van Parys JAP (1987) Controlled release carbamazepine: Cognitive side effects in patients with epilepsy. *Epilepsia, 28,* 507–514.

Alexander DA (1973a) Attention dysfunction in senile dementia. *Psychological Reports, 32,* 229–230.

Alexander DA (1973b) Some tests of intelligence and learning for elderly psychiatric patients: A validation study. *British Journal of Social and Clinical Psychology, 12,* 188–193.

Alexander GE, DeLong MR, Strick PL (1986) Parallel organization of functionally segregated circuits linking basal ganglia and cortex. *Annual Review of Neuroscience, 9,* 357–381.

Alpherts WCJ (1986) Personal communication, quoted in Brons K, Arts B (1987) *Cognitieve stoornissen bij epilepsie.* Projektverslag Klinische Psychologie, Rijksuniversiteit, Groningen, Netherlands.

Alpherts WCJ, Aldenkamp AP (1990) *FEPSY—The Iron Psyche.* Information Bulletin, Instituut voor Epilepsiebestrijding, Heemstede.

Amabile G, Cordischi MV, D'Alessio C, Foti A, Giunti P, Fattaposta F (1991) A possible dopaminergic influence on the P-3 component of the oddball ERP: A study in Parkinsonian patients. *Electroencephalography and Clinical Neurophysiology, 79,* S-2.

Anderson SW, Damasio H, Dallas Jones R, Tranel D (1991) Wisconsin Card Sorting Test Performance as a measure of frontal lobe damage. *Journal of Clinical and Experimental Neuropsychology, 13,* 909–922.

Atkinson RL, Atkinson RC, Smith EE, Bem DJ (1990) *Introduction to Psychology.* Harcourt Brace Jovanovich, San Diego, CA.

Babinski J (1914) Contribution a l'etude des troubles mentaux dans l'hémiplégie organique cérébrale (anosognosie). *Revue Neurologique, 27,* 845–848.

Bachmann T (1984) The process of perceptual retouch: Nonspecific afferent activation dynamics in explaining visual masking. *Perception and Psychophysics, 35,* 69–84.

Baddeley A (1976) *The Psychology of Memory*. Harper & Row, New York.

Baddeley A (1986) *Working Memory*. Oxford University Press, London.

Baddeley A (1990) *Human Memory: Theory and Practice*. Allyn & Bacon, Boston.

Baddeley AD (1993) Working Memory or Working Attention? To appear in Baddeley AD and Weiskrantz L (eds.), *Attention: Selection, Awareness and Control. A Tribute to Donald Broadbent*. Oxford University Press, Oxford.

Baddeley A, Hitch G (1974) Working memory. In: Bower GA (ed.), *Recent Advances in Learning and Motivation*, vol. 8, Academic Press, New York.

Baddeley AD, Lieberman K (1980) Spatial working memory. In: Nickerson RS (ed.), *Attention and Performance*, vol. 8, pp. 521–539. Lawrence Erlbaum, Hillsdale, NJ.

Baddeley A, Logie R, Bressi S, Della Salla S, Spinnler H (1986) Dementia and working memory. *Quarterly Journal of Experimental Psychology*, *38A*, 603–618.

Baker EL, Letz R, Fidler S, Shalat S, Plantamura D, Lyndon M (1985) Computer-based neurobehavioral testing for occupational and environmental epidemiology. *Neurobehavioral Toxicology and Teratology*, *7*, 369–378.

Ball K, Owsley C (1991) Identifying correlates of accident involvement for the older driver. *Human Factors*, *33*, 583–595.

Barlow HB (1985) The twelfth Bartlett memorial lecture: The role of single neurons in the psychology of perception. *Quarterly Journal of Experimental Psychology*, *37A*, 121–145.

Barry P, Riley JM (1987) Adult norms for the Kaufman Hand Movement Test and a single-subject design for acute brain injury rehabilitation. *Journal of Clinical and Experimental Neuropsychology*, *9*, 449–455.

Barth JT, Alves WM, Ryan TV, Macciocchi SN, Rimel RW, Jane JA, Nelson WE (1989) Mild head injury in sports: Neuropsychological sequelae and recovery of function. In: Levin HS, Eisenberg HM, Benton AL (eds.), *Mild Head Injury*. Oxford University Press, New York.

Bayles KA, Boone DR (1982) The potential of language tasks for identifying senile dementia. *Journal of Speech and Hearing Disorders*, *47*, 210–217.

Benecke R, Rothwell JC, Dick JPR, Day BL, Marsden CD (1986) Performance of simultaneous movements in patients with Parkinson's disease. *Brain*, *109*, 739–757.

Benson DF, Geschwind N (1975) Psychiatric conditions associated with focal lesions of the central nervous system. In: Arieti S, Reiser M (eds.), *American Handbook of Psychiatry*, vol. 4, pp. 208–243. Basic Books, New York.

Benton AL (1986) Reaction time in brain disease: Some reflections. *Cortex*, *22*, 129–140.

Benton AL, Joynt RJ (1958) Reaction time in unilateral cerebral disease. *Confinia Neurologica*, *19*, 247–256.

Benton AL, Sutton S, Kennedy JA, Brokaw JR (1962) The crossmodal retardation in reaction time of patients with cerebral disease. *Journal of Nervous and Mental Disease*, *136*, 413–418.

Ben-Yishay Y, Piasetsky EB, Rattock J (1987) A systematic method for ameliorating disorders in basic attention. In: Meyer MJ, Benton AL, Diller L (eds.), *Neuropsychological Rehabilitation*. Churchill Livingstone, Edinburgh.

Berg IJ, Koning-Haanstra M, Deelman BG (1991) Long-term effects of memory rehabilitation: A controlled study. *Neuropsychological Rehabilitation*, *1*, 97–111.

Berrol S (1990) Issues in cognitive rehabilitation. *Archives of Neurology*, *47*, 219–220.

Betts TA (1982) Psychiatry and epilepsy. In: Laidlaw J, Richens A (eds.), *A Textbook of Epilepsy*, pp. 227–268. Churchill Livingstone, Edinburgh.

Bhutani GE, Montaldi D, Brooks DN, McCulloch J (1992) A neuropsychological investigation into frontal lobe involvement in dementia of the Alzheimer type. *Neuropsychology*, 6, 211–224.

Bisiach E, Luzatti C (1978) Unilateral neglect of representational space. *Cortex*, 14, 29–33.

Blackburn HL, Benton AL (1955) Simple and choice reaction time in cerebral disease. *Confinia Neurologica*, 15, 327–338.

Bloxham CA, Dick DJ, Moore M (1987) Reaction times and attention in Parkinson's disease. *Journal of Neurology, Neurosurgery and Psychiatry*, 50, 1178–1183.

Bloxham CA, Mindel TA, Frith CD (1984) Initiation and execution of predictable and unpredictable movements in Parkinson's disease. *Brain*, 107, 371–384.

Bodis-Wollner I, Yahr MD, Mylin LH (1984) Nonmotor functions of the basal ganglia. *Advances in Neurology*, 40, 289–298.

Boff KR, Kaufman L, Thomas JP (1986) *Handbook of Perception and Human Performance, vol. 1*. Wiley, New York.

Bohnen NI (1991) *Mild Head Injury and Postconcussive Sequelae*. [Doctoral Dissertation]. Rijksuniversiteit Limburg, Maastricht, Netherlands.

Bondareff W, Mountjoy CQ, Roth M (1982) Loss of neurons of origin of the adrenergic projection to cerebral cortex (nucleus locus coeruleus) in senile dementia. *Neurology*, 32, 164–168.

Bourdon B (1895) Observations comparatives sur la reconnaissance, la discrimination et l'association. *Revue Philosophique*, 40, 153–185.

Bradley VA, Welch JL, Dick DJ (1989) Visuospatial working memory in Parkinson's disease. *Journal of Neurology, Neurosurgery and Psychiatry,* 52, 1228–1235.

Brain WR (1941) Visual disorientation with special reference to lesions of the right cerebral hemisphere. *Brain*, 64, 244–272.

Braun CMJ, Baribeau JMG, Ethier M, Daigneault S, Proulx R (1989a) Processing of pragmatic and facial affective information by patients with closed head injuries. *Brain Injury*, 3, 5–17.

Braun CMJ, Bartolini G, Bouchard A (1985) *Cognitive Rehabilitation Software*. Université de Quebec à Montréal.

Braun CMJ, Daigneault S, Champagne D (1989b) Information processing deficits as indexed by reaction time parameters in severe closed head injury. *International Journal of Clinical Neuropsychology*, 11, 167–176.

Brickenkamp R (1981) *Test d-2, Aufmerksamkeits-Belastungstet*. Hogrefe-Verlag, Göttingen, Germany.

Brickenkamp R, Rump G (1966) Die Stabilität des Aufmerksamkeits-Belastungs-Test d-2 über längere Zeitabschnitte. *Diagnostica*, 12, 17–24.

Broadbent DE (1958) *Perception and Communication*. Pergamon Press, London.

Broadbent DE (1971) *Decision and Stress*. Academic Press, London.

Brons K, Arts B (1987) *Cognitieve Stoornissen bij Epilepsie*. Projectverslag Klinische Psychologie, Rijksuniversiteit, Groningen, Netherlands.

Brooks DN (1984) *Closed Head Injury: Psychological, Social and Family Consequences*. Oxford University Press, Oxford.

Brooks DN (1987) Measuring neuropsychological and functional recovery. In: Levin HS, Grafman J, Eisenberg HM (eds.), *Neurobehavioral Recovery from Head Injury*, pp. 57–72. Oxford University Press, New York.

Brooks DN, Deelman BG, van Zomeren AH, van Dongen H, van Harskamp F, Aughton ME (1984) Problems in measuring cognitive recovery after acute brain injury. *Journal of Clinical Neuropsychology*, 6, 71–85.

Brooks N (1990) Head injury: Rehabilitation of behavioural and mental changes. In: von Wild K, Janzik HH (eds.), *Neurologische Frührehabilitation*, Zuckschwerdt Verlag, München.

Brooks N McKinlay W Symington C, Beattie A, Campsie L (1987) Return to work within the first seven years of severe head injury. *Brain Injury*, *1*, 5–19.

Brouwer WH (1985) *Limitations of Attention After Closed Head Injury*. [Doctoral Dissertation]. University of Groningen, Netherlands.

Brouwer WH, Lakke JPWF (1983) The effect of foreknowledge concerning time and place of appearance on the speed of execution of a goal directed steering movement in severely hypokinetic Parkinson patients. [Abstract]. *Proceedings of the Congress on Restorative Neurology in the Central and Peripheral Nervous System*, Venice, May 1983.

Brouwer WH, Van Wolffelaar PC (1985) Sustained attention and sustained effort after closed head injury. *Cortex*, *21*, 111–119.

Brouwer WH, Ickenroth JGM, Ponds RWHM, Van Wolffelaar PC (1990) Divided attention in old age: Difficulty in integrating skills. In: Drenth PJD, Sergeant JA, Takens RJ (eds.), *European Perspectives in Psychology*, vol. 2, pp. 335–348. Wiley, New York.

Brouwer WH, Ponds RWHM, Van Wolffelaar PC, Van Zomeren AH (1989) Divided attention 5 to 10 years after closed head injury. *Cortex*, *25*, 219–230.

Brouwer WH, Rothengatter JA, Van Wolffelaar PC (1988) Compensatory potential in elderly drivers. In: Rothengatter JA, De Bruin RA (eds.), *Road User Behaviour: Theory and Research*, pp. 296–301. Van Gorcum, Assen.

Brouwer WH, Rothengatter JA, Van Wolffelaar PC (1992) Older drivers and road traffic informatics. In: Bouma H, Graafmans JAM (eds.), *Gerontechnology*, pp. 317–328. IOS Press, Amsterdam.

Brouwer WH, Waterink W, Van Wolffelaar PC, Rothengatter JA (1991) Divided attention in experienced young and older drivers: Lane tracking and visual analysis in a dynamic driving simulator. *Human Factors*, *33*, 573–582.

Brown RG, Marsden CD (1984) How common is dementia in Parkinson's disease. *The Lancet*, *1*, 1262–1265.

Brown RG, Marsden CD (1987) Neuropsychology and cognitive function in Parkinson's disease: An overview. In: Marsden CD, Fahn S (eds.), *Movement Disorders*, pp. 99–123. Butterworth, New York.

Brown RG, Marsden CD (1988) Internal versus external cues and the control of attention in Parkinson's disease. *Brain*, *111*, 323–345.

Browne TR, Penry JK, Porter RJ, Dreifuss FE (1974) Responsiveness before, during and after spike-wave paroxysms. *Neurology*, *24*, 659–665.

Bruhn P (1970) Disturbances of vigilance in subcortical epilepsy. *Acta Neurologica Scandinavica*, *46*, 442–454.

Bruhn P, Parsons OA (1971) Continuous reaction time in brain damage. *Cortex*, *7*, 278.

Bruhn P, Parsons OA (1977) Reaction time variability in epileptic and brain-damaged patients. *Cortex*, *13*, 373–384.

Bruins R, Van Nieuwenhuizen CH (1990) *PASAT is PVSAT?* Projectverslag, Internal Report, Department of Neuropsychology, State University of Groningen, Netherlands.

Brunia CHM, Damen (1988) Distribution of slow brain potentials related to motor preparation and stimulus anticipation in a time estimation task. *Electroencephalography and Clinical Neurophysiology*, *69*, 234–243.

Brunia CHM, Vingerhoets AJJM (1981) The central and peripheral recording of motor preparation in man. Internal report, University of Tilburg, Netherlands.

Buchtel HA (1987) Attention and vigilance after head trauma. In: Levin HS, Grafman J, Eisenberg HM (eds.), *Neurobehavioral Recovery from Head Injury*. Oxford University Press, New York.

Buchtel HA, Guitton D (1980) Saccadic eye movements in patients with discrete unilateral frontal-lobe removals. *Abstracts of the Society of Neurosciences*, 6, 316.

Buchwald JS, Erwin RJ, Read S, Van Lancker D, Cummings JL (1989) Midlatency auditory evoked responses: Differential abnormality of P-1 in Alzheimer's disease. *Electroencephalography and Clinical Neurophysiology*, 74, 378–384.

Burke WH, Wesolowski MD, Buyer DM, Zawlocki RJ (1990) The rehabilitation of adolescents with traumatic brain injury: Outcome and follow-up. *Brain Injury*, 4, 371–378.

Burke WH, Zencius AH, Wesolowski MD, Doubleday F (1991) Improving executive function disorders in brain-injured clients. *Brain Injury*, 5, 241–252.

Caltagirone C, Carlesimo A, Nocenti U, Vicari S (1989) Defective concept formation in parkinsonians is independent from mental deterioration. *Journal of Neurology, Neurosurgery and Psychiatry*, 52, 334–337.

Campbell K, Houle S, Lorrain D, Deacon-Elliot D, Proulx G (1986) Event-related potentials as an index of functioning in head-injured out-patients. In: McCallum WC, Zappoli R, Denoth F (eds.), *Cerebral Psychophysiology: Studies in Event-Related Potentials*. Elsevier, Amsterdam.

Cant BR, Gronwall DMA, Burgess R (1975) Recovery process of the slow auditory response following head injury. *Revue de Laryngologie*, 96, 199–205.

Caplan B (1987) Assessment of unilateral neglect: A new reading test. *Journal of Clinical and Experimental Neuropsychology*, 9, 359–364.

Carpenter MB (1976) Anatomical organization of the corpus striatum and related nuclei. In: Yahr MD (ed.), *The Basal Ganglia*. Raven Press, New York.

Cerella J (1990) Aging and information processing rate. In: Birren JE, Warner Schaie K (eds.), *Handbook of the Psychology of Aging*, pp. 201–221. Academic Press, San Diego, CA.

Chadwick O, Rutter M, Brown G, Shaffer D, Traub M (1981) A prospective study of children with head injuries: II. Cognitive sequelae. *Psychological Medicine*, 11, 49–61.

Cohen J (1957) Factor-analytically based rationale for Wechsler Adult Intelligence Scale. *Journal of Consulting Psychology*, 21, 451–457.

Cohen RM, Semple WE, Gross WE, Holcomb HJ, Dowling SM, Nordahl TE (1988) Functional localization of sustained attention. *Neuropsychology and Behavioral Neurology*, 1, 3–20.

Conkey RC (1938) Psychological changes associated with head injuries. *Archives of Psychology*, 33, 232.

Cools AR, Van den Bercken JHL, Horstink MWI, Van Spaendonck KPM, Berger HJC (1984) Cognitive and motor shifting aptitude disorder in Parkinson's disease. *Journal of Neurology, Neurosurgery and Psychiatry*, 47, 443–453.

Corrigan JD, Dickerson J, Fisher E, Meyer P (1990) The Neurobehavioral Rating Scale: Replication in an acute, inpatient rehabilitation setting. *Brain Injury*, 4, 215–222.

Corsellis JAN (1970) The limbic areas in Alzheimer's disease and other conditions associated with dementia. In: Wolstenhome GEW, O'Connor M (eds.), *Alzheimer's Disease and Related Conditions*. Churchill, London.

Coslett HB, Bowers D, Heilman KM (1987) Reduction in cerebral activation after right hemisphere stroke. *Neurology*, 37, 957–962.

Cossa FM, Della Sala S, Spinnler H (1989) Selective visual attention in Alzheimer and Parkinson patients: Memory- and data-driven control. *Neuropsychologia*, 27, 887–892.

Côté L, Crutcher MD (1985) Motor functions of the basal ganglia and diseases of transmitter metabolism. In: Kandel ER, Schwartz JH (eds.), *Principles of Neuroscience*, pp. 521–535. Elsevier, New York.

Craik FIM, Lockhart RS (1972) Levels of processing: A framework for memory research. *Journal of Verbal Learning and Verbal Behavior*, *11*, 671–684.

Crepeau F (1992) Problemsolving following traumatic brain injury: A work simulation evaluation. [Abstract]. *Proceedings of the Second International Congress on Objective Assessment in Rehabilitation Medicine*, Montreal, October 1992.

Cummings JL (1988) Intellectual impairments in Parkinson's disease: Clinical, pathologic and biochemical correlates. *Journal of Geriatric Psychiatry and Neurology*, *1*, 24–36.

Curry SH (1981) Event-related potentials as indicants of structural and functional damage in closed head injury. *Progress in Brain Research*, *54*, 507–515.

Curry SH (1984) Contingent Negative Variation and slow waves in a short interstimulus interval GO/NO GO task situation. *Annals of New York Academy of Sciences*, *425*, 171–176.

Damasio AR, Damasio H, Chang Chui H (1980) Neglect following damage to frontal lobe or basal ganglia. *Neuropsychologia*, *18*, 123–132.

Davies A (1968) The influence of age on Trailmaking Test performance. *Journal of Clinical Psychology*, *24*, 96–98.

Davies DR, Jones DM, Taylor A (1984) Selective and sustained-attention tasks: Individual and group differences. In: Parasuraman R, Davies DR (eds.), *Varieties of Attention*, pp. 395–447. Academic Press, Orlando, FL.

Davies P (1979) Neurotransmitter-related enzymes in senile dementia of the Alzheimer type. *Brain Research*, *138*, 385–392.

Davies RD, Davies D, Avory M, Quaife P (1966) *Dedicated Follower of Fashion*. Pye Records, 7N17064A.

Dee HL, Van Allen MW (1973) Speed of decision making processes in patients with unilateral cerebral disease. *Archives of Neurology*, *28*, 163–166.

Deelman BG (1972) *Etudes in de Neuropsychologie*. [Doctoral Dissertation]. University of Groningen, Netherlands.

Deelman BG, Saan RJ (1990) Memory deficits: Assessment and recovery. In: Deelman BG, Saan RJ, Van Zomeren AH (eds.), *Traumatic Brain Injury: Clinical, Social and Rehabilitational Aspects*. Swets and Zeitlinger, Amsterdam.

Deelman BG, Brouwer WH, Van Zomeren AH, Saan RJ (1980) Functiestoornissen na trauma capitis. In: Jennekens-Schinkel A, Diamant JJ, Diesfeldt HFA, Haaxma R (eds.), *Neuropsychologie in Nederland*, pp. 253–282. Van Loghum Slaterus, Deventer, Netherlands.

De Jong PF (1991) *Het Meten van Aandacht*. [Doctoral Dissertation]. Free University, Amsterdam.

DeKosky ST, Heilman KM, Bowers D, Valenstein E (1980) Recognition and discrimination of emotional faces and pictures. *Brain and Language*, *9*, 206–214.

Deland N, Vanier M, Lambert J, Provost J (1992) A study on focused attention in severely head-injured patients. *Proceedings of the Conference on Attention: Theoretical and Clinical Perspectives*. Baycrest Centre, Toronto, Canada.

DeLong MR (1974) Motor functions of the basal ganglia: Single unit activity during movement. In: Schmitt FO, Worden FG (eds.), *The Neurosciences, Third Study Program*. MIT Press, Cambridge, MA.

Dencker SJ, Löfving B (1958) A psychometric study of identical twins discordant for closed head injury. *Acta Psychiatrica Neurologica Scandinavica*, *33*, suppl. 122.

Denny-Brown D (1962) *The Basal Ganglia*, Oxford University Press, London.

Denny-Brown D, Fischer EG (1976) Physiological aspects of visual perception: The subcortical visual direction of behavior. *Archives of Neurology*, *33*, 228–243.

Denny-Brown D, Yanigisawa N (1976) The role of the basal ganglia in the initiation of movement. In: Yahr MD (ed.), *The Basal Ganglia*. Raven Press, New York.

DeRenzi E, Faglioni P (1965) The comparative efficiency of intelligence and vigilance tests in detecting hemispheric cerebral damage. *Cortex*, *1*, 410–433.

Deutsch G, Papanicolaou AC, Bourbon T, Eisenberg HM (1988) Cerebral blood flow evidence of right cerebral activation in attention demanding tasks. *International Journal of Neurosciences*, *36*, 23–28.

Deutsch JA, Deutsch D (1963) Attention: Some theoretical considerations. *Psychological Review*, *70*, 80–90.

De Vries H, van Houte LR, Lindeboom J, van Eijk JM, de Haan M (1992) Optellen onder tijdsdruk: Een neuropsychologische test voor het verdelen van aandacht. *Tijdschrift voor Gerontologie en Psychiatrie*, *23*, 147–156.

Dikmen S, Matthews CG (1977) Effect of major motor seizure frequency upon cognitive-intellectual functions in adults. *Epilepsia*, *18*, 21–29.

Dikmen S, Temkin N (1987) Determination of the effects of head injury and recovery in behavioral research. In: Levin HS, Grafman J, Eisenberg HM (eds.), *Neurobehavioral Recovery from Head Injury*. Oxford University Press, New York.

Dikmen S, Matthews CG, Harley JP (1975) The effect of early versus late onset of major motor epilepsy upon cognitive-intellectual performance. *Epilepsia*, *16*, 73–81.

Dikmen S, McLean A, Temkin N (1986) Neuropsychological and psychosocial consequences of minor head injury. *Journal of Neurology, Neurosurgery and Psychiatry*, *49*, 1227–1232.

Diller L, Weinberg J (1977) Hemi-inattention in rehabilitation: The evolution of a rational remediation program. *Advances in Neurology*, *18*, 63–82.

Diller L, Ben-Yishay Y, Gerstman LJ, Goodkin R, Gordon W, Weinberg J (1974) *Studies of Cognition and Rehabilitation in Hemiplegia*. Rehabilitation Monograph no. 50, New York University Medical Center, New York.

Dodrill CB (1978) A neuropsychological battery for epilepsy. *Epilepsia*, *19*, 611–623.

Dodrill CB, Wilensky AJ (1992) Neuropsychological abilities before and after 5 years of stable antiepileptic drug therapy. *Epilepsia*, *33*, 327–334.

Dolgushkin NI, Freed DM, Zemansky M, Schneider LS (1989) Selective attention in Alzheimer's disease: Further evidence for subgroups of patients. *Journal of Clinical and Experimental Neuropsychology*, *11*, 19–20.

Donchin E (1984) *Attention and Performance*. Appleton & Lange, E. Norwalk, CT.

Dorff JE, Mirsky A, Mishkin M (1965) Effects of unilateral temporal lobe removals on tachistoscopic recognition in the left and right visual fields. *Neuropsychologia*, *3*, 39–51.

Downes JJ, Roberts AC, Sahakian BJ, Evenden JL, Morris RG, Robbins TW (1989) Impaired extra-dimensional shift performance in medicated and unmedicated Parkinson's disease: Evidence for a specific attentional dysfunction. *Neuropsychologia*, *27*, 1329–1343.

Dreifuss FE, Bancaud J, Henriksen O, Rubio-Donnadieu F, Seino M, Pentry JK (1981) Proposal for revised clinical and electroencephalographic classification of epileptic seizures. *Epilepsia*, *22*, 489–501.

Droogleever-Fortuyn J (1979) On the neurology of perception. *Clinical Neurology and Neurosurgery*, *81*, 97–107.

Dyer FN (1973) The Stroop phenomenon and its use in the study of perceptual, cognitive and response processes. *Memory and Cognition*, *1*, 106–120.

Egan V (1988) PASAT: Observed correlations with IQ. *Personal and Individual Differences*, *9*, 179–180.

Elsass L, Kinsella G (1987) Social interaction following severe closed head injury. *Psychological Medicine*, *17*, 67–78.

Elting R, Brouwer WH, Van Zomeren AH (1988) *Aandacht na Contusio Cerebri: Meer dan Traagheid Alleen?* [Doctoral Dissertation]. Rijksuniversiteit Groningen, Netherlands.

Elting R, Van Zomeren AH, Brouwer WH (1989) Flexibility of attention after severe head injury. *Journal of Clinical and Experimental Neuropsychology*, *11*, 370.

Engel FL (1977) Visual conspicuity, visual search and fixation tendencies of the eye. *Vision Research*, *17*, 95–108.

Engum ES, Cron L, Hulse CK, Pendergrass TM, Lambert W (1988a) Cognitive Behavioral Driver's Inventory. *Cognitive Rehabilitation*, September/October, pp. 34–50.

Engum ES, Lambert EW, Scott K (1990) Criterion-related validity of the Cognitive Behavioral Driver's Inventory: brain-injured patients versus normal controls. *Cognitive Rehabilitation*, March/April, pp. 20–26.

Engum ES, Lambert EW, Womac J, Pendergrass T (1988b) Norms and decision making rules for the Cognitive Behavioral Driver's Inventory. *Cognitive Rehabilitation*. November/December, pp. 12–18.

Etcoff NL (1991) The recognition of emotion. In: Boller F, Grafman J (eds.), *Handbook of Neuropsychology*, vol. 3, pp. 363–382. Elsevier, Amsterdam.

Evarts EV, Teravainen H, Calne DB (1981) Reaction times in Parkinson's disease. *Brain*, *104*, 167–186.

Finger S, Stein DG (1982) *Brain Damage and Recovery: Research and Clinical Perspectives.* Academic Press, New York.

Flowers KA, Robertson C (1985) The effect of Parkinson's disease on the ability to maintain a mental set. *Journal of Neurology, Neurosurgery and Psychiatry*, *43*, 517–529.

Fodor JA (1983) *The Modularity of Mind.* MIT Press, Cambridge, MA.

Folstein MF, Folstein SE, McHugh PR (1975) Mini Mental State: A practical method for grading the cognitive status of patients for the clinician. *Journal of Psychiatric Research*, *12*, 189–198.

Fountain AJ, Lewis JR, Heck AF (1983) Driving with epilepsy: A contemporary perspective. *Southern Medical Journal*, *76*, 481–484.

Fox GK, Bashford GM; Caust SL (1992) Identifying safe versus unsafe drivers following brain impairment: The Coorabel Programme. *Disability and Rehabilitation*, *14*, 140–145.

Freed DM, Corkin S, Growdon JH, Nissen MJ (1988) Selective attention in Alzheimer's disease: CSF correlates of behavioral impairments. *Neuropsychologia*, *26*, 895–902.

Freed DM, Corkin S, Growdon JH, Nissen MJ (1989) Selective attention in Alzheimer's disease: Characterizing cognitive subgroups of patients. *Neuropsychologia*, *27*, 325–339.

Freedman M (1990) Object alternation and orbitofrontal system dysfunction in Alzheimer's and Parkinson's disease. *Brain and Cognition*, *14*, 134–143.

Friedland RP, Koss E, Kumar A, Gaine S, Metzler D, Haxby JV, Moore A (1988) Motor vehicle crashes in dementia of the Alzheimer type. *Annals of Neurology*, *24*, 782–786.

Fuster JM (1980) *The Prefrontal Cortex: Anatomy, Physiology and Neuropsychology of the Frontal Lobe.* Raven Press, New York.

Gaillard A (1978) *Slow Brain Potentials Preceding Task Performance*. Academische Pers, Amsterdam.

Gardner H (1983) *Frames of Mind: The Theory of Multiple Intelligences*. Basic Books, New York.

Gastaut H, Zifkin BG (1987) The risk of automobile accidents with seizures occurring while driving. *Neurology, 37*, 1613–1616.

Gauggel S, Von Cramon D, Schuri U (1991) Zum Zusammenhang zwischen Lern- und Gedachtnisleistungen und der Informationsverarbeitungsgeschwindigkeit bei hirngeschadigten Patienten. *Zeitschrift für Neuropsychologie, 2*, 91–99.

Gauthier L, Dehaut F, Joannette Y (1989) The Bells Test: A quantitative and qualitative test for visual neglect. *International Journal of Clinical Neuropsychology, 11*, 49–54.

Geissler H (1909) *Moderne Verirrungen auf philosophisch-mathematische Gebieten: Kritische und selbstgebende Untersuchungen*. Ebikon, Luzern.

Geschwind N (1982) Disorders of attention: A frontier in neuropsychology. *Philosophical Transactions of the Royal Society of London, 298*, 173–185.

Glas S, Brouwer W, Brand B, Engels M (1992) Hemi-inattentie: Literatuurstudie en een onderzoek naar het effect van training. Doctoraalscriptie, Rijksuniversiteit van Groningen, Netherlands.

Gloor P, Pellegrini A, Kostopoulos GK (1979) Effects of changes in cortical excitability upon the epileptic bursts in generalized penicillin epilepsy in the cat. *Electroencephalography and Clinical Neurophysiology, 46*, 274.

Godfrey HPD, Knight RG, Marsh NV, Moroney B, Bishara SN (1989) Social interaction and speed of information processing following very severe head injury. *Psychological Medicine, 9*, 175–182.

Goldenberg G, Lang W, Podreka I, Deecke L (1990) Are cognitive deficits in Parkinson's disease caused by frontal lobe dysfunction? *Journal of Psychophysiology, 4*, 137–144.

Goldman-Rakic PS (1988) Topography of cognition: Parallel distributed networks in primate association cortex. *Annual Review of Neurosciences, 11*, 137–156.

Goodglass H, Kaplan EF (1979) Assessment of cognitive defect in the brain-injured patient. In: Gazzaniga MS (ed.), *Handbook of Behavioral Neurobiology, vol. 2: Neuropsychology*, pp. 3–22. Plenum, New York.

Goodin DS, Aminoff MJ (1987) Electrophysiological differences between demented and non-demented patients with Parkinson's disease. *Annals of Neurology, 21*, 90–94.

Goodin DS, Squires KC, Henderson B, Starr A (1978) Age-related variations in evoked potentials to auditory stimuli in normal human subjects. *Journal of Electroencephalography and Clinical Neurophysiology, 54*, 447–458.

Goodrich S, Henderson L, Kennard C (1989) On the existence of an attention-demanding process peculiar to simple reaction time: Converging evidence from Parkinson's disease. *Cognitive Neuropsychology, 6*, 309–331.

Gordon W, Hibbard MR, Egelko S, Diller L, Shaver P, Lieberman A, Ragnarson L (1985) Perceptual remediation in patients with right brain damage: A comprehensive program. *Archives of Physical Medicine and Rehabilitation, 66*, 353–359.

Gorman LL, Roberts RJ, Varney NR, Hines ME (1990) Dichotic listening is more sensitive than standard EEG to cerebral dysfunction in patients with multiple seizure symptoms. *Journal of Clinical and Experimental Neuropsychology, 12*, 76.

Gotham AM, Brown RG, Marsden CD (1988) "Frontal" cognitive function in patients with Parkinson's disease "on" and "off" levadopa. *Brain, 111*, 299–321.

Gottschaldt K (1928) Ueber den Einfluss der Erfahrung auf die Wahrnehmung von Figuren. *Psychologische Forschungen*, *8*, 18–317.

Gouvier W, Bua B, Blanton P, Urey J (1987) Behavioural changes following visual scanning training: Observation of five cases. *International Journal of Clinical Neuropsychology*, *9*, 74–80.

Gouvier WD, Cottam G, Webster JS, Beissel GF, Wofford J (1984) Behavioral interventions with stroke patients for improving wheelchair navigation. *International Journal of Clinical Neuropsychology*, *6*, 186–190.

Gouvier WD, Maxfield MW, Schweitzer JR, Horton CR, Shipp M, Nielson K, Hale PN (1989) Psychometric prediction of driving performance among the disabled. *Archives of Physical Medicine and Rehabilitation*, *70*, 745–750.

Grady CL, Grimes AM, Patronas N, Sunderland T, Foster NL, Rapoport SI (1989) Divided attention, as measured by dichotic speech performance, in dementia of the Alzheimer type. *Archives of Neurology*, *48*, 317–320.

Grady CL, Haxby JV, Horwitz B, Sundaram M, Berg G, Schapiro M, Friedland RP, Rapoport SI (1988) Longitudinal study of the early neuropsychological and cerebral metabolic changes in dementia of the Alzheimer type. *Journal of Clinical and Experimental Neuropsychology*, *10*, 576–596.

Grafman J, Litvan I, Gomez C, Chase TN (1990) Frontal lobe function in progressive supranuclear palsy. *Archives of Neurology*, *47*, 553–558.

Gray JM (1990) The remediation of attentional disorders following brain injury of acute onset. In: Wood RL, Fussey I (eds.), *Cognitive Rehabilitation in Perspective*. Taylor and Francis, London.

Gray JM, Robertson I, Pentland B, Anderson S (1992) Microcomputer-based attentional retraining after brain damage: A randomised group controlled trial. *Neuropsychological Rehabilitation*, *2*, 97–115.

Greber R, Perret E (1985) Attention and short-term memory disorders after brain stem lesions. *Proceedings of an EBBS Workshop*, Zurich.

Gregory S (1989) Functional evaluation of the driver with acquired brain damage. In: Anderson V, Bailey M (eds.), *Theory and Function: bridging the gap*, pp. 43–46. ASSBI, Melbourne, Australia.

Grewel F (1953) Le test de Bourdon-Wiersma. *Folia Psychiatrica Neurologica Neurochirurgica Neerlandica,* *56*, 694.

Grisell JL, Levin SM, Cohen BD, Rodin EA (1964) Effects of subclinical seizure activity on overt behavior. *Neurology*, *14*, 133–135.

Gronwall D (1977) Paced Auditory Serial Addition Task: A measure of recovery from concussion. *Perceptual and Motor Skills*, *44*, 367–373.

Gronwall D (1987) Advances in the assessment of attention and information processing after head injury. In: Levin HS Grafman J, Eisenberg HM (eds.), *Neurobehavioral Recovery from Head Injury*. Oxford University Press, New York.

Gronwall D (1991) Minor head injury. *Neuropsychology*, *5*, 253–265.

Gronwall D, Sampson H (1974) *The Psychological Effects of Concussion*. Auckland University Press, Auckland.

Gronwall D, Wrightson P (1974) Delayed recovery of intellectual function after minor head injury. *Lancet*, *2*, 995–997.

Gronwall D, Wrightson P (1981) Memory and information processing capacity after closed head injury. *Journal of Neurology, Neurosurgery and Psychiatry*, *44*, 889–895.

Gross Y, Schutz LE (1986) Invervention models in neuropsychology. In: Uzzell BP, Gross Y (eds.), *The Clinical Neuropsychology of Intervention*. Nijhoff, Boston.

Gurd JM, Ward CD (1988) Retrieval from semantic and letter initial categories in patients with Parkinson's disease. *Neuropsychologia*, *27*, 743–746.

Hachinski V (1990) Cognitive rehabilitation. *Archives of Neurology*, *47*, 224.

Haider M (1964) Neuropsychology of attention, expectation and vigilance. In: Mostofsky DI (ed.), *Attention: Contemporary Theory and Analysis*. Appleton & Lange, E. Norwalk, CT.

Hallett M, Khoshbin S (1980) A physiological mechanism of bradykinesia. *Brain*, *103*, 301–304.

Halligan PW, Cockburn J, Wilson BA (1991) The behavioural assessment of visual neglect. *Neuropsychological Rehabilitation*, *1*, 5–32.

Hanley JR, Dewick HC, Davies ADM, Playfer J, Turnbull C (1990) Verbal fluency in Parkinson's disease. *Neuropsychologia*, *28*, 737–741.

Hannay HJ, Levin HS, Grossman RG (1979) Impaired recognition memory after head injury. *Cortex*, *15*, 269–283.

Hansch EC, Syndulko K, Coehn SN, Goldberg, ZI, Potvin AR, Tourtelette WW (1982) Cognition in Parkinson's disease: An event-related potential perspective. *Annals of Neurology*, *11*, 599–607.

Hansotia P, Broste SK (1991) The effect of epilepsy or diabetes mellitus on the risk of automobile accidents. *New England Journal of Medicine*, *343*, 22–26.

Harris JE, Sunderland A (1981) A brief survey of the management of memory disorders in rehabilitation units in Britain. *International Rehabilitation Medicine*, *3*, 206–209.

Hart S (1985) *Explorations of cognitive dysfunction in dementia of Alzheimer type*. [Doctoral Dissertation]. University of London.

Hart S, Semple JM (1990) *Neuropsychology and the dementias*. Taylor and Francis, London.

Hart T, Plenger PM, Helffenstein DA, Hayden ME (1985) Neuropsychological correlates and qualitative features of vocational performance after severe closed head injury. *Journal of Clinical and Experimental Neuropsychology*, *7*, 148.

Hartje W, Pach R, Willmes K, Hannen P, Weber E (1991a) Driving ability of brain-damaged patients. *Zeitschrift für Neuropsychologie*, *2*, 100–114.

Hartje W, Willmes K, Pach R, Hannen P, Weber E (1991b) Driving ability of aphasic and non-aphasic brain-damaged patients. *Neuropsychological Rehabilitation*, *1*, 161–174.

Hassler R (1978) Striatal control of locomotion, intentional actions and of integrating and perceptive activity. *Journal of the Neurological Sciences*, *36*, 187–224.

Hauser WA (1978) Epidemiology of epilepsy. *Advances in Neurology*, *19*, 313–338.

Heaton RK (1981) *Wisconsin Card Sorting Test Manual*. Psychological Assessment Resources, Odessa, FL.

Hebb DO (1958) *A Textbook of Psychology*. WB Saunders, Philadelphia.

Heilman KM, Van den Abell T (1979) Right hemisphere dominance for mediating cerebral activation. *Neuropsychologia*, *17*, 315–321.

Heilman KM, Watson RT, Valenstein E (1985) Neglect and related disorders. In: *Clinical Neuropsychology*. Oxford University Press, New York.

Heinze HJ, Münte TF, Gobiet W, Niemann H, Ruff AM (1992) Parallel and serial visual search after closed head injury: Electrophysiological evidence for perceptual dysfunction. *Neuropsychologia*, *30*, 495–514.

Hicks L, Birren JE (1970) Aging, brain damage and psychomotor slowing. *Psychological Bulletin*, *74*, 377–396.

Hietanen M, Teräväinen H (1986) Cognitive performance in early Parkinson's disease. *Acta Neurologica Scandinavica*, *73*, 151–159.

Hinkeldey NS, Corrigan JD (1990) The structure of head-injured patients' neurobehavioral complaints: A preliminary study. *Brain Injury*, *4*, 115–134.

Hockey GRJ, Gaillard AWK, Coles MGH (1986) *Energetics and Human Information Processing.* Nijhoff, Dordrecht, Netherlands.

Hopewell CA, Van Zomeren AH (1990) Neuropsychological aspects of motor vehicle operation. In: Tupper DE, Cicerone KD (eds.), *The Neuropsychology of Everyday Life.* Kluwer, Boston.

Hopewell CA, Burke WH, Wesolowski M, Zawlocki R (1990) Behavioural learning therapies for the traumatically brain-injured patient. In: Wood RL, Fussey I (eds.), *Cognitive Rehabilitation in Perspective.* Taylor and Francis, London.

Horstink MWIM, Berger HJC, Van Spaendonck KPM, Van den Bercken JHL, Cools AR (1990) Bimanual simultaneous motor performance and impaired ability to shift attention in Parkinson's disease. *Journal of Neurology, Neurosurgery and Psychiatry, 53*, 685–690.

Howes D, Boller F (1975) Simple reaction time: Evidence for focal impairments from lesions of the right hemisphere. *Brain, 98*, 317–332.

Hutt SJ (1972) Experimental analysis of brain activity and behavior in children with "minor" seizures. *Epilepsia, 13*, 520–534.

Hutt SJ, Denner S, Newton J (1977) Auditory thresholds during evoked spike-wave activity in epileptic patients. *Cortex, 12*, 249–257.

Hutt SJ, Jackson PM, Belsham A, Higgins G (1968) Perceptual motor behavior in relation to phenobarbitone blood level: A preliminary report. *Developmental Medicine and Child Neurology, 10*, 626–632.

Hyman BT, van Hoesen GW, Damasio AR, Barnes CL (1984) Alzheimer's disease: Cell specific pathology isolates the hippocampal formation. *Science, 225*, 1168–1170.

Inglis J (1965) Immediate memory, age and brain function. In: Welford AT, Birren JE (eds.), *Behavior, Aging and the Nervous System.* CC Thomas, Springfield, IL.

Inglis J (1970) Memory disorder. In: Costello CG (ed.), *Symptoms of Psychopathology.* Wiley, New York.

James W (1890) *The Principles of Psychology*, vol. 1. Holt & Co., New York.

Jasper HH (1954) Functional properties of the thalamic reticular system. In: The Council for International Organization of Medical Sciences (eds.), *Brain Mechanisms and Consciousness.* Blackwell, Oxford.

Jeeves MA, Dixon NF (1970) Hemisphere differences in response rates to visual stimuli. *Psychonomic Science, 20*, 249–251.

Jennett B (1982) Post-traumatic epilepsy. In: Laidlaw J, Richens A (eds.), *A Textbook of Epilepsy*, pp. 146–154. Churchill Livingstone, Edinburgh.

Jones R, Tranel D, Benton A, Paulsen J (1992) Differentiating dementia from "pseudodementia" early in the clinical course: Utility of neuropsychological tests. *Neuropsychology, 6*, 13–22.

Jorm AF (1986) Controlled and automatic information processing in senile dementia: A review. *Psychological Medicine, 16*, 77–88.

Jung R, Hassler R (1960) The extrapyramidal motor system. In: Field J, Magoun W, Hall VE (eds.), *Handbook of Physiology, Section I: Neurophysiology*, vol. 2. Williams & Wilkins, Baltimore.

Kahneman D (1973) *Attention and Effort.* Prentice Hall, Englewood Cliffs, NJ.

Kahneman D, Ben-Ishai R, Lotan M (1973) Relation of a test of attention to road accidents. *Journal of Applied Psychology, 58*, 113–115.

Kalska H (1991) Cognitive changes in epilepsy: A ten year follow-up. Dissertation, University of Helsinki.

Karyandis F (1989) Parkinson's disease: A conceptualization of neuropsychological deficits within an information-processing framework. *Biological Psychology, 29*, 149–179.

Kasteleyn-Nolst Trenité DGA, Riemersma JBJ, Binnie CD, Smit AM, Meinardi H (1987) The influence of subclinical epileptiform EEG discharges on driving behaviour. *Clinical Neurophysiology*, 67, 167–170.

Kasteleyn-Nolst Trenité DGA, Siebelink BM, Smit AM, Klepper J, Meinardi H (1993) Epilepsy and driving: clinical and neurophysiological aspects. (submitted).

Kaszniak AW, Keyl PM, Albert MS (1991) Dementia and the older driver. *Human Factors*, 33, 527–537.

Kaszniak AW, Nussbaum P, Allender JA (1990) Driving in elderly patients with dementia or depression. Paper presented at *Annual Meeting of the American Psychological Association*, Boston.

Kertesz A, Polk M, Carr T (1990) Cognition and white matter changes on magnetic resonance imaging in dementia. *Archives of Neurology*, 47, 387–391.

Kewman DG, Yanus B, Kirsch N (1988) Assessment of distractability in auditory comprehension after traumatic brain injury. *Brain Injury*, 2, 131–137.

Kinsbourne M (1970) The cerebral basis of lateral asymmetries in attention. *Acta Psychologica*, 33, 193–201.

Kinsbourne M (1987) Mechanisms of unilateral neglect. In: Jeannerod M (ed.), *Neurophysiological and Neuropsychological Aspects of Spatial Neglect*. North-Holland, New York.

Kinsbourne M, Hicks RE (1978) Functional cerebral space: A model for overflow transfer and interference effects in human performance. In: Requin J (ed.), *Attention and Performance VII*, pp. 81–97. Erlbaum, Hillsdale, NJ

Kolb B, Whishaw IQ (1990) *Fundamentals of Human Neuropsychology*. Freeman, New York.

Koning-Haanstra M, Berg IJ, Deelman BG (1990) Training memory strategies: Description of a method. In: Deelman BG, Saan RJ, Van Zomeren AH (eds.), *Traumatic Brain Injury: Clinical, Social and Rehabilitational Aspects*, pp. 145–168. Swets and Zeitlinger, Amsterdam.

Korteling JE (1988) Reaction time and driving capabilities of brain injured and elderly drivers. In: Rothengatter JA, De Bruin R (eds.), *Road User Behavior: Theory and Research*. Van Gorcum, Assen.

Korteling JE (1990) Perception-response speed and driving capabilities of brain-damaged and older drivers. *Human Factors*, 32, 95–108.

Koss E, Ober BA, Delis DC (1984) The Stroop Color Word Test: Indicator of dementia severity. *International Journal of Neuroscience*, 24, 53–61.

Kreutzer JS (1993) Improving the prognosis for return to work after brain injury. In: Frommelt P, Wiedmann KD (eds.), *Neurorehabilitation: A Perspective for the Figure*, pp. 26–29. Deggendorf Conference.

Kreutzer JS, Devany CW, Myers SL, Marwitz JH (1991) Neurobehavioral outcome following traumatic brain injury: Review, methodology, and implications for cognitive rehabilitation. In: Kreutzer JS, Wehmann P (eds.), *Cognitive Rehabilitation for Persons with Traumatic Brain Injury: A Functional Approach*. Brookes, Baltimore.

Kulig BM (1980) The evaluation of the behavioral effects of antiepileptic drugs in animals and man. In: Kulig BM, Meinardi H, Stores G (eds.), *Epilepsy and Behavior*, pp. 48–61. Swets and Zeitlinger, Lisse.

Kwak HW, Dagenbach D, Egeth HE (1991) Further evidence for a time independent shift of the focus of attention. *Perception and Psychophysics*, 49, 473–480.

LaBerge D, Brown V (1986) Theory of attentional operations in shape identification. *Psychological Review*, 96, 101–124.

Lachman R, Lachman JL, Butterfield EC (1979) *Comparative Psychology and Information Processing: An Introduction.* Wiley, New York.

Ladavas E (1992) The rehabilitation of visual neglect: A dissociation between automatic and voluntary orienting of attention. *Proceedings of the Conference on Attention: Theoretical and Clinical Perspectives,* Baycrest Centre, 26–27 March, Toronto, Canada.

Laidlaw J, Richens AL (1982) *A Textbook of Epilepsy.* Churchill Livingstone, Edinburgh.

Lambert EW, Engum ES (1992) Construct validity of the cognitive Behavioral Driver's Inventory: Age, diagnosis and driving ability. *Journal of Cognitive Rehabilitation,* May/June, p. 12–18.

Langston JW, Irwin I, Finnegan KT (1989) Using neurotoxicants to study aging and Parkinson's disease. In: Calne DB, Comi G, Crippa D, Horowski R, Trabucchi M (eds.), *Parkinsonism And Aging,* pp. 145–153. Raven Press, New York.

Lansdell H, Mirsky AF (1964) Attention in focal and centrencephalic epilepsy. *Experimental Neurology, 9,* 463–469.

LaRue A (1992) *Aging and Neuropsychological Assessment.* Plenum, New York.

Lawson IR (1962) Visual-spatial neglect in lesions of the right cerebral hemisphere. *Neurology, 12,* 23–33.

Leahey TH (1980) *A History of Psychology.* Prentice Hall, Englewood Cliffs.

Leibniz GW (1765) *New Essays Concerning Human Understanding.* [Translated by W. Langley, 1916.] Open Court, London.

Lesser RP, Lüders H, Wyllie E, Dinner DS, Morris HH (1986) Mental deterioration in epilepsy. *Epilepsia, 27 (suppl. 2),* 105–123.

Levin HS (1990) Cognitive rehabilitation: Unproved but promising. *Archives of Neurology, 47,* 223–224.

Levin HS, Grafman J, Eisenberg HM (eds.) (1987) *Neurobehavioral Recovery from Head Injury.* Oxford University Press, New York.

Levin HS, High WM, Goethe KE (1987b) The neurobehavioral rating scale: Assessment of the behavioral sequelae of head injury by the clinician. *Journal of Neurology, Neurosurgery and Psychiatry, 50,* 183–193.

Lewis R, Kupke T (1977) The Lafayette Clinic repeatable neuropsychological test battery. Paper presented at the Southeastern Psychological Association, Hollywood, FL.

Lezak MD (1982) The problems of assessing executive functions. *International Journal of Psychology, 17,* 281–297.

Lezak MD (1983) *Neuropsychological Assessment.* Oxford University Press, New York.

Lines CR, Dawson C, Preston GC, Reich S, Foster C, Traub M (1991) Memory and attention in patients with senile dementia of the Alzheimer type and in normal elderly subjects. *Journal of Clinical and Experimental Neuropsychology, 13,* 691–702.

Lishman WA (1978) *Organic Psychiatry.* Blackwell, Oxford.

Livingstone M, Hubel D (1988) Segregation of form, color, movement and depth: Anatomy, physiology and perception. *Science, 240,* 740–749.

Longley WA, Sulway MR, Broe GA, Creasey H, Korten A (1990) Deficits in executive function in mild Alzheimer's disease patients may suggest early frontal lobe dysfunction. *Journal of Clinical and Experimental Neuropsychology, 12,* 424.

Loring D (1982) 40-Hz EEG and Alzheimer's Disease, multi-infarct dementia and normal aging. Unpublished doctoral dissertation, University of Houston, TX.

Lucas-Blaustein MJ, Filipp L, Dungan Ch, Tune L (1988) Driving in patients with dementia. *Journal of the American Geriatric Society, 36,* 1087–1091.

Luria AR (1963) *Restoration of Function After Brain Injury.* Pergamon Press, Oxford.

Luria AR (1966) *Higher Cortical Functions in Man.* Tavistock, London.

Luria AR (1971) Memory disturbances in local brain lesions. *Neuropsychologia*, 9, 367–376.

Luria AR (1973) *The Working Brain*. Penguin Press, London.

Luria AR, Homskaya ED (1970) Frontal lobes and the regulation of activation processes. In: Mostofsky D (ed.), *Attention: Contemporary Theory and Analysis*. Appleton and Lange, E. Norwalk, CT.

MacFlynn G, Montgomery EA, Fenton GW, Rutherford W (1984) Measurement of reaction time following minor head injury. *Journal of Neurology, Neurosurgery and Psychiatry*, 47, 1326–1331.

Mackworth JF (1970) *Vigilance and Attention: A Signal-Detection Approach*. Penguin Books, Harmondsworth.

Mackworth NH (1950) Researches in the measurement of human performance. MRC Special Report 268. In: Sinaiko HA (ed.), 1961, *Selected Papers on Human Factors in the Design and Use of Control Systems*, pp. 174–331. Dover, London.

Malec J (1984) Training the brain-injured client in behavioral self-management skills. In: Edelstein BA, Couture ET (eds.), *Behavioral Assessment and Rehabilitation of the Traumatically Brain-Damaged*. Plenum, New York.

Malec J, Rao N, Jones R, Stubbs K (1984) Video game practice effects on sustained attention in patients with craniocerebral trauma. *Cognitive Rehabilitation*, 2, 18–23.

Mandleberg IA, Brooks DN (1975) Cognitive recovery after severe head injury. I. Serial testing on the Wechsler Adult Intelligence Scale. *Journal of Neurology, Neurosurgery and Psychiatry*, 38, 1121–1126.

Marsden CD (1982) The mysterious motor function of the basal ganglia: The Robert Wartenberg lecture. *Neurology (NY)*, 32, 514–539.

Martin A, Brouwers P, Lalonde F, Cox C, Teleska P, Fedio P, Foster NL, Chase PN (1986) Towards a behavioral typology of Alzheimer's patients. *Journal of Clinical and Experimental Neuropsychology*, 8, 594–610.

Mattis S (1976) Mental status examination for organic mental syndrome in the elderly patient. In: Bellak L, Karasu TB (eds.), *Geriatric Psychiatry*, pp. 77–121. Grune & Stratton, Orlando, FL.

Maurer K, Ihl R, Dierks T (1988) Topography of P-300 in psychiatry: Cognitive P-300 fields in dementia. *EEG EMG*, 19, 26–29.

McClelland JL, Rumelhart DE (1985) Distributed memory and the representation of general and specific information. *Journal of Experimental Psychology*, 114, 159–188.

McComas JC (1922) A measure of attention. *Journal of Experimental Psychology*, 5, 1–18.

McFarland RA, Moore RC, Warren AB (1954) *Human Variables in Motor Vehicle Accidents: A Review of the Literature*. Harvard School of Public Health, Cambridge, MA.

McGlinchey-Berroth R, Kilduff PT, Grande L, Verfaellie M, Milberg WP, Alexander M (1992) Semantic priming by words and pictures in the neglected field. Paper presented at the Baycrest Centre conference *Attention, Theoretical and Clinical Perspectives*, Toronto, Canada, 1992 (26–27 March).

McGlynn SM (1990) Behavioral approaches to neuropsychological rehabilitation. *Psychological Bulletin*, 108, 420–441.

McKenna FP, Duncan J, Brown ID (1986) Cognitive abilities and safety on the road: A reexamination of individual differences in dichotic listening and search for embedded figures. *Ergonomics*, 29, 649–663.

McKhann G, Drachman D, Folstein M, Katzman R, Price D, Stadlan EM (1984) Clinical diagnosis of Alzheimer's disease: Report of the NINCDS/ADRDA work group under the auspices of the Department of Health and Human Services task force on Alzheimer's disease. *Neurology*, *34*, 939–944.

McLean A, Dikmen S, Temkin N, Wyler AR, Gale JL (1984) Psychosocial functioning at 1 month after head injury. *Neurosurgery*, *14*, 393–399.

Meichenbaum D (1977) *Cognitive Behavior Modification: An Integrative Approach*. Plenum, New York.

Mesulam MM (1981) A cortical network for directed attention and unilateral neglect. *Annals of Neurology*, *10*, 309–325.

Mesulam MM (1985) *Principles of Behavioral Neurology*. FA Davis, Philadelphia.

Michon JA (1979) Dealing with danger: Summary report of a workshop in the Traffic Research Centre, State University, Groningen.

Michon JA, Eijckman EGJ, De Klerk LFW (1976) Inleiding. In: *Handboek der Psychonomie*, pp. 3–13. Van Loghum Slaterus, Deventer, NL.

Miller E (1970) Simple and choice reaction time following severe head injury. *Cortex*, *6*, 121–127.

Miller E (1977) *Abnormal Ageing*. Wiley, London.

Miller E (1984) Verbal fluency as a measure of verbal intelligence and in relation to different types of cerebral pathology. *British Journal of Clinical Psychology*, *23*, 53–57.

Miller E, Cruzat A (1980) A note on the effects of irrelevant information on task performance after mild and severe head injury. *British Journal of Social and Clinical Psychology*, vol. 20, 69–70.

Milner B (1963) Some effects of frontal lobectomy in man. In Warren JM, Akert K (eds.), *The Frontal Granular Cortex and Behaviour*, pp. 313–331. McGraw-Hill, New York.

Minderhoud JM, Boelens MEM, Huizenga J, Saan RJ (1980) Treatment of minor head injuries. *Clinical Neurology and Neurosurgery*, *82*, 127–140.

Mirsky AF, Van Buren JM (1965) On the nature of the "absence" in centrencephalic epilepsy: A study of some behavioral, electroencephalographic and autonomic factors. *Electroencephalography and Clinical Neurophysiology*, *18*, 334–348.

Mirsky AF, Primac DW, Marsan CA, Rosvold HE, Stevens JR (1960) A comparison of the psychological test performance of patients with focal and nonfocal epilepsy. *Experimental Neurology*, *2*, 75–89.

Moerland MC, Aldenkamp AP, Alpherts WCJ (1986) A neuropsychological test battery for the Apple II-E. *International Journal for Man-Machine Studies*, *25*, 453–467.

Montaldi D, Brooks DN, McColl JH, Wyper D, Patterson J, Barron E, McCulloch J (1990) Measurements of rCBF and cognitive performance in Alzheimer's disease. *Journal of Neurology, Neurosurgery and Psychiatry*, *53*, 33–38.

Moray N (1969) *Attention: Selective Processes in Vision and Hearing*. Hutchinson Educational, London.

Morgan SF, Wheelock J (1992) Digit symbol and symbol digit modalities tests: Are they directly interchangeable? *Neuropsychology 6*, 327–330.

Morris RG, Downes JJ, Sahakian BJ, Evenden JL, Heald A, Robbins TW (1988) Planning and spatial working memory in Parkinson's disease. *Journal of Neurology, Neurosurgery and Psychiatry*, *51*, 757–766.

Moruzzi I, Magoun HW (1949) Brain stem reticular formation and activation of the EEG. *Electroencephalography and Clinical Neurophysiology*, *1*, 455–473.

Müller G, Richter RA, Weisbrod S, Klingberg F (1991) Reaction time prolongation in the early stage of presenile onset Alzheimer's disease. *European Archives of Psychiatry and Clinical Neurosciences*, *241*, 46–48.

Muskens JP (1993) The course of dementia: an explorative longitudinal study in general practice. Thesis, Catholic University of Nijmegen.

Myerson J, Hale S, Wagstaff D, Poon LW, Smith GA (1990) The information-loss model: A mathematical theory of age-related cognitive slowing. *Psychological Review*, 97, 475–487.

Näätänen R (1988) Implications of ERP data for psychological theories of attention. *Biological Psychiatry*, 26, 117–163.

Nauta HJW (1979) A proposed conceptual reorganization of the basal ganglia and telencephalon. *Neuroscience*, 4, 1875–1881.

Nauta WJ (1964) Some efferent connections of the prefrontal cortex in the monkey. In: Warren JM, Akert K (eds.), *Frontal Granular Cortex and Behavior*. McGraw-Hill, New York.

Nebes RD, Brady CB (1989) Focused and divided attention in Alzheimer's disease. *Cortex*, 25, 305–315.

Nebes RD, Brady CB (1992) Generalized cognitive slowing and severity of dementia in Alzheimer's disease: Implications for the interpretation of response-time data. *Journal of Clinical and Experimental Neuropsychology*, 14, 317–326.

Neisser U (1967) *Cognitive Psychology*. Appleton and Lange, E. Norwalk, CT.

Nelson HE (1976) A modified card sorting test sensitive to frontal lobe damage. *Cortex*, 12, 313–324.

Nestor PG, Parasuraman R, Haxby JV (1991a) Speed of information processing and attention in early Alzheimer's dementia. *Developmental Neuropsychology*, 7, 243–256.

Nestor PG, Parasuraman R, Haxby JV, Grady CL (1991b) Divided attention and metabolic brain dysfunction in mild dementia of the Alzheimer type. *Neuropsychologia*, 29, 279–288.

Newcombe F (1982) The psychological consequences of closed head injury: assessment and rehabilitation. *Injury*, 14, 111–136.

Newell A, Simon HA (1972) *Human Problem Solving*. Prentice-Hall, Englewood Cliffs, NJ.

Niemann H, Ruff RM, Baser CA (1990) Computer-assisted attention retraining in head-injured individuals: A controlled efficacy study of an outpatient program. *Journal of Consulting and Clinical Psychology*, 58, 811–817.

Nissen MJ, Corkin S, Growdon JH (1981) Attentional focusing in amnesia and Alzheimer's disease. Paper presented to the American Aging Association, New York.

Norman DA (1969) *Memory and Attention: An Introduction to Human Information Processing*. Wiley, New York.

Norrman B, Svahn K (1961) A follow-up study of severe brain injuries. *Acta Psychiatrica Scandinavica*, 37, 236–264.

Obersteiner H (1874) Ueber eine neue einfache Methode zur Bestimmung der psychischen Leistungsfähigkeit des Gehirnes Geisteskranker. *Virchows Archive*, 14, 427–459.

Obersteiner H (1879) Experimental researches on attention. *Brain*, 1, 439–453.

O'Connor KP (1980a) Slow potential correlates of attention dysfunction in senile dementia: I. *Biological Psychology*, 11, 193–202.

O'Connor KP (1980b) Slow potential correlates of attention dysfunction in senile dementia: II. *Biological Psychology*, 11, 203–216.

O'Shaughnessy EJ, Fowler RS, Reid V (1984) Sequelae of mild closed head injuries. *Journal of Family Practice*, 18, 391–394.

Osterrieth PA (1944) Le test de copie d'une figure complexe. *Archives de Psychologie*, 30, 206–356.

Owen A, Downes JJ, Sahakian BJ, Polkey CE, Robbins TW (1990) Planning and spatial working memory following frontal lobe lesions in man. *Neuropsychologia, 28,* 1021–1034.

Papanicolaou AC (1987) Electrophysiological methods for the study of attentional deficits in head injury. In: Levin HS, Grafman J, Eisenberg HM (eds.), *Neurobehavioral Recovery from Head Injury*. New York, Oxford University Press.

Papanicolaou AC, Levin HS, Eisdenberg HM, Moore BD, Goethe KE, High WM (1984) Evoked potential correlates of posttraumatic amnesia after closed head injury. *Neurosurgery, 14,* 676–678.

Parasuraman R, Davies DR (1977) A taxonomic analysis of vigilance performance. In: Mackie RR (ed.), *Vigilance, Theory, Operational Performance and Physiological Correlates*. Plenum, New York.

Parasuraman R, Davies DR (1984) *Varieties of Attention*. Academic Press, Orlando, FL.

Parasuraman R, Nestor P (1986) Energetics of attention and Alzheimer's disease. In: Hockey GRJ, Gaillard A, Coles MGH (eds.), *Energetics and Human Information Processing*. Nijhoff, Dordrecht.

Parasuraman R, Nestor PG (1991) Attention and driving skills in aging and Alzheimer's disease. *Human Factors, 33,* 539–557.

Parasuraman R, Mutter SA, Molloy R (1991) Sustained attention following mild closed head injury. *Journal of Clinical and Experimental Neuropsychology, 13,* 789–811.

Parasuraman R, Nestor P, Haxby J (1985) Patterns of attentional loss in aging and early Alzheimer's disease. *Technical Report CNL-85-1*. Cognitive Neuroscience Laboratory, Catholic University, Washington, DC.

Peeters S (1986) Automatic and controlled processing in lexical decision and recognition following closed head injury. *Journal of Clinical and Experimental Neuropsychology, 8,* 123.

Penfield W (1952) Memory mechanisms. *AMA Archives of Neurology and Psychiatry, 67,* 178–191.

Petersen SE, Fox PT, Posner MI, Mintun M, Raichle ME (1988) Positron emission tomographic studies of the cortical anatomy of single word processing. *Nature, 331,* 585–589.

Petersen SE, Robinson DL, Morris JD (1987) Contributions of the pulvinar to visual spatial attention. *Neuropsychologia, 25,* 97–105.

Pillsbury WB (1908) *Attention*. London.

Plum F, Posner JB (1980) *The Diagnosis of Stupor and Coma*. FA Davis, Philadelphia.

Pollock VE, Schneider LS, Chui HC, Henderson V, Zemansky M, Sloane RB (1989) Visual evoked potentials in dementia: A meta-analysis and empirical study of Alzheimers disease patients. *Biological Psychiatry, 25,* 1003–1013.

Ponds RWHM, Brouwer WH, Van Wolffelaar PC (1988) Age differences in divided attention in a simulated driving task. *Journal of Gerontology, 43,* 151–156.

Ponsford J (1990) The use of computers in the rehabilitation of attention disorders. In: Wood RL, Fussey I (eds.), *Cognitive Rehabilitation in Perspective*. Taylor and Francis, London.

Ponsford JL, Kinsella G (1988) Evaluation of a remedial programme for attentional deficits following closed head injury. *Journal of Clinical and Experimental Neuropsychology, 10,* 693–708.

Ponsford J, Kinsella G (1991) The use of a rating scale of attentional behaviour. *Neuropsychological Rehabilitation, 1,* 241–257.

Ponsford J, Kinsella G (1992) Attentional deficits following closed head injury. *Journal of Experimental and Clinical Neuropsychology, 14,* 822–838.

Poppelreuter WL (1917) *Die psychischen Schaedigungen durch Kopfschuss im Kreig 1914–1916; Die Störungen der niederen und hoheren Leistungen durch Verletzungen des Oksipitalhirns.* vol. I. Leopold Voss, Leipzig.

Porter RJ, Penry JK, Dreifuss FE (1973) Responsiveness at the onset of spike-wave bursts. *Electroencephalography and Clinical Neurophysiology*, 34, 239–245.

Portin R, Rinne UK (1980) Neuropsychological responses of parkinsonian patients to long-term levodopa treatment. In: Rinne UK, Klinger M, Stamm G (eds.), *Parkinson's Disease: Current Progress, Problems and Management*, pp. 271–304. Elsevier/North Holland, Amsterdam.

Posner MI (1975) The psychobiology of attention. In: Gazzaniga MS, Blakemore C (eds.), *Handbook of Psychobiology*, pp. 441–480. Academic Press, New York.

Posner MI (1980) Orienting of attention. *Quarterly Journal of Experimental Psychology*, 32, 3–25.

Posner MI (1988) Structures and functions of selective attention. In: Boll T, Bryant B (eds.), *Clinical Neuropsychology and Brain Function*, Master lectures, pp. 173–202. American Psychology Association, Washington, DC.

Posner MI (1989) *Foundations of Cognitive Science*. MIT Press, Cambridge, MA.

Posner MI (1992) Attention as a cognitive and anatomical system. Conference Proceedings *Attention: Theoretical and Clinical Perspectives*, Baycrest Centre, Toronto, Canada.

Posner MI, Cohen Y (1984) Components of performance. In: Bouma H, Bouwhuis D (eds.), *Attention and Performance*, pp. 531–556. Erlbaum, Hillsdale, NJ.

Posner MI, Petersen SE (1990) The attention system of the human brain. *Annual Review of Neurosciences*, 13, 182–196.

Posner MI, Rafal RD (1987) Cognitive theories of attention and the rehabilitation of attentional deficits. In: Meier MJ, Benton A, Diller L (eds.), *Neuropsychological Rehabilitation*. Churchill Livingstone, New York.

Posner MI, Cohen A, Rafal R (1982) Neural systems control of spatial orienting. *Philosophical Transactions of the Royal Society*, 298, 187–198.

Posner M, Nissen M, Ogden W (1978) Attended and unattended processing modes: The role of set for spatial location. In: Pick H, Saltzman E (eds.), *Modes of Perceiving and Processing Information*, Erlbaum, Hillsdale, NJ.

Posner MI, Petersen SE, Fox PT, Raichle ME (1988) Localization of cognitive operations in the human brain. *Science*, 240, 1627–1631.

Powell GE (1981) *Brain Function Therapy*. Gower-Aldershot, Hants.

Prasher D, Findley L (1991) Dopaminergic induced changes in cognitive and motor processing in Parkinson's disease: An electrophysiological investigation. *Journal of Neurology, Neurosurgery and Psychiatry*, 54, 603–609.

Prechtl HFR, Boeke PE, Schut T (1961) The electroencephalogram and performance in epileptic patients. *Neurology*, 11, 296–302.

Pribram KH, McGuinness D (1975) Arousal, activation and effort in the control of attention. *Psychological Review*, 82, 116–149.

Price DL, Whitehouse PJ, Strubble RG (1986) Cellular pathology in Alzheimer's disease and Parkinson's disease. *Trends in the Neurosciences*, 9, 29–33.

Prigatano GP (1985) *Neuropsychological Rehabilitation after Brain Injury*. Johns Hopkins University Press, Baltimore.

Prigatano GP (1987) Psychiatric aspects of head injury: Problem areas and suggested guidelines for research. In: Levin HS, Grafman J, Eisenberg HM (eds.), *Neurobehavioral Recovery from Head Injury*. Oxford University Press, New York.

Rafal RD, Posner MI, Walker JA, Friedrich FJ (1984) Cognition and the basal ganglia. *Brain*, 107, 1083–1094.

Rao SM, Bieliauskas LA (1983) Cognitive rehabilitation two-and-one-half years post right temporal lobectomy. *Journal of Clinical Neuropsychology*, *5*, 313–320.

Raskin S, Borod J, Tweedy J (1990) Neuropsychological aspects of Parkinson's disease. *Neuropsychology Review*, *1*, 185–221.

Rattok J, Ben-Yishay Y, Ezrachi O, Lakin PH, Piasetsky E, Ross B, Silver S, Vakil E, Zide E, Diller L (1992) Outcome of different treatment mixes in a multidimensional neuropsychological rehabilitation program. *Neuropsychology*, *6*, 395–415.

Rebok GW, Bylsma FW, Keyl P (1990) The effects of Alzheimer's disease on elderly drivers. Paper presented at the *annual meeting of the Gerontological Society of America*, Boston.

Reinvang I, Bjartveit S, Johannessen SI, Hagen OP, Larsen S, Fagerthun H, Gjerstad L (1991) Cognitive function and time-of-day variation in serum carbamazepine concentration in epileptic patients treated with monotherapy. *Epilepsia*, *32*, 116–121.

Reitan RM (1958) Validity of the Trailmaking Test as an indication of organic brain damage. *Perceptual and Motor Skills*, *8*, 271–276.

Reitan RM (1966) A research program on the psychological effects of brain lesions in human beings. In: Ellis NR (ed.), *International Review of Research in Mental Retardation*, vol. 1, pp. 153–218. Academic Press, New York.

Remond A, Bouhours P (1988) Memory, attention and evoked potentials during aging and in Alzheimer type senile dementia. *Neurophysiologie Clinique*, *18*, 153–160.

Reuter-Lorenz PA, Kinsbourne M, Moscovitch M (1990) Hemispheric control of spatial attention. *Brain and Cognition*, *12*, 240–266.

Rey ER, Bueckart G, Oldigs J (1983) Aufmerksamkeits-veränderungen bei Hirntraumatikern: Eine experimentalpsychologische Untersuchung mit Hilfe von Reaktionszeitaufgaben. Paper read at the *20. Tagung Deutsche Gesellschaft für Hirntraumatologie und Klinische Hirnpathologie*, Mannheim.

Reynolds EH (1983) Mental effects of antiepileptic medication: A review. *Epilepsia, 24, suppl. 2*, 85–95.

Reynolds JR (1861) *Epilepsy: Its symptoms, treatment and relation to other chronic convulsive diseases*. Churchill, London.

Rizzo PA, Amabile C, Caporali M, Spadaro M, Zanasi M, Morocutti C (1978) A CNV study in a group of patients with traumatic head injuries. *Electroencephalography and Clinical Neurophysiology*, *45*, 281–285.

Roberts RJ, Varney NR, Paulsen JS, Richardson ED (1990) Dichotic listening and complex partial seizures. *Journal of Clinical and Experimental Neuropsychology*, *12*, 448–458.

Robertson IH, Cashman E (1991) Auditory feedback for walking difficulties in a case of unilateral neglect: A pilot study. *Neuropsychological Rehabilitation*, *1*, 175–183.

Robertson IH, North N (1992a) Unilateral limb activation in unilateral left neglect: Three single case studies of its therapeutic effects. *Journal of Clinical and Experimental Neuropsychology*, *14*, 38.

Robertson I, North N (1992b) Spatio-motor cueing in unilateral left neglect: The role of hemispace, hand and motor activity. *Neuropsychologia*, *30*, 553–563.

Robertson I, Gray J, McKenzie S (1988) Micro-computer-based·cognitive rehabilitation of visual neglect: Three multiple baseline single-case studies. *Brain Injury*, *2*, 151–163.

Robertson I, Gray J, Pentland B, Waite L (1990) Microcomputer-based rehabilitation of unilateral left visual neglect: A randomised controlled trial. *Archives of Physical Medicine and Rehabilitation*, *71*, 663–668.

Robertson IH, North NT, Geggie C (1992) Spatio-motor cueing in unilateral left neglect: three single-case studies of its therapeutic effects. *Journal of Neurology, Neurosurgery and Psychiatry 55*, 799–805.

Rodin EA (1968) *The Prognosis of Patients with Epilepsy*. Thomas, Springfield, IL.

Rosenboom B, Brouwer WH (1989) *Lange-termijn gevolgen van ernstige hersenletsels in relatie tot planning*. [Doctoral Dissertation]. Internal Report 8936, State University, Groningen.

Rosvold HE, Schwarcbart MK (1964) Neural structures involved in delayed response performance. In: Warren JM, Akert K (eds.), *The Frontal Granular Cortex and Behavior*. McGraw-Hill, New York.

Rosvold HE, Mirsky AF, Sarason I, Bransome ED, Beck LH (1956) A Continuous Performance Test of brain damage. *Journal of Consulting Psychology, 20*, 343–350.

Rosvold HE, Mishkin M, Szwarcbart MK (1958) Effects of subcortical lesions in monkeys on visual discrimination and single alternation performance. *Journal of Comparative and Physiological Psychology, 51*, 437–444.

Roth M, Tym E, Mountjoy CQ, Huppert FA, Hendrie H, Verma S, Goddard R (1986) CAMDEX: A standardized instrument for the diagnosis of mental disorder in the elderly with special reference to the early detection of dementia. *British Journal of Psychiatry, 149*, 698–709.

Rubin E (1921) Die Nicht-Existenz der Aufmerksamkeit. Cited in Sanders, 1963.

Rudel RG, Denckla MB (1974) Relation of forward and backward digit repetition to neurological impairment in children with learning disabilities. *Neuropsychologia, 12*, 109–118.

Ruesch J (1944a) Intellectual impairment in head injuries. *American Journal of Psychiatry, 100*, 480–496.

Ruesch J (1944b) Dark adaptation, negative after images, tachistoscopic examination and reaction time in head injuries. *Journal of Neurosurgery, 1*, 243–251.

Rugg MD (1992) Event-related potentials in clinical neuropsychology. In: Crawford JE, Parker DM, McKinlay WW (eds.), *A Handbook of Neuropsychological Assessment*. Lawrence Erlbaum Associates, Hove, England.

Rugg MD, Cowan CP, Nagy ME, Milner AD, Jacobson I, Brooks DN (1988) Event-related potentials from closed head injury patients in an auditory odd-ball task: Evidence of dysfunction in stimulus categorization. *Journal of Neurology, Neurosurgery and Psychiatry, 51*, 691–698.

Rugg MD, Cowan CP, Nagy ME, Milner AD, Jacobson I, Brooks DN (1989) CNV abnormalities following closed head injury. *Brain, 112*, 489–506.

Russell EW (1981) The pathology and clinical examination of memory. In: Filskov SB, Boll TJ (eds.), *Handbook of Clinical Neuropsychology*, p. 304. Wiley, New York.

Russell WR (1934) The after-effects of head injury. *Edinburgh Medical Journal, 41*, 129–131.

Russell WR (1971) *The Traumatic Amnesias*. Oxford University Press, London.

Saan RJ (1994) Recovery of cognitive functions after severe head injury. [Doctoral Dissertation]. State University of Groningen (in preparation).

Sagar HJ, Sullivan EV, Gabriel JDE, Corkin S, Growdon JH (1988) Temporal ordering and short-term memory deficits in Parkinson's disease. *Brain, 111*, 525–539.

Sahakian BJ, Morris RG, Evenden JL, Heald A, Levy R, Philpot M, Robbins TW (1988) A comparative study of visuospatial memory and learning in Alzheimer-type dementia and Parkinson's disease. *Brain, 111*, 695–718.

Salazar AM, Grafman JH, Vance SC, Weingartner H, Dillon JD, Ludlow C (1986) Consciousness and amnesia after penetrating head injury: Neurology and anatomy. *Neurology, 36*, 178–187.

Salthouse TA (1982) *Adult Cognition*. Springer-Verlag, New York.

Salthouse TA (1988) Initiating the formalization of theories of cognitive aging. *Psychology and Aging*, *3*, 3–16.

Sanders AF (1963) *The Selective Process in the Functional Visual Field*. Van Gorcum, Assen, NL.

Sanders AF (1983) Towards a model of stress and human performance. *Acta Psychologica*, *53*, 61–97.

Saper CB (1988) Chemical Neuroanatomy of Alzheimer's Disease. In: Inversen SD, Iversen LL, Snyder SH (eds.), *Handbook of Psychopharmacology*, vol. 20, pp. 131–156. Plenum, New York.

Schacter DL, Crovitz HF (1977) Memory function after closed head injury: A review of quantitative research. *Cortex*, *13*, 150–176.

Schmitter-Edgecombe ME, Marks W, Fahy JF, Long CJ (1992) Effects of severe closed head injury on three stages of information processing. *Journal of Clinical and Experimental Neuropsychology*, *14*, 717–737.

Schneider W (1987) Connectionism: Is it a paradigm shift for psychology? *Behavior, Research Methods, Instruments and Computers*, *19*, 73–83.

Schwab RS, Chafetz ME, Walker S (1954) Control of two simultaneous voluntary motor acts in normals and parkinsonism. *Archives of Neurology*, *72*, 591–598.

Schwartz ML (1987) Focal cognitive deficits in dementia of the Alzheimer type. *Neuropsychology*, *1*, 27–35.

Seashore CE, Lewis D, Saetviet JG (1960) *Seashore Measures of Musical Talents: Manual*. Psychological Corporation, New York.

Segalowitz SJ, Unsal A, Dywan J (1992) CNV Evidence for the distinctiveness of frontal and posterior neural processes in a traumatic brain-injured population. *Journal of Clinical and Experimental Neuropsychology*, *14*, 545–565.

Serafetinides EA, Hoare RD, Drive MV (1965) Intracarotid sodium amylobarbitone and cerebral dominance for speech and consciousness. *Brain*, *88*, 107–132.

Shallice T (1982) Specific impairments of planning. In: Broadbent DE, Weiskrantz L (eds.), *The Neuropsychology of Cognitive Function*, pp. 199–209. The Royal Society, London.

Shallice T (1988) *From Neuropsychology to Mental Structure*. Cambridge University Press, Cambridge, England.

Sharpe MH (1990) Patients with early Parkinson's disease are not impaired on spatial orientation of attention. *Cortex*, *26*, 515–524.

Sharpe MH (1992) Auditory attention in early Parkinson's disease: An impairment in focused attention. *Neuropsychologia*, *30*, 101–106.

Sharpless S, Jasper H (1956) Habituation of the arousal reaction. *Brain*, *79*, 655–680.

Sheer DE, Schrock B (1986) Attention. In: Hannay HJ (ed.), *Experimental Techniques in Human Neuropsychology*, pp. 95–137. Oxford University Press, New York.

Shiffrin RM, Schneider W (1977) Controlled and automatic human information processing: II: Perceptual learning, automatic attending and a general theory. *Psychological Review*, *84*, 127–190.

Shorvon SD (1984) *Epilepsy*. Update Publications Ltd., London.

Shum DHK, McFarland K, Bain JD, Humphreys MS (1990) Effects of closed head injury on attentional processes: An information-processing stage analysis. *Journal of Clinical and Experimental Neuropsychology*, *12*, 247–264.

Shyi GC-W, Chen SW (1992) The size of attentional focus and the speed of attentional movement. *Proceedings of the Baycrest Centre conference on Attention: Theoretical and Clinical Perspectives*, Toronto, Canada, 26–27 March, 1992.

Simms B (1986) Learner drivers with spina bifida and hydrocephalus: The relationship between perceptual-cognitive deficit and driving performance. *Zeitschrift für Kinderchirurgie*, *41*, *suppl. 1*, 51–55.

Sivak M, Hill CS, Olson PL (1984a) Computerized video tasks as training techniques for driving-related perceptual deficits of persons with brain damage: A pilot evaluation. *International Journal of Rehabilitation Research*, *7*, 389–398.

Sivak M, Hill CS, Henson DL, Butler BP, Silber SM, Olson PL (1984b) Improved driving performance following perceptual training in persons with brain damage. *Archives of Physical Medicine and Rehabilitation*, *65*, 163–167.

Sivak M, Olson PL, Kewman DG, Won H, Henson DL (1981) Driving and perceptual/cognitive consequences of brain-damage. *Archives of Physical Medicine and Rehabilitation*, *62*, 476–483.

Smith A (1967) The serial sevens subtraction test. *Archives of Neurology*, *17*, 78–80.

Smith A (1982) *Symbol Digit Modalities Test: Manual*. Western Psychological Services, Los Angeles.

Smith EE (1968) Choice reaction time: An analysis of the major theoretical positions. *Psychological Bulletin*, *69*, 77–110.

Smolensky P (1988) On the proper treatment of connectionism. *The Behavioral and Brain Sciences*, *11*, 1–74.

Snoek JW (1990) The pathophysiology of head injuries. In: Deelman BG, Saan RJ, Van Zomeren AH (eds.), *Traumatic Brain Injury: Clinical, Social and Rehabilitational Aspects*. Swets and Zeitlinger, Lisse.

Sohlberg MM, Mateer CA (1987) Effectiveness of an attention training program. *Journal of Experimental and Clinical Neuropsychology*, *19*, 117–130.

Somberg BL, Salthouse TA (1982) Divided Attention abilities in young and old adults. *Journal of Experimental Psychology*, *8*, 651–663.

Stankov L (1983) Attention and intelligence. *Journal of Educational Psychology*, *4*, 471–490.

Stankov L (1988) Aging, attention and intelligence. *Psychology and Aging*, *4*, 59–74.

Starkstein SE, Preziosi TJ, Berthier ML, Bolduc PL, Mayberg HS, Robinson RG (1989) Depression and cognitive impairment in Parkinson's disease. *Brain*, *112*, 1141–1153.

Stelmach GE, Phillips JG, Chau AW (1989) Visuo-spatial processing in parkinsonians. *Neuropsychologia*, *27*, 485–493.

Sternberg RJ (1985) General intellectual ability. In: Sternberg RJ (ed.), *Human Abilities: An information-processing approach*, pp. 5–29. Freeman and Co., New York.

Sternberg S (1969) The discovery of processing stages: Extensions of Donders' method. *Acta Psychologia*, *30*, 276–315.

Sternberg S (1975) Memory scanning: New findings and current controversies. *Quarterly Journal of Experimental Psychology*, *27*, 1–32.

Stokx LC, Gaillard AWK (1986) Task and driving performance of patients with a severe concussion of the brain. *Journal of Clinical and Experimental Neuropsychology*, *8*, 421–436.

Strauss ME, Allred LJ (1987) Measurement of differential cognitive deficits after head injury. In: Levin HS, Grafman J, Eisenberg HM (eds.), *Neurobehavioral Recovery from Head Injury*. Oxford University Press, New York.

Strich SJ (1961) Shearing of nerve fibers as a cause of brain damage due to head injury. *Lancet*, *ii*, 443–448.

Stroop JR (1935) Studies of interference in serial verbal reactions. *Journal of Experimental Psychology*, *18*, 643–662.

Strub RL, Black FW (1985) *The Mental Status Examination in Neurology.* FA Davis, Philadelphia.

Sturm W, Willmes K (1991) Efficacy of a reaction training on various attentional and cognitive functions in stroke patients. *Neuropsychological Rehabilitation, 1,* 242–259.

Sturm W, Dahmen W, Hartje W, Willmes K (1983) Ergebnisse eines Trainingprogramms zur Verbesserung der visuellen Auffassungsschnelligkeit und Konzentrationsfähigkeit bei Hirngeschädigten. *Archive für Psychiatrie und Nervenkrankheiten, 233,* 9–22.

Sturm W, Hartje W, Orgass B, Willmes K (1993) Computer-assisted rehabilitation of attention impairments. In: Stachowiak F (ed.), *Developments in the Assessment and Rehabilitation of Brain-damaged Patients.* Narr, Tübingen, Germany.

Sturm W, Reul J, Willmes K (1989) Is there a generalized right hemisphere dominance for mediating cerebral activation? Evidence from a choice reaction experiment with lateralized simple warning stimuli. *Neuropsychologia, 27,* 747–751.

Stuss DT, Benson DF (1984) Neuropsychological studies of the frontal lobes. *Psychological Bulletin, 95,* 3–28.

Stuss DT, Benson DF (1986) *The Frontal Lobes.* Raven Press, New York.

Stuss DT, Ely P, Hugenholtz H, Richard MT, Larochelle S, Poirier CA, Bell I (1985) Subtle neuropsychological deficits in patients with good recovery after closed head injury. *Neurosurgery, 17,* 41–47.

Stuss DT, Stethem LL, Hugenholtz H, Picto T, Pivik J, Richard MT (1989) Reaction time after head injury: Fatigue, divided and focused attention, and consistency of performance. *Journal of Neurology, Neurosurgery and Psychiatry, 52,* 742–748.

Stuss DT, Stethem LL, Pelchat F (1988) Three tests of attention and rapid information processing: An extension. *Clinical Neuropsychologist, 2,* 246–250.

Stuss DT, Stethem LL, Poirier CA (1987) Comparison of three tests of attention and rapid information processing across six age groups. *Clinical Neuropsychologist, 1,* 139–152.

Talland GA (1963) Manual skill in Parkinson's disease. *Geriatrics, 18,* 613–620.

Talland GA (1965) *Deranged Memory.* Academic Press, New York.

Talland GA, Schwab RS (1964) Performance with multiple sets in Parkinson's disease. *Neuropsychologia, 2,* 45–53.

Tariot PN, Sunderland T, Weingartner H, Murphy DL, Welkowitz JA, Thompson K, Cohen RM (1987) Cognitive effects of L-deprenyl in Alzheimer's disease. *Psychopharmacology, 91,* 489–495.

Tartaglione A, Bino G, Manzino M, Sapdavecchia L, Favale E (1986) Simple reaction time changes in patients with unilateral brain damage. *Neuropsychologia, 24,* 649–658.

Taylor AE, Saint-Cyr JA, Lang AE (1986) Frontal lobe dysfunction in Parkinson's disease: The cortical focus of neostriatal outflow. *Brain, 109,* 845–883.

Taylor AE, Saint-Cyr JA, Lang AE (1987) Parkinson's disease: Cognitive changes in relation to treatment response. *Brain, 110,* 35–51.

Taylor AE, Saint-Cyr JA, Lang AE (1990) Memory and learning in early Parkinson's disease: evidence for a "frontal lobe syndrome." *Brain and Cognition, 13,* 211–232.

Teuber HL (1976) Complex functions of basal ganglia. In: Yahr MD (ed.), *The Basal Ganglia.* Raven Press, New York.

Teuber HL, Battersby WS, Bender MB (1960) *Visual Field Defects After Penetrating Missile Wounds of the Brain.* Published for the Commonwealth Fund by Harvard University Press, Cambridge, MA.

Theeuwis J (1992) *Selective Attention in the Visual Field*. [Doctoral Dissertation]. Vrije Universiteit, Amsterdam.

Theios J (1975) The components of response latency in simple human information processing tasks. In: Rabbitt PMA, Dornic S (eds.), *Attention and Performance*, vol. 5. Academic Press, New York.

Thomas C (1977) *Deficits of Memory and Attention Following Closed Head Injury*. [Master's Dissertation]. University of Oxford.

Thompson PJ, Huppert FA (1980) Problems in the development of measures to test cognitive performance in adult epileptic patients. In: Kulig BM, Meinardi H, Stores G (eds.), *Epilepsy and Behavior*. Swets and Zeitlinger, Lisse.

Thompson PJ, Trimble MR (1981) Sodium valproate and cognitive functioning in normal volunteers. *British Journal of Clinical Pharmacology*, *12*, 819–824.

Thompson PJ, Huppert FA, Trimble MR (1981) Phenytoin and cognitive function: Effects on normal volunteers and implications for epilepsy. *British Journal of Clinical Psychology*, *20*, 155–162.

Thomsen IV (1974) The patient with severe head injury and his family. *Scandinavian Journal of Rehabilitation Medicine*, *6*, 18–183.

Thurstone LL (1944) *A Factorial Study of Perception*. University of Chicago Press, Chicago.

Titchener EB (1908) *Lectures on the Elementary Psychology of Feeling and Attention*. Macmillan, New York.

Towle D, Lincoln N (1991) Use of the indented paragraph test with right hemisphere-damaged stroke patients. *British Journal of Clinical Psychology*, *30*, 37–45.

Transportation in an Aging Society, vol. 1 & 2 (1988) Transportation Research Board of the National Research Council, Washington, DC.

Treisman AM (1964) Verbal cues, language and meaning in selective attention. *American Journal of Psychology*, *77*, 206–219.

Treisman AM, Gelade G (1980) A feature-integration of attention. *Cognitive Psychology*, *12*, 97–136.

Trimble MR (1988) Cognitive hazards of seizure disorders. *Epilepsia*, *29, suppl. 1*, 19–24.

Trimble MR, Thompson PJ (1983) Anticonvulsant drugs, cognitive function, and behavior. *Epilepsia*, *24, suppl. 1*, 55–63.

Tromp E (1993) De wereld gehalveerd: De neuropsycholoog en het hemispatieel neglect. *De Psycholoog*, *28*, 1–5.

Valley V, Broughton R (1983) The physiological (EEG) nature of drowsiness and its relation to performance deficits in narcoleptics. *Electroencephalography and Clinical Neurophysiology*, *55*, 243–251.

Van der Heiden AHC (1991) *Selective Attention in Vision*, Routledge, London.

Van der Lugt PJM (1975) Traffic accidents caused by epilepsy. *Epilepsia*, *16*, 747–751.

Vanier M, Gauthier L, Lambert J, Pepin E, Robillard A, Dubouloz CJ, Gagnon R, Joannette Y (1990) Evaluation of left visuospatial neglect: Norms and discrimination power of two tests. *Neuropsychology*, *4*, 87–96.

Van Vreden W (1986) *Aandacht voor de Basale Ganglia*, unpublished master's thesis, Neuropsychology Dept. of Univ. of Groningen.

Van Wolffelaar PC, Brouwer WH, Van Zomeren AH (1990) Driving ability 5 to 10 years after severe head injury. In: Benjamin T (ed.), *Driving Behaviour in a Social Context*, pp. 564–574. Paradigme, Caen, France.

Van Wolffelaar PC, Rothengatter JA, Brouwer WH (1991) Elderly drivers' traffic merging decisions. In: Gale A (ed.), *Vision in Vehicles*, vol. 3, pp. 247–255. Amsterdam.

Van Wolffelaar P, van Zomeren AH, Brouwer WH, Rothengatter T (1988) Assessment of fitness to drive of brain-damaged persons. In: Rothengatter T, De Bruin R (eds.), *Road User Behaviour: Theory and Research*, pp. 302–309. Van Gorcum, Assen.

Van Zomeren AH (1981) *Reaction Time and Attention After Closed Head Injury*. Swets Publishing, Lisse.

Van Zomeren AH (1989) The comeback of attention in neuropsychology. In: Anderson V, Bailey M (eds.), *Theory and Function: Bridging the Gap*, pp. 9–17, ASSBI, Melbourne.

Van Zomeren AH, Brouwer WH (1987) Head injury and concepts of attention. In: Levin HS, Grafman J, Eisenberg HM (eds.), *Neurobehavioral Recovery from Head Injury*. Oxford University Press, New York.

Van Zomeren AH, Deelman BG (1976) Differential effects of simple and choice reaction after closed head injury. *Clinical Neurology and Neurosurgery*, *79*, 81–90.

Van Zomeren AH, Deelman BG (1978) Long-term recovery of visual reaction time after closed head injury. *Journal of Neurology, Neurosurgery and Psychiatry*, *41*, 452–457.

Van Zomeren AH, Fasotti L (1992) Impairments of attention and approaches to rehabilitation. In: Von Cramon D, Pöppel E, Von Steinbüchel N (eds.), *Brain Damage and Rehabilitation: A Neuropsychological Approach*. Springer-Verlag, Heidelberg.

Van Zomeren AH, Van den Burg W (1985) Residual complaints of patients two years after severe head injury. *Journal of Neurology, Neurosurgery and Psychiatry*, *48*, 21–28.

Van Zomeren AH Brouwer WH, Deelman BG (1984) Attentional deficits: The riddles of selectivity, speed and alertness. In: Brooks DN (ed.), *Closed Head Injury, Psychological, Social and Family Consequences*, pp. 74–107. Oxford University Press, Oxford.

Van Zomeren AH, Brouwer WH, Minderhoud JM (1987) Acquired brain damage and driving: A review. *Archives of Physical Medicine and Rehabilitation*, *68*, 697–705.

Van Zomeren AH, Brouwer WH, Rothengatter JA, Snoek JW (1988) Fitness to drive a car after recovery from severe head injury. *Archives of Physical Medicine and Rehabilitation*, *69*, 90–96.

Veltman JC, Brouwer WH, Van Zomeren AH (1990) *Verdeelde aandacht 3 tot 6 maanden na contusio cerebri*. [Doctoral Dissertation]. Internal report nr. 9032, State University, Groningen.

Verfaellie M, Bowers D, Heilman KM (1988) Hemispheric asymmetries in mediating intention, but not selective attention. *Neuropsychologia*, *26*, 521–531.

Villardita C, Smirni P, Zappala G (1983) Visual neglect in Parkinson's disease. *Archives of Neurology*, *40*, 737–739.

Volpe BT, McDowell FH (1990) The efficacy of cognitive rehabilitation in patients with traumatic brain injury. *Archives of Neurology*, *47*, 220–222.

Von Cramon DY, Matthes-von Cramon G, Mai N (1991) Problem-solving deficits in brain-injured patients: A therapeutic approach. *Neuropsychological Rehabilitation*, *1*, 45–64.

Wade DT, Wood VA, Langton Hewer R (1988) Recovery of cognitive function soon after stroke: A study of visual neglect, attention span and verbal recall. *Journal of Neurology, Neurosurgery and Psychiatry*, *51*, 10–13.

Waller JA (1967) Cardiovascular disease, aging, and traffic accidents. *Journal of Chronic Diseases*, *20*, 615–620.

Walsh KW (1978) *Neuropsychology: A Clinical Approach*. Churchill Livingstone, Edinburgh.

Walter WG, Cooper R, Aldridge V, McCallum WC, Winter AL (1964) Contingent negative variation: An electric sign of sensorimotor association and expectancy in the human brain. *Nature, 203,* 380–384.

Watson RT, Miller BD, Heilman KM (1978) Nonsensory neglect. *Annals of Neurology, 3,* 505–508.

Weber AM (1988) A new clinical measure of attention: The Attentional Capacity Test. *Neuropsychology, 2,* 59–71.

Webster JS, Scott RR (1983) The effects of self-instructional training on attentional deficits following head injury. *Clinical Neuropsychologist, 5,* 69–74.

Webster JS, Jones S, Blanton P, Gross R, Beissel GF, Wofford J (1984) Visual scanning training with stroke patients. *Behavior Therapy, 15,* 129–143.

Wechsler D (1955) *The Measurement of Adult Intelligence.* Williams & Wilkins, Baltimore.

Wechsler D (1981) *WAIS-R Manual.* The Psychological Corporation (Harcourt Brace Jovanovich, Publishers), New York.

Weinberg J, Diller L, Gordon W, Gerstman L, Lieberman A, Lakin P, Hodges G, Ezrachi O (1977) Visual scanning training effect on reading-related tasks in acquired right brain damage. *Archives of Physical Medicine and Rehabilitation, 58,* 479–486.

Weinberg J, Diller L, Gordon W, Gerstman L, Lieberman A, Lakin P, Hodges G, Ezrachi O (1979) Training sensory awareness and spatial organisation in people with right brain damage. *Archives of Physical Medicine and Rehabilitation, 60,* 491–496.

Weingartner H, Kaye W, Smallberg SA, Ebert MH Gillin JC, Sitaram N (1981) Memory failures in progressive idiopathic dementia. *Journal of Abnormal Psychology, 90,* 187–196.

Welford AT (1962) On changes of performance with age. *Lancet, 1,* 335.

Welford AT (1981) Signal, noise, performance and age. *Human Factors, 23,* 97–109.

Wells FL, Kelly M, Murphy G (1921) On attention and simple reactions. *Journal of Experimental Psychology, 4,* 391–398.

Whyte J (1992) Quantification of attention-related behaviors in traumatic brain injury. *Proceedings of the Conference on Attention: Theoretical and Clinical Perspectives.* Baycrest Centre, Toronto, Canada.

Wickens CD (1984) Processing resources in attention. In: Parasuraman R, Davis DR (eds.), *Varieties of Attention,* pp. 63–102. Academic Press, New York.

Wickens CD, Mountford SJ, Schreiner W (1981) Multiple resources, task hemispheric integrity and individual differences in time-sharing. *Human Factors, 23,* 211–229.

Wilkins AJ, Shallice T, McCarthy R (1987) Frontal lesions and sustained attention. *Neuropsychologia, 25,* 359–365.

Wilson B, Cockburn J, Baddeley AL (1985) *The Rivermead Behavioural Memory Test.* Thames Valley Test Co., Reading, PA.

Wilson BA, Cockburn J, Halligan P (1987) The development of a behavioral test of visuospatial neglect. *Archives of Physical Medicine and Rehabilitation, 68,* 98–102.

Wilson C, Robertson IH (1992) A home based intervention for attentional slips during reading following head injury: A single case study. *Neuropsychological Rehabilitation 2,* 193–205.

Wilson RS, Kaszniak AW, Klawans HL, Garron DC (1980) High speed memory scanning in parkinsonism. *Cortex, 16,* 67–72.

Wittenborn JR (1943) Factorial equations for tests of attention. *Psychometrica, 8,* 19–35.

Wolters EC, Calne DB (1989) Is Parkinson's disease related to aging? In: Calne DB, (eds.), *Parkinsonism and Aging*, pp. 125–132. Raven Press, New York.

Wood RL (1987) *Brain Injury Rehabilitation: A Neurobehavioural Approach*. Croom Helm, London.

Wood RL, Fussey I (1987) Computer-based cognitive retraining: A controlled study. *International Disability Studies*, 9, 149–153.

Woodrow H (1939) The common factors in fifty-two mental tests. *Psychometrica*, 4, 99–108.

Wrightson P, Gronwall D (1981) Time off work and symptoms after minor head injury. *Injury*, 12, 445–454.

Yahr MD, Sciarra D, Carter S, Merritt HH (1952) Evaluation of standard anticonvulsants therapy in three hundred nineteen patients. *Journal of the American Medical Association*, 150, 663–667.

Yates FA (1966) *The Art of Memory*. University of Chicago Press, Chicago.

Yokoyama K, Jennings R, Ackles P, Hood P, Boller F (1987) Lack of heart rate changes during an attention-demanding task after right hemisphere lesion. *Neurology*, 37, 624–630.

Zimmermann P, Fimm B (1989) A computerized neuropsychological assessment of attention deficits. *Internal Report*, Psychologisches Institut der Universität, Freiburg.

Zimmermann P, Sprengelmeyer R, Fimm B, Wallesch CW (1992) Cognitive slowing in decision tasks in early and advanced Parkinson's disease. *Brain and Cognition*, 18, 60–69.

Index